Biomaterials and Bioengineering Handbook

Biomaterials and Bioengineering Handbook

Contributors

Kris N. J. Stevens, Yvette B. J. Aldenhoff et al.

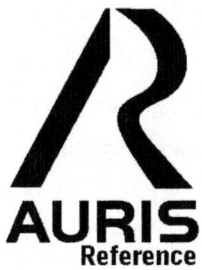

AURIS
Reference

www.aurisreference.com

Biomaterials and Bioengineering Handbook

Contributors: Kris N. J. Stevens, Yvette B. J. Aldenhoff et al.

Published by Auris Reference Limited

www.aurisreference.com

United Kingdom

Biomaterials and Bioengineering Handbook

ISBN: 978-1-78154-840-0

British Library Cataloguing in Publication Data
A CIP record for this book is available from the British Library

Printed in the United Kingdom

Exclusively distributed by CBS Publishers & Distributors Pvt. Ltd.

Sales & Distribution Rights only for India, Pakistan, Bangladesh, Sri Lanka, Nepal and Bhutan. This book is not to be sold outside these territories.

Contents

List of Abbreviations

AMI	Acute myocardial infarction
AFSC	Amniotic Fluid Stem Cells
AWGC	apatite-wollastonite glass ceramic
AFM	Atomic force microscopy
BMC	Bone marrow cells
BCNT	boron-neutron capture therapy
BET	Brunauer-Emmett-Teller
CF	carbon fibres
CNT	carbon nanotube
CSC	Cardiac Stem Cells
CPB	Cardiopulmonary bypass
CDC	Cardiosphere derived cells
CVD	Cardiovascular diseases
CTAD	Citrate, theophylline, adenosine, dipyridamole
CHD	coronary heart diseases
DSC	differential scanning calorimetric
DCG	discontinuous crack growth
DMEM	Dulbecco's Modified Eagle's Medium
DMA	dynamic mechanical analysis
ESC	Embryonic Stem Cells
EC	endothelial cells
ELISA	enzyme-linked immunosorbent assay
ECM	extracellular matrix
FCS	fetal calf serum
FTIR	Fourier Transform Infrared spectroscopy
SEM	scanning electron micrographs
SEM	scanning electron microscope
SWCNT	single-walled nanotube
SM	Skeletal Myoblasts
SIS	Small intestinal submucosa
SD	standard deviation
UCBC	Umbilical Cord Blood Cells
VSMC	vascular smooth muscle cells
XRD	X - ray diffraction

List of Contributors

Kris N. J. Stevens
Department of Cardiothoracic Surgery, Academic Hospital Maastricht, P.O. Box 5800, Maastricht 6200 MD, The Netherlands

Yvette B. J. Aldenhoff
Centre for Biomaterials Research, University of Maastricht, P.O. Box 616, Maastricht 6200 MD, The Netherlands

Frederik H. van der Veen
Department of Cardiothoracic Surgery, Academic Hospital Maastricht, P.O. Box 5800, Maastricht 6200 MD, The Netherlands

Jos G. Maessen
Department of Cardiothoracic Surgery, Academic Hospital Maastricht, P.O. Box 5800, Maastricht 6200 MD, The Netherlands

Leo H. Koole
Department of Cardiothoracic Surgery, Academic Hospital Maastricht, P.O. Box 5800, Maastricht 6200 MD, The Netherlands

Sudip Mondal
Centre for Advanced Material Processing, Central Mechanical Engineering Research Institute,Mahatma Gandhi Avenue, Durgapur-713209, India
Department of Biotechnology, National Institute of Technology, Mahatma Gandhi Avenue Durgapur-713209, India

Biswanath Mondal
Centre for Advanced Material Processing, Central Mechanical Engineering Research Institute,Mahatma Gandhi Avenue, Durgapur-713209, India

Apurba Dey
Department of Biotechnology, National Institute of Technology, Mahatma Gandhi Avenue Durgapur-713209, India

Sudit S. Mukhopadhyay
Department of Biotechnology, National Institute of Technology, Mahatma Gandhi Avenue Durgapur-713209, India

Yang Cao
College of Biological and Environmental Engineering, Jiangsu University of Science and Technology, Zhenjiang Jiangsu 212018, P.R. China

Bochu Wang
College of Biological and Environmental Engineering, Jiangsu University of Science and Technology, Zhenjiang Jiangsu 212018, P.R. China
College of Bioengineering, Chongqing University, Chongqing 400030, P.R. China

Mustafa Türk
Department of Biology, Faculty of Arts and Sciences, Kırıkkale University, Yahşihan, Turkey

Gülten Kahraman
Sarayköy Nuclear Research and Training Center, Turkish Atomic Energy Authority, Ankara, Turkey

Sevda A. Khalilova
Scientific Research Institute of Medicinal Prophylaxis, Ministry of Public Health, Baku, Azerbaijan

Zakir M. O. Rzayev
Institute of Science & Engineering, Division of Nanoscience and Nanomedicine, Hacettepe University, Ankara, Turkey

Serpil Oguztüzün
Department of Biology, Faculty of Arts and Sciences, Kırıkkale University, Yahşihan, Turkey

Modesto T. Lopez-Lopez
Department of Applied Physics, Faculty of Sciences, University of Granada, Granada, Spain, and Instituto de Investigación Biosanitaria ibs.GRANADA, Granada, Spain

Giuseppe Scionti
Department of Histology, Faculty of Medicine, University of Granada, Granada, Spain, and Instituto de Investigación Biosanitaria ibs.GRANADA, Granada, Spain

Ana C. Oliveira
Department of Histology, Faculty of Medicine, University of Granada, Granada, Spain, and Instituto de Investigación Biosanitaria ibs.GRANADA, Granada, Spain

Juan D. G. Duran
Department of Applied Physics, Faculty of Sciences, University of Granada, Granada, Spain, and Instituto de Investigación Biosanitaria ibs.GRANADA, Granada, Spain

Antonio Campos
Department of Histology, Faculty of Medicine, University of Granada, Granada, Spain,

and Instituto de Investigación Biosanitaria ibs.GRANADA, Granada, Spain

Miguel Alaminos
Department of Histology, Faculty of Medicine, University of Granada, Granada, Spain, and Instituto de Investigación Biosanitaria ibs.GRANADA, Granada, Spain

Ismael A. Rodriguez
Department of Histology, Faculty of Medicine, University of Granada, Granada, Spain, and Instituto de Investigación Biosanitaria ibs.GRANADA, Granada, Spain
Department of Histology, School of Dentistry, National University of Cordoba, Cordoba, Argentina

Naresh Kasoju
Department of Biomaterials and Bioanalogous Polymer Systems, Institute of Macromolecular Chemistry, Academy of Sciences of the Czech Republic, v.v.i., Prague, Czech Republic

Dana Kubies
Department of Biomaterials and Bioanalogous Polymer Systems, Institute of Macromolecular Chemistry, Academy of Sciences of the Czech Republic, v.v.i., Prague, Czech Republic

Marta M. Kumorek
Department of Biomaterials and Bioanalogous Polymer Systems, Institute of Macromolecular Chemistry, Academy of Sciences of the Czech Republic, v.v.i., Prague, Czech Republic

Jan Kříž
Laboratory of Islets of Langerhans, Institute for Clinical and Experimental Medicine, Prague, Czech Republic

Eva Fábryová
Laboratory of Islets of Langerhans, Institute for Clinical and Experimental Medicine, Prague, Czech Republic

Lud'ka Machová
Department of Biomaterials and Bioanalogous Polymer Systems, Institute of Macromolecular Chemistry, Academy of Sciences of the Czech Republic, v.v.i., Prague, Czech Republic

Jana Kovářová
Department of Polymer Processing, Institute of Macromolecular Chemistry, Academy of Sciences of the Czech Republic, v.v.i., Prague, Czech Republic

František Rypáček
Department of Biomaterials and Bioanalogous Polymer Systems, Institute of Macromolecular Chemistry, Academy of Sciences of the Czech Republic, v.v.i., Prague, Czech Republic

George Z. Kyzas
Laboratory of General & Inorganic Chemical Technology, Department of Chemistry, Aristotle University of Thessaloniki, Thessaloniki GR 541 24, Greece
Department of Petroleum and Natural Gas Technology, Technological Educational Institute of Kavala, Kavala GR 654 04, Greece

Jie Fu
Environmental Engineering Program, Department of Civil Engineering, Auburn University, Auburn, AL 36849, USA

Kostas A. Matis
Laboratory of General & Inorganic Chemical Technology, Department of Chemistry, Aristotle University of Thessaloniki, Thessaloniki GR 541 24, Greece

M. Arnal-Pastor
Center for Biomaterials and Tissue Engineering, Universitat Politècnica de València, Cno. de Vera s/n, Valencia, Spain

J. C. Chachques
Department of Cardiovascular Surgery, Laboratory of Biosurgical Research, Georges Pompidou European Hospital, Paris, France

M. Monleón Pradas
Center for Biomaterials and Tissue Engineering, Universitat Politècnica de València, Cno. de Vera s/n, Valencia, Spain
Networking Research Center on Bioengineering, Biomaterials and Nanomedicine (CIBER-BBN), Valencia, Spain

A. Vallés-Lluch
Center for Biomaterials and Tissue Engineering, Universitat Politècnica de València, Cno. de Vera s/n, Valencia, Spain

Nicholas Dunne
School of Mechanical & Aerospace Engineering, Queen's University of Belfast, Ashby Building, Belfast, UK

Ross W. Ormsby
School of Mechanical & Aerospace Engineering, Queen's University of Belfast, Ashby Building, Belfast, UK

Preface

Biomaterials are materials used in close or direct contact with the body to augment or replace faulty materials. Bioengineering is the application of the life sciences, physical sciences, mathematics and engineering principles to define and solve problems in biology, medicine, health care and other fields. The text Biomaterials and Bioengineering Handbook examines both research and clinical issues surrounding traditional and emerging biomaterials from a variety of professional perspectives. First chapter reports a systematic evaluation of two commercial cardiopulmonary bypass (CPB) tubings, each with a hemocompatible coating, and one uncoated control. In second chapter, we present the synthesis and characterization of HAp materials from different sources like bovine bone and fish scales and their application in tissue engineering. Third chapter focuses on silk-based biomaterials and reviews the degradation behaviors of silk materials. Fourth chapter presents the synthesis and characterization of organoboron, PEO branched and FA complexed derivatives of PPA and investigation of their antitumor activity toward HeLa and Fibroblast cells by using a combination of various biochemical, statistical and microscopy methods. The aim of fifth chapter is to generate magnetic biomaterials whose mechanical properties can be controlled by noncontact magnetic forces. In sixth chapter, we demonstrate a TIPS-based efficient, facile and adaptable methodology, hereby termed as Dip TIPS, to obtain the polymer foams with a controlled shape, size and pore design. Seventh chapter aims to gather and report the bioengineering insights regarding the rebinding (adsorption) using MIPs along with discussion for the importance of the models for fitting. Eighth chapter focuses on biomaterials for cardiac tissue engineering. Last chapter discusses the use of carbon nanotube (CNT) based nanocomposites for biomedical applications, particularly in the area of orthopaedic bone cement used in joint replacement surgery.

Chapter 1

BIOENGINEERING OF IMPROVED BIOMATERIALS COATINGS FOR EXTRACORPOREAL CIRCULATION REQUIRES EXTENDED OBSERVATION OF BLOOD-BIOMATERIAL INTERACTION UNDER FLOW

Kris N. J. Stevens,[1] Yvette B. J. Aldenhoff,[2] Frederik H. van der Veen,[1] Jos G. Maessen,[1] and Leo H. Koole[1]

[1]Department of Cardiothoracic Surgery, Academic Hospital Maastricht, P.O. Box 5800, Maastricht 6200 MD, The Netherlands

[2]Centre for Biomaterials Research, University of Maastricht, P.O. Box 616, Maastricht 6200 MD, The Netherlands

ABSTRACT

Extended use of cardiopulmonary bypass (CPB) systems is often hampered by thrombus formation and infection. Part of these problems relates to imperfect hemocompatibility of the CPB circuitry. The engineering of biomaterial surfaces with genuine long-term hemocompatibility is essentially virgin territory in biomaterials science. For example, most experiments with the well-known Chandler loop model, for evaluation of blood-biomaterial interactions under flow, have been described for a maximum duration of 2 hours only. This study reports a systematic evaluation of two commercial CPB tubings, each with a hemocompatible coating, and one uncoated control. The experiments comprised (i) testing over 5 hours under flow, with human whole blood from 4 different donors; (ii) measurement of essential blood parameters of hemocompatibility; (iii) analysis of the luminal surfaces by scanning electron microscopy and thrombin generation time measurements. The dataset indicated differences in hemocompatibility of the tubings. Furthermore, it appeared that discrimination between biomaterial coatings can be made only after several hours of blood-biomaterial contact. Platelet counting, myeloperoxidase quantification, and scanning electron microscopy proved to be the most useful methods. These findings are believed to be relevant with respect to the bioengineering of extracorporeal devices that should function in contact with blood for extended time.

INTRODUCTION

Cardiopulmonary bypass (CPB) technology represents one of the most striking examples of progress in biomedical engineering. Procedures in cardiac surgery that rely on CPB can nowadays be regarded as safe, that is, they are associated with a low incidence of mortality [1–3]. These developments resulted, to a significant extent, from improvements in the polymeric biomaterials that constitute the inner surface of CPB circuits. Within CPB circuits, there is extensive blood contact with the tubing, the pump, and, particularly, the oxygen/carbon dioxide exchange membrane. It is well known that cellular components of the blood (particularly, leukocytes and platelets) may become activated, and that four different but partially overlapping plasma protein cascades will go into operation (intrinsic and extrinsic clotting cascade, complement system, and fibrinolytic protein system) [4]. For more than 4 decades, heparin has been used as the standard "anticoagulant" to counterbalance these effects. Improvements resulted from the use of surface coatings exposing heparin at the blood-biomaterial interface. These coatings reduce coagulation, inflammation, complement activation, and platelet activation [2, 4]. More recently, CPB equipment has been coated with poly(2-methoxy-ethylacrylate) (PMEA), based on the hypothesis that this material leads to improved blood compatibility compared to uncoated surfaces. PMEA is cheap compared to heparin-exposing coatings and was postulated to provide a useful alternative for patients with heparin-associated disorders [5–7].

However, serious complications may arise if extracorporeal circulation has to be sustained, that is, for several days. The most frequent problems stem from bacterial infection, hemolysis, thrombus formation within the circuit, and formation of circulating thrombotic emboli [8–10]. We became intrigued by these problems, since they relate to long-term hemocompatibility of polymeric materials, which is in fact unexplored territory in biomaterials science. Indeed, we noticed that the literature on blood compatibility of CPB circuits merely contains experimental data that correspond to short testing periods. For example, Weber et al. extensively studied hemocompatibility of 4 different biomaterials in a CPB model, but only up to 120 minutes [11]. We adhere to the idea that successful development of novel biomaterials or biomaterial coatings for CPB will depend on robust evaluation models in which the blood-biomaterial contact is maintained for several hours at least.

Herein we report a systematic methodological study in which two commercial surface-coated CPB tubings (heparin-coated tubings and PMEA-coated tubings) and one uncoated control were evaluated in contact with human whole blood under flow, for a period of 5 hours. We calculated that 5 hours of experimentation implies a level of blood-biomaterial contact that corresponds to at least 9 hours of operation in a typical CPB system (vide infra). Several assays were used to evaluate the blood (platelet counts and assays to determine hemolysis, platelet activation, leukocyte activation, and activation of the complement system). Scanning electron microscopy (SEM) was used to study deposition of blood components at the surface of the tubings. A full set of data was acquired for the three different materials, four donors and five time points (0, 75, 150, 225, and 300 minute). The three materials showed clear differences, in general pointing towards an inferior hemocompatibility of the PMEA coating. Moreover, two points with respect to bioengineering of improved coatings for long-term CPB emerged as follows: (i) since most of the differences between the three surfaces did not become apparent during the first 2 hours of experimentation, long-term (e.g., 5 hour) testing of blood-biomaterial interactions under flow is required; (ii) preferably, parallel tests with blood from several different donors should be performed, since the results from several assays appeared to be clearly donor-dependent.

MATERIALS AND METHODS

Materials

Polyvinyl chloride (PVC) tubings with a coating of PMEA were a generous gift of Terumo Europe NV (Leuven, Belgium). The internal diameter of the tubings was 0.476 cm. The same company also provided the uncoated tubings with identical internal diameter, which were used as controls. Tubings with a coating of heparin were obtained from Maquet Cardiopulmonary AG (Hirrlingen, Germany). The internal diameter was also 0.476 cm. All tubings were received in a sterile package and cut to length of (42.5 cm) immediately prior to the experiments. Lepirudin (Refludan) was purchased from Pharmion (Windsor Berkshire, UK). Bovine serum albumin (BSA), Na-citrate, ethylenediaminetetraacetic acid (EDTA), and Zymosan A were from Sigma-Aldrich Chemie B.V. (Zwijndrecht, The Netherlands). 4-(2-hydroxyethyl)-1-piperazineethanesulfonic acid (HEPES), NaCl, KCl, and Glutaraldehyde 25% were from Acros Organics (Geel, Belgium). Na2HPO4 and KH2PO4 were from Janssen Chimica (Beerse, Belgium). Ethanol 100% was from Merck KGaA (Darmstadt, Germany). The chromogenic substrate S2238 was synthesized according to Rijkers et al. [12]. The following solutions were prepared: a lepirudin stock solution (lepirudin 200 µg/mL, NaCl 9 g/L), a

HEPES/EDTA stock solution (HEPES 100 mM, EDTA 40 mM, pH 7.4), a phosphate-buffered saline (PBS) solution (NaCl 8 g/L, KCl 0.2 g/L, Na_2HPO_4 1.44 g/L, KH_2PO_4 0.24 g/L, pH 7.4), a $CaCl_2$ stock solution (0.5 M $CaCl_2$), a Na-citrate stock solution (Na-citrate 0.13 M), an S2238 stock solution (S2238 2 mM), and a stop buffer (NaCl 140 mM, HEPES 20 mM, EDTA 20 mM, BSA 1 mg/mL, S2238 stock solution 1/10, pH 7.5). Citrate, theophylline, adenosine, dipyridamole (CTAD) stock solution (BD Vacutainer CTAD Tubes) was a product from Becton Dickinson (Alphen aan den Rijn, The Netherlands). The enzyme-linked immunosorbent assay (ELISA) for β-thromboglobulin (β-TG) (Asserachrom β-TG) was purchased from Diagnostica Stago (Asnieres sur Seine, France) and ELISA kits for terminal ` complement complex (TCC) and myeloperoxidase (MPO) were from Hycult biotechnology B.V. (Uden, The Netherlands).

Equipment

Experiments were performed on a modified Chandler loop system, which was equipped with a broad wheel with a diameter of 13 cm [13]. On this wheel, 12 tubes could be rotated simultaneously. The rotating speed was set at 32 per minute. The rotating wheel and the mounted tubes were immersed in a water bath that was kept at 37∘C throughout the entire experiment. The Chandler loop device was made by the mechanical workshop of the Instrument Development Engineering & Evaluation of the University Maastricht. Centrifugation was performed with an Eppendorf Centrifuge 5417C (Eppendorf, Hamburg, Germany). Platelets were counted on an automatic cell counter (Coulter AC-T diff, Beckman Coulter, Miami, Fl, USA). The absorbance of plasmafree hemoglobin (Hb) was determined on a spectrophotometer (Multiskan Spectrum Microplate Spectrophotometer, Thermo Labsystems, Vantaa, Finland). Microtiter plates were heated on a plate warmer (Single Micro-Hywel, Chromogenix, Milano, Italy). For both the ELISA assays and the thrombin generation time assay, the absorbances of the microtiter plates were determined spectrophotometrically on a microplate reader (ELx808 Absorbance Microplate Reader, BioTek Instruments, Inc., Vt, USA). Samples for SEM were coated with gold on a sputter coater (Sputter coater 108 auto/SE, Cressington Scientific Instruments Ltd., Watford, UK) and then analyzed with a scanning electron microscope (Philips XL30 Scanning Electron Microscope, Philips, Eindhoven, The Netherlands).

Experiments under Flow Conditions: The Chandler Loop Model

This study was approved by the Ethical Committee of the University of Maastricht. Four healthy male blood donors (further indicated by their initials as WW, KS, SB, and JB) aged between 20 and 25 years old were included in this study. They were all nonsmokers and did not take any haemostasisinfluencing medicines at least 10 days before the experiment. Each donor visited our laboratories twice and donated blood for two different experiments; there were at least 7 days between the two visits.

Hemocompatibility Analysis by Platelet Counting and Assessment of Hemolysis (Performed After the First Visit of Each Donor)

Blood was withdrawn by venipuncture and immediately anticoagulated with lepirudin stock solution (1 part lepirudin stock solution and 9 parts whole blood), following recommendations made by Kopp et al. [14]. Directly after blood collection, 1.35 mL of blood was sampled and processed as described further to obtain baseline values. Next, three different tubes (one heparin-coated tube, one PMEA-coated tube, and one uncoated control tube) were each filled with 6.7 mL whole blood, which corresponds to a degree of filling of 88%. The tubes were then closed end-to-end using silicon sleeves, mounted on the rotating wheel, and rotated in a water bath at 37∘C and 32 rpm.

From each tube, 1.35 mL blood was withdrawn after 75, 150, 225, and 300 minutes of incubation; note that in the tubes, the degree of filling gradually dropped from 88%, via 70% and 53%, to 35%. Immediately after withdrawal from the tube, each blood sample was mixed with 150 µL HEPES/EDTA stock solution. One third of this mixture (500 µL) was used for platelet counting; these counts were performed intriplicate. The other part of the HEPES/EDTA-mixed blood sample (1 mL) was processed for assessment of hemolysis. The percentage of plasma-free Hb was used as an indicator for hemolysis. 25 µL of HEPES/EDTA-mixed blood sample was diluted 40 times with 975 µL deionized water to achieve total hemolysis. The other 975 µL of HEPES/EDTA-mixed blood sample was kept undiluted. Both the diluted and undiluted parts were centrifuged (3220 g, 20 minutes, 4∘C) to obtain plasma. Subsequently, the absorbance was measured at three wavelengths (560, 576, and 592 nm) in plasma of both the diluted and undiluted parts of the HEPES/EDTA-mixed blood sample. The percentage of plasma-free Hb was then calculated for each blood sample according to the procedure of Cripps [15].

Hemocompatibility Analysis by Quantification of Blood Activation Markers via ELISA and SEM of the Tube Inner Surfaces (Performed After the Second Visit of Each Donor)

Blood was withdrawn by venipuncture and immediately anticoagulated with lepirudin stock solution (1 part lepirudin stock solution and 9 parts whole blood), following recommendations made by Kopp et al. [14]. Immediately after blood collection, a 4.5 mL and 1.8 mL blood sample were isolated and processed as described further to obtain baseline values. Next, twelve tubes (four heparin-coated tubes, four PMEA-coated tubes, and four uncoated control tubes) were each filled with 6.7 mL whole blood, which corresponds to a degree of filling of 88%. The tubes were then closed endto-end using silicon sleeves, mounted on the rotating wheel, and rotated in a water bath at 37∘C and 32 rpm.

After 75, 150, 225, and 300 minutes of incubation, each time three tubes (one heparin-coated tube, one PMEAcoated tube and, an one uncoated control tube) were removed from the rotating wheel. Two blood samples were isolated from each tube: 4.5 mL blood was withdrawn and immediately mixed with 0.5 mL CTAD stock solution, and 1.8 mL of blood was withdrawn and immediately mixed with 0.2 mL HEPES/EDTA stock solution. Both the CTAD-mixed and HEPES/EDTA-mixed blood were incubated on ice for 15 minutes. Then, plasma was isolated by two subsequent centrifugation steps (2550 g, 20 minutes, 4∘C). The plasma was aliquoted and stored at −80∘C until further analysis. ELISA was used to evaluate activation of leukocytes, complement, and platelets. As a marker for leukocyte activation the levels of MPO were quantified in HEPES/EDTAstabilized plasma. The concentration of β-TG in CTADstabilized plasma served as a marker for platelet activation. Complement activation was investigated by measuring plasma concentrations of TCC in HEPES/EDTA-stabilized plasma. Zymosan A activated whole blood was used as a positive control for complement activation.

Following isolation of the blood samples, each tube was prepared for SEM analysis. Nonadherent blood components were washed away by rinsing the tubes extensively with 25 volumes of PBS solution. Next, adherent blood components were fixed by incubating the tubes overnight in 2.5% glutaraldehyde at 2–8∘C. Fixed samples were dehydrated by immersion in an ethanol series (50, 70, 80, 95, and 100% ethanol). Following dehydration, the samples were air-dried. For each time point, three pieces of air-dried tubing with a length of 1 cm were cut out. The pieces were then cut lengthwise for analysis of the inner surface. This was done for all donors. Finally, the samples were sputter coated with gold and imaged with a scanning electron microscope.

Experiments under Static Conditions: Thrombin Generation Time Assay

This assay was carried out as described previously [16– 19]. Briefly, blood was withdrawn by venipuncture from a healthy, nonsmoking male blood donor who did not take any haemostasis-influencing medicines at least 10 days before the experiment. The blood was immediately anticoagulated with citrate stock solution (1 part citrate stock solution and 9 parts whole blood) and kept at 37°C until the start of the experiment. Uncoated, heparin-coated and PMEAcoated PVC tubes were cut to a length of 5.5 cm. These pieces were closed at one end with a tube clamp. At the start of the experiment, blood was recalcified with 40 µL CaCl2 stock solution per mL blood. Subsequently, 750 µL of blood was added to each tube sample and the tube samples were incubated at 37°C under static conditions. After 5 minutes of incubation, 17.5 µL of blood was taken from each tube sample and mixed with 282.5 µL stop buffer. Sampling was done every 5 minutes until 24 minutes of incubation, from then samples were taken every 2 minutes. Blood samples were kept on ice until further handling. At the end of the experiment, the blood samples were centrifuged at 10621 g for 5 minutes. Next, 200 µL plasma of each sample was loaded onto a microtiter plate that was kept on ice. After loading, the microtiter plate was heated for 5 minutes at 37°C. Finally, thrombin concentrations were measured using absorption spectrophotometry at 405 nm.

Statistics

Statistical analysis was performed using Mann-Whitney analysis for between-group comparisons and the Wilcoxon test for paired observations for comparison within groups. A P-value less than .05 (two-tailed) was considered significant.

RESULTS AND DISCUSSION

Analysis of the Blood Samples

Platelet Counts

Figure 1 compiles the results on the platelet count experiments; note that data referring to the three different biomaterials, based on blood from four different donors and measured at five time points, are combined. This format is used consistently throughout this article. At the start of the experiment, the donors had platelet counts between 75,000 and 180,000 per µL, which is within the normal range. Some increased spreading is noted, especially in the counts that were measured after 225 or 300 minutes. The heparin-coated specimens and the uncoated controls show invariant platelet counts as a function of time. The PMEA coating, on the other hand, induces a decrease in the concentration of circulating platelets. For donor JB, this effect can be noticed already after 75 min, and the decrease goes on during the entire experiment. For the other donors, platelet counts start to decline only after 150 minutes (KS and SB), or after 225 minutes (WW). The largest drop in platelet count was found with the blood from donor JB in the PMEA-coated tube; the concentration of circulating platelets decreased by almost 60%, from ca. 140,000 per µL to ca. 60,000 per µL. At the end of the experiment, the concentration of circulating platelets was significantly lower in the PMEA-coated tubes compared to the heparin-coated tubes (79,917 ± 6,304 platelets/µL blood for PMEA-coated tubes versus 135,333 ± 10,623 platelets/µL blood for heparin-coated tubes (mean ± sem), see Table 1 (supplementary material), P = .001) and the uncoated controls (79,917 ± 6,304 platelets/µL blood for PMEA-coated tubes versus 133,833 ± 10,650 platelets/µL blood for uncoated controls (mean ± sem), see Table 1 (supplementary material), P = .001). This indicated that the PMEA coating has a propensity to activate contacting platelets. This is, most probably, not a direct effect, but an effect of plasma proteins adsorbed onto the PMEA surface. Activated platelets are known to adhere to adsorbed fibrinogen, von Willebrand factor, vitronectin, and fibronectin [20]. Consequently, this results in lower platelet counts.

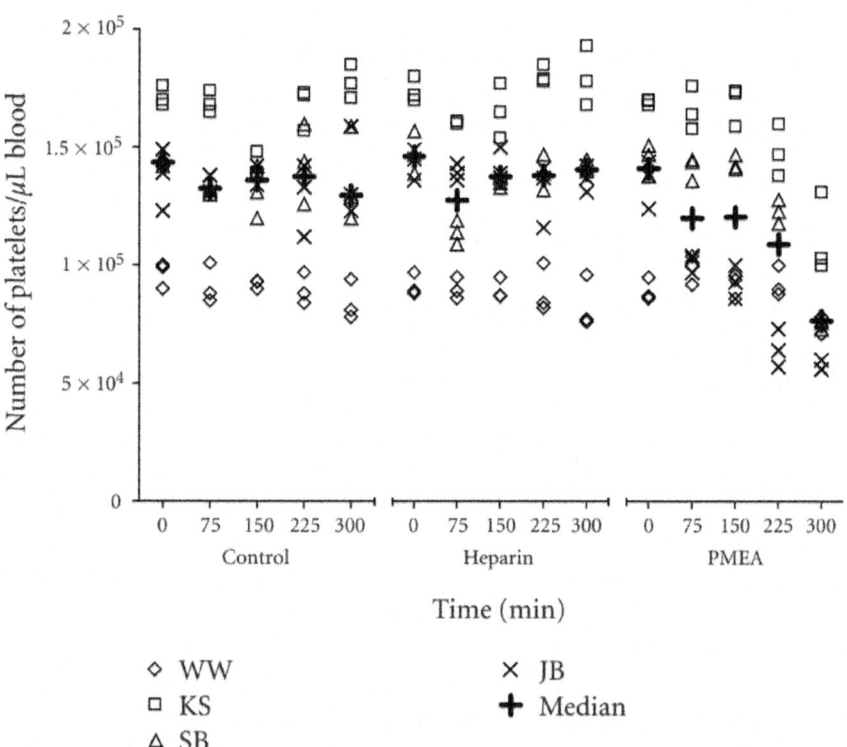

Figure 1: Platelet counts for the individual donors. Data are shown at five time points for each tubing surface tested. Measurements were performed in triplicate.

In addition, activated platelets adhere to each other via fibrinogen bridges, anchored by GPIIb/IIIa receptors [21]. Activated platelets also adhere to circulating leukocytes [22, 23]. Some of the surface-attached platelets partially detach, leaving adherent membrane fragments [24]. Other platelets are damaged by shear forces [25]. Recently, platelet counts were also used in a clinical study to evaluate hemocompatibility of heparinand PMEA-coated CPB circuits. Kutay et al. reported a more significant depletion of circulating platelets in PMEA-coated circuits compared to heparin-coated circuits [26].

Hemolysis

Figure 2 shows the dataset resulting from our concentration measurements of extracellular (free) Hb. Rupture of erythrocytes (hemolysis) (e.g., due to collisions with the lumen of the tubes) leads to release of Hb into the plasma. The vertical axis in Figure 2 depicts the ratio free Hb : total Hb, expressed as a percentage. Clearly, hemolysis is very low, that is, most of the erythrocytes remained intact in all cases. Even in the most extreme situation (donor JB, PMEA coating, 300 minutes circulation), only 1 out of every 400 molecules Hb is free. Despite the occurrence of little hemolysis, it is clear that the level of free Hb in the plasma increases with circulation time, which was expected. The three coatings do not perform differently in this respect. No significant differences in the levels of plasma-free Hb were found between the different tubes. The hemolysis assay applied in this study was based on the Cripps method to measure levels of plasma-free Hb [15]. In a study by Malinauskas [27], this method was shown to be more precise and accurate than the chemical addition methods to measure levels of plasma-free Hb.

Activation of Platelets: β-thromboglobulin

Figure 3 provides an overview of the concentration measurements of β-TG, which is a soluble marker for platelet activation [28]. Activated platelets release β-TG from their α-granules.

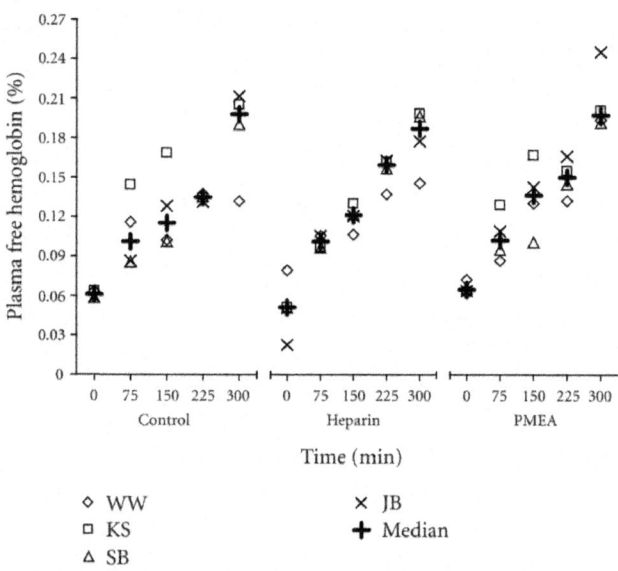

Figure 2: Percentage of plasma-free Hb for the individual donors. Data are shown at five time points for each tubing surface tested.

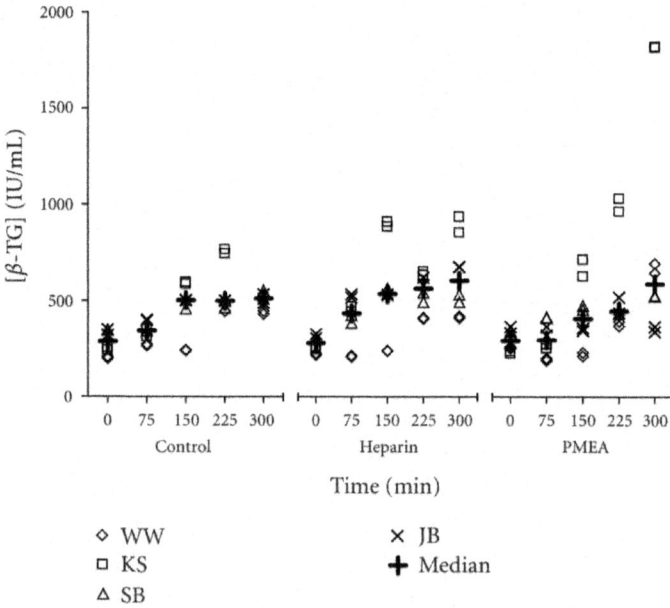

Figure 3: Concentrations of β-thromboglobulin for the individual donors. Data are shown at five time points for each tubing surface tested. Measurements were performed in duplicate.

The β-TG concentration versus time profiles show an increasing trend, revealing that platelet activation progresses with time. With the blood of the donors WW and SB, this is found consistently for all coatings. The blood of donor JB follows this pattern, except in contact with PMEA: the concentration of β-TG then remains virtually unchanged. This is remarkable, since the platelet counts for this donor and this coating were found to decrease sharply (see Figure 1). Most likely, platelets of this donor adhere to PMEA without subsequent release of the granular contents. Donor KS is slightly aberrant. The levels of β-TG are relatively high, throughout all experiments, but it must be kept in mind that this donor also had the highest platelet counts (see Figure 1). In contact with the PMEA coating, a steep increase of the concentration of β-TG is found after 150 minutes of incubation. However, there were no significant differences in platelet activation levels between uncoated, heparin-coated, and PMEAcoated tubes. This indicates that immobilization of heparin or coating with PMEA does not help to reduce platelet activation within blood that contacts a PVC surface.

Activation of Leukocytes: Myeloperoxidase

During ECC, contact between the blood and artificial surfaces is known to induce an inflammatory response characterized by the activation of various leukocyte cell types [23, 29]. Of the various leukocytes, neutrophils are the most abundant; they play a central role in the inflammatory response to CPB [27]. MPO is a glycoprotein abundantly present in the primary granules of neutrophils; activated neutrophils release MPO by degranulation [23, 30, 31].

Figure 4 presents the data of the concentration measurements of MPO. A clear pattern emerging from the data is that for every donor, the concentration of MPO increases continuously. The rise in MPO levels was the highest in PMEA-coated tubes. This resulted in significantly higher levels of MPO compared to heparin-coated tubes, at time points 225 minute (163 ± 11.6 ng/mL for PMEA-coated tubes versus 131.5 ± 4.8 ng/mL for heparin-coated tubes (mean ± sem), see Table 1 (supplementary material), P = .01) and 300 minute (222.3±11.5 ng/mL for PMEA-coated tubes versus 157.7 ± 3.6 ng/mL for heparin-coated tubes (mean ± sem), see Table 1 (supplementary material), P = .001), and to uncoated controls, at time point 300 minute (222.3 ± 11.5 ng/mL for PMEA-coated tubes versus 176.8±9.8 ng/mL for uncoated controls (mean ± sem), see Table 1 (supplementary material), P = .01). These data indicate that the PMEA coating induces MPO release more abundantly as compared to both other surfaces. It is of interest to compare our data with a recent study of Lappegard et al. who also used ° the Chandler loop model to investigate neutrophil activation after blood-artificial surface contact [23, 29]. After 4 hours of blood circulation they found significantly lower levels of MPO release in heparin-coated tubes compared to uncoated controls. Lappegard et al., however, used a heparin coating ° based on covalently end point-attached heparin [29], while the heparin coating used in our experiments involved both covalent and ionic interactions of heparin with the surface.

Our results appear to be in line with a recent clinical study by Kutay et al. who compared the hemocompatibility of PMEA- and heparin-coated CPB [26]. MPO levels at the end of CPB were significantly higher in the PMEA-coated circuits compared to the heparin-coated circuits. Besides MPO, plasma levels of interleukin-8, a proinflammatory cytokine, were also quantified by ELISA. In the three different tubes, plasma levels of interleukin-8 remained undetectable until 225 minutes of incubation. At the end of the experiment, interleukin-8 generation did not differ significantly between the three tubes and plasma levels never exceeded 90 pg/mL (data not shown).

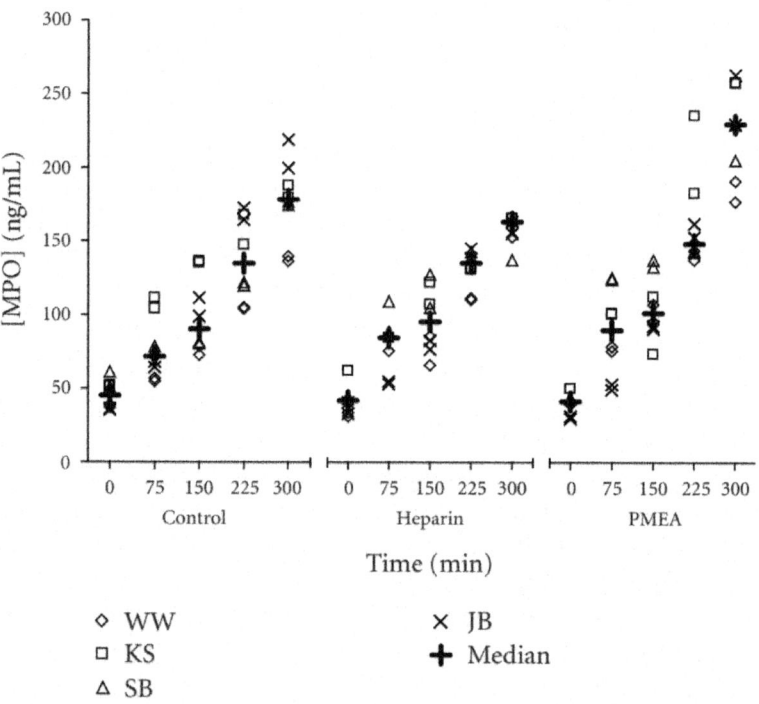

Figure 4: Concentrations of myeloperoxidase for the individual donors. Data are shown at five time points for each tubing surface tested. Measurements were performed in duplicate.

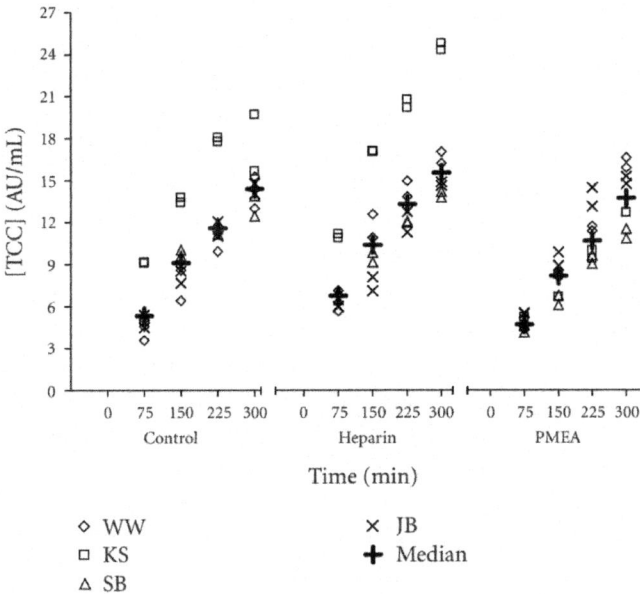

Figure 5: Concentrations of terminal complement complex for the individual donors. Data are shown at five time points for each tubing surface tested. Measurements were performed in duplicate. As can be seen, TCC was undetectable in all samples at time point 0 hour.

Apparently, 5 hours of blood-biomaterial contact in our model are not sufficient to use interleukin-8 as a discriminating marker for inflammatory responses.

Activation of the Complement System: Terminal Complement Complex

Complement activation has been studied extensively as a marker for hemocompatibility of artificial surfaces. Different components of the complement activation cascade can be used [31]. However, in a study by Gong et al. [32], generation of complement activation products in the Chandler loop model displayed component-specific responsiveness to the size of the gas surface and the biomaterial surface. Of the complement activation markers evaluated, generation of TCC was least influenced by the size of the gas surface and mainly dependent on the biomaterial surface. This prompted us to use TCC as a complement activation marker in our study. Figure 5 depicts the data of the concentration measurements of TCC. The levels of TCC were undetectable at the start of the experiments but increased steadily in all tubes throughout the experiment. At several time points, significantly higher levels of TCC could be detected in heparin-coated tubes compared to PMEA-coated tubes (at 75 minute: 7.5 ± 0.8 AU/mL for heparin-coated tubes versus 4.8 ± 0.2 AU/mL for PMEA-coated tubes (mean ± sem), see Table 1 (supplementary material), $P = .001$; at 150 minute: 11.5 ± 1.4 AU/mL for heparin-coated tubes versus 7.9 ± 0.4 AU/mL for PMEA-coated tubes (mean ± sem), see Table 1 (supplementary material), $P = .024$; at 225 minute: 14.7 ± 1.3 AU/mL for heparin-coated tubes versus 11.1 ± 0.7 AU/mL for PMEA-coated tubes (mean ± sem), see Table 1 (supplementary material), $P = .027$) and uncoated controls (at 75 minute: 7.5 ± 0.8 AU/mL for heparin-coated tubes versus 5.9 ± 0.7 AU/mL for uncoated controls (mean ± sem), see Table 1 (supplementary material), $P = .036$). This suggests that TCC generation proceeds faster in heparin-coated tubes compared to PMEA-coated tubes and uncoated controls. Several in vitro studies using the Chandler loop model reported prevention of TCC generation by heparin-coated PVC compared to uncoated PVC [20, 23, 29, 33]. However, none of these studies had blood circulation times of more than two hours. Also, these studies used heparin coatings which were structurally different from the heparin coating evaluated in our study. Weber et al. compared covalently heparin-coated tubes from four different manufacturers and also found marked differences in hemocompatibility [11].

Analysis of the Inner Surface

Scanning Electron Microscopy

A set of scanning electron micrographs was recorded (3 different materials, 4 donors, 5 different times of circulation in the Chandler loop system, and three samples of every tube were examined). In general, we observed that adhesion of blood components developed slowly and gradually as the experiments proceeded. However, the SEM data revealed a striking difference between uncoated PVC and heparincoated PVC on one hand, and the PMEA-coated PVC on the other hand. Four micrographs, taken after 5 hours of blood circulation over the surfaces, are shown in Figure 6 to illustrate this difference. The uncoated PVC and heparin-coated PVC surfaces showed a remarkable resemblance. These surfaces were, to an extent of approximately 80%, devoid of any visible adherent blood components. There were, however, island-like regions, usually small (e.g., 10×10 μm) but sometimes larger (e.g., 100×200 μm). Enlarged images of these islands (see Figures 6(a) and 6(b)) revealed a flat patch-like structure, presumably composed of fibrin threads.

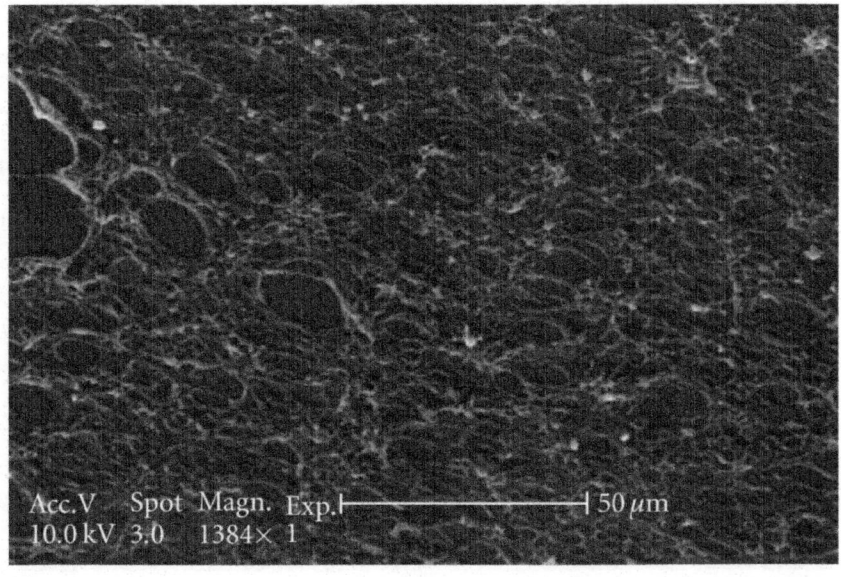

Acc.V Spot Magn. Exp.|————————————|50 μm
10.0 kV 3.0   1384× 1

(a)

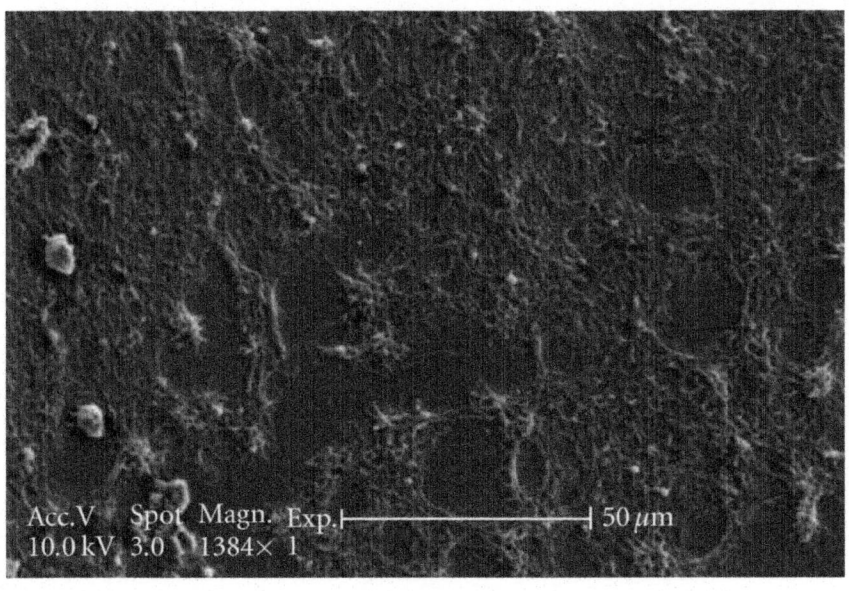

Acc.V Spot Magn. Exp.|————————————|50 μm
10.0 kV 3.0   1384× 1

(b)

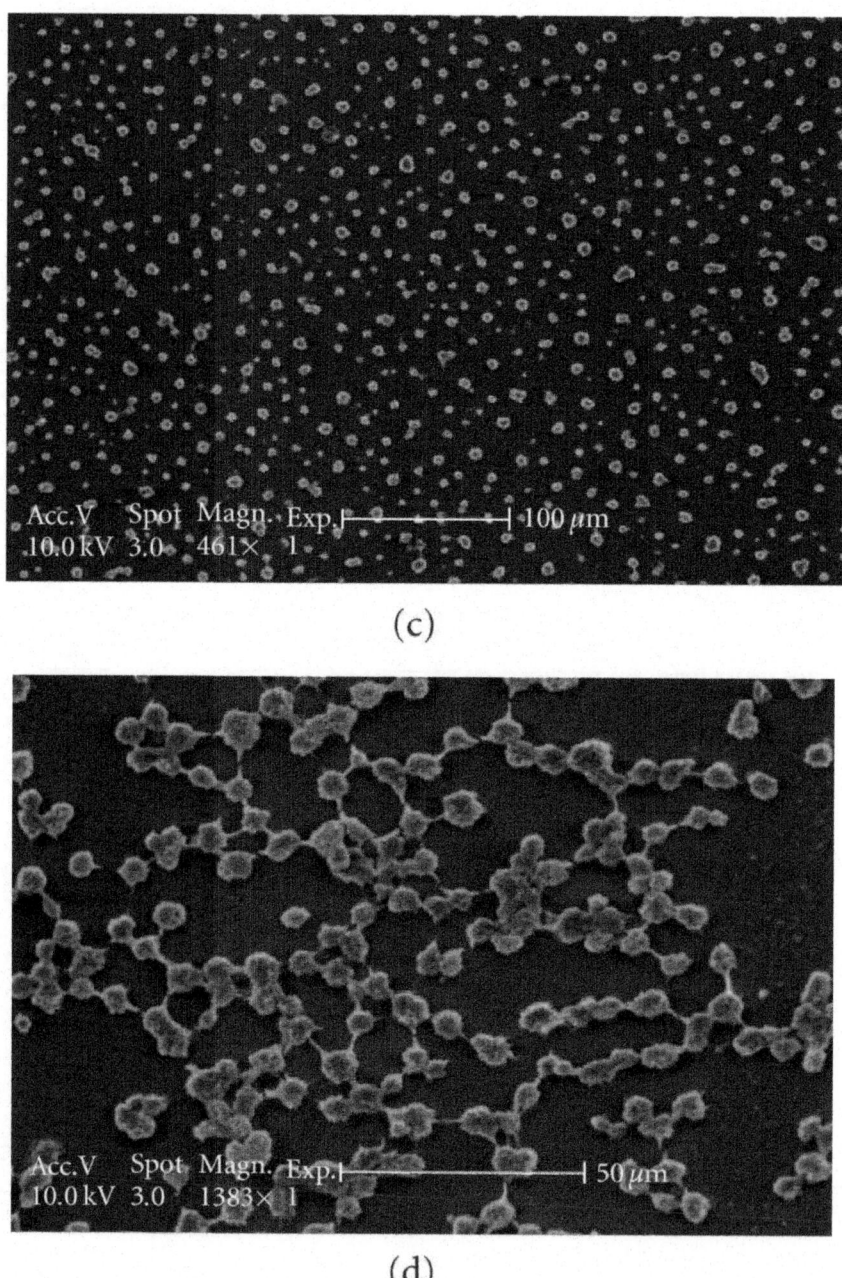

(c)

(d)

Figure 6: (a) Scanning electron micrograph of a typical island structure on the inner surface of the uncoated (control) tube, after 5 hours contact with full human blood in the Chandler loop model. A patch-like structure is seen, which is, presumably, composed of fibrin threads, which adhered to the surface. (b) Scanning electron micro-graph of a typical island structure on the inner surface of the heparin-coated tube (same conditions). The patch-like structures in (a) and (b) are similar; note that platelets as well as cells (presumably leukocytes) are seen in (b). (c) Scanning electron micrograph of the PMEA-coated surface, after 5 hours of experimentation in the Chandler loop. Adhered cells are observed, either individually, or in small aggregates of 2 or 3 cells. Cells and aggregates are, to a good approximation, evenly spread over the surface, although regions of relatively high cell density could be discerned. (d) Close-up on a region of relatively high cell density. Note that most of the adherent cells are engaged into cell-cell contacts through pseudopodia.

Some blood platelets were entrapped in the patch, in the case of the uncoated surface (see Figure 6(a)). For the heparin-coated surface, platelets as well as larger cells (presumably leukocytes) were entrapped in or adhered to the patch structure (see Figure 6(b)). Evaluation of the inner surface of the PMEA-coated tubing showed radically different pictures as can be seen in Figures 6(c) and 6(d). Fibrin formation is evident on the uncoated and heparin-coated surfaces, but not for the PMEA-coating. Scattered over the PMEA-coated surface, we encountered isolated cells, or ensembles of a small number of cells (typically 2 or 3 cells). Presumably, the adhered cells are leukocytes; the diameter of these cells is 10–15 μm. Figure 6(d) shows a detailed SEM micrograph of a region that was relatively densely populated with adherent cells. It is seen that most of the cells extend pseudopodia, through which they are connected to one or more neighbors. Leukocyte activation induced by surface contact, leading to pseudopodia (see Figure 6(d)), can also explain why the MPO concentration was highest for the PMEA-coated PVC tube as compared to the other two tubes (see Figure 4).

Measurement of Thrombin Generation Times

In view of the differences between these coatings encountered after prolonged blood contact in the Chandler loop, we decided to subject the surfaces also to the well-known thrombin generation assay [16–19]. Contact activation of the blood coagulation system is accompanied by a sudden increase of thrombin levels, after a lag-time that varies between approximately 5 minutes for highly thrombogenic materials to approximately 60 minutes for materials with extremely low thrombogenicity. Figure 7 shows the thrombin generation curves measured in triplicate with the uncoated, heparincoated, and PMEA-coated PVC tubes. Thrombin generation occurred between 30 and 40 minutes in the uncoated PVC tubes. Coating of the PVC with immobilized heparin prolonged the thrombin generation time until 60 minutes. This clearly indicates the better antithrombogenic properties of the heparin-coated PVC tubes compared to uncoated PVC tubes. A remarkable finding, however, was that coating of PVC tubes with PMEA resulted in thrombin generation times comparable to those of the uncoated PVC tubes. Note that, in the case of the heparin-coated PVC, the thrombin concentration remains heparin-coated PVC.

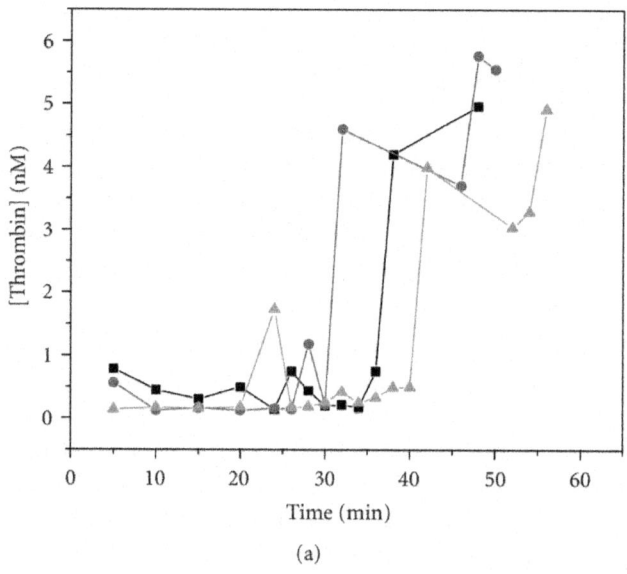

(a)

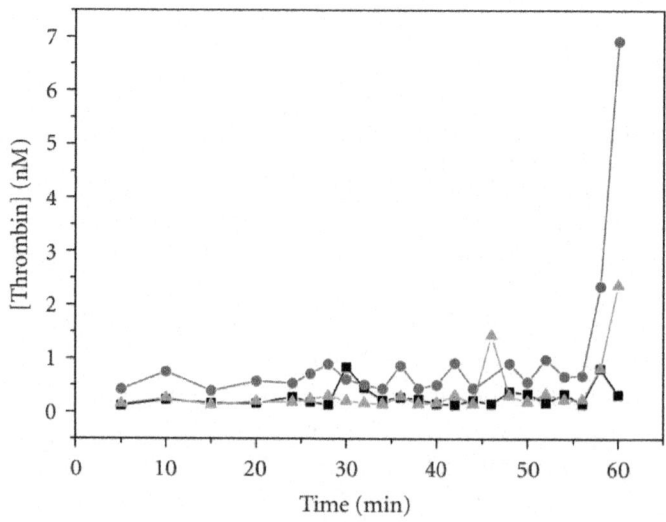

(b)

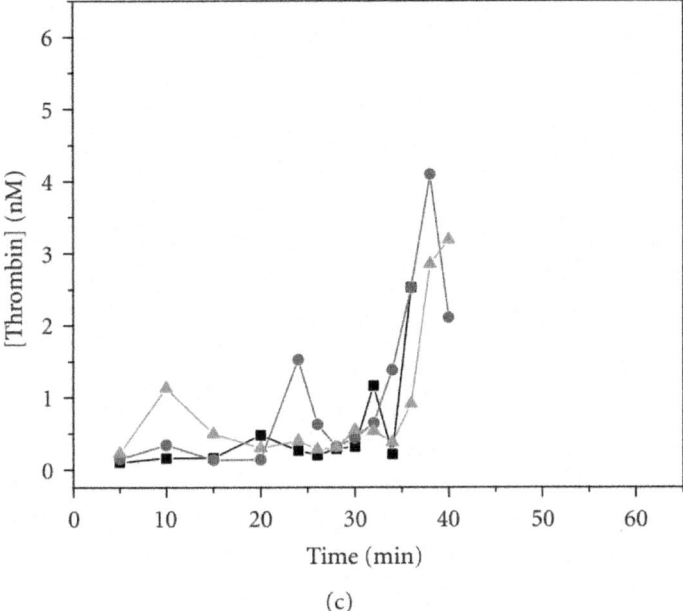

(c)

Figure 7: Thrombin generation curves measured for uncoated PVC (a), heparin-coated PVC (b), and PMEA-coated PVC (c) incubated with recalcified blood under static conditions. Experiments were performed in triplicate, that is, every blood sample was analyzed three times.

The Chandler Loop Model

After collecting all data, we wondered whether any correlation could be defined between the intensity of bloodbiomaterial contact in the Chandler loop system, and that in real-life extracorporeal circulation in CPB. Assuming that the level of blood-biomaterial contact (Q) is proportional to the surface area of the artificial material (S) and the time of blood-biomaterial contact (t), and inversely proportional to the blood volume (V), it can be calculated for the Chandler loop system (with S = 40 cm², V = 7 mL, t = 5 h), that Q = 28.6 h/cm. For a typical CPB system (with S = 25,000 cm², V = 8,000 mL (6 L of blood + 2 L of priming fluid)), it then follows that t = (28.6 × 8,000)/25,000 ≈ 9 h. In other words, this simple model indicates that 5 hours of experimentation in the Chandler loop corresponds with a level of bloodbiomaterial contact that corresponds to at least 9 hours of operation in a typical CPB system. Most probably, the estimated 9 hours is an underestimation, since the blood cells in real-life CPB are oxygenated and the blood resides mostly within the patient's vasculature. This probably implies that some recuperation of blood cells occurs during real-life CPB, while this is evidently not the case in our model system.

Noteworthy, the extent of hemolysis encountered in our experiments was very low, that is,

CONCLUSION

Systematic evaluation of the blood biomaterial contact for the three different tubings, using relatively long periods of blood-biomaterial contact, was performed. The three different surfaces were as follows: uncoated PVC, heparincoated PVC, and PMEA-coated PVC; the latter two are already in clinical use, as tubings in extracoporeal circulation equipment. Clear differences with respect to platelet counts, leukocyte activation (MPO release), and deposition of blood components at the inner surfaces were found. Most of these differences became apparent only after the first 2– 3 hours of experimentation. This underlines the importance of extended evaluation of blood-contacting biomaterials that are to be used in long-term applications, such as extended CPB. It is noteworthy that the PMEA-coated tubes showed a relatively low level of hemocompatibility. Compared with uncoated PVC and heparin-coated PVC, (i) a substantial drop of the platelet counts, (ii) activation of leukocytes and marked adherence of leukocytes at the inner surface, and (iii) a thrombogenicity comparable to uncoated PVC were observed. The present results lead to two important conclusions.

1. The Chandler loop system is the most useful method for the evaluation of blood-biomaterial interactions, which is most probably relevant for the development of equipment for extracorporeal circulation. Extended experimentation times (e.g., 5 hours) are mandatory, since differences for various materials may masquerade during the first few hours.

2.. PMEA biomaterial is probably not optimal for use in extracorporeal circulation equipment; further improvements are necessary.

ACKNOWLEDGMENTS

The help of H. Jussen and F. Spee (Instrument Development Engineering and Evaluation, University of Maastricht) is gratefully acknowledged. This study was financed within the framework of the Bioterials program, a 4-years privatepublic joint effort of the Dutch Ministry of Economic Affairs, the Province of Dutch Limburg, DSM Research BV (Geleen, the Netherlands), the Academic Hospital Maastricht, and the University of Maastricht. Bioterials runs in the period April 2005–April 2009.

REFERENCES

1. S. C. Skinner, R. B. Hirschl, and R. H. Bartlett, "Extracorporeal life support," Seminars in Pediatric Surgery, vol. 15, no. 4, pp. 242–250, 2006.

2. O. Mangoush, S. Purkayastha, S. Haj-Yahia, et al., "Heparinbonded circuits versus nonheparin-bonded circuits: an evaluation of their effect on clinical outcomes," European Journal of Cardio-Thoracic Surgery, vol. 31, no. 6, pp. 1058–1069, 2007.

3. F. D. Rubens, "Cardiopulmonary bypass technology transfer: musings of a cardiac surgeon," Journal of Biomaterials Science, Polymer Edition, vol. 13, no. 4, pp. 485–499, 2002.

4. H. P. Wendel and G. Ziemer, "Coating-techniques to improve the hemocompatibility of artificial devices used for extracorporeal circulation," European Journal of Cardio-Thoracic Surgery, vol. 16, no. 3, pp. 342–350, 1999.

5. D. Baykut, F. Bernet, J. Wehrle, K. Weichelt, P. Schwartz, and H. R. Zerkowski, "New surface biopolymers for oxygenators: an in vitro hemocompatibility test of poly(2- methoxyethylacrylate)," European Journal of Medical Research, vol. 6, no. 7, pp. 297–305, 2001.

6. X. M. Mueller, D. Jegger, M. Augustburger, J. Horisberger, and L. K. von Segesser, "Poly 2-methoxyethylacrylate (PMEA) coated oxygenator: an ex vivo study," International Journal of Artificial Organs, vol. 25, no. 3, pp. 223–229, 2002.

7. M. Ninomiya, K. Miyaji, and S. Takamoto, "Influence of PMEA-coated bypass circuits on perioperative inflammatory response," Annals of Thoracic Surgery, vol. 75, no. 3, pp. 913– 917, 2003.

8. J. O'Neill, G. Schutze, M. Heulitt, P. Simpson, and B. Taylor, "Nosocomial infections during extracorporeal membrane oxygenation," Intensive Care Medicine, vol. 27, no. 8, pp. 1247– 1253, 2001.

9. D. P. Mason, D. J. Boffa, S. C. Murthy, et al., "Extended use of extracorporeal membrane oxygenation after lung transplantation," Journal of Thoracic and Cardiovascular Surgery, vol. 132, no. 4, pp. 954–960, 2006.

10. K. Sung, Y. T. Lee, P. W. Park, et al., "Improved survival after cardiac arrest using emergent autopriming percutaneous cardiopulmonary support," Annals of Thoracic Surgery, vol. 82, no. 2, pp. 651–656, 2006.

11. N. Weber, H. P. Wendel, and G. Ziemer, "Quality assessment of heparin

coatings by their binding capacities of coagulation and complement enzymes," Journal of Biomaterials Applications, vol. 15, no. 1, pp. 8–22, 2000.

12. D. S. Rijkers, S. J. H. Wielders, G. I. Tesser, and H. C. Hemker, "Design and synthesis of thrombin substrates with modified kinetic parameters," Thrombosis Research, vol. 79, no. 5-6, pp. 491–499, 1995.

13. A. B. Chandler, "In vitro thrombotic coagulation of the blood; a method for producing a thrombus," Laboratory Investigation, vol. 7, no. 2, pp. 110–114, 1958.

14. R. Kopp, R. Bensberg, A. Kashefi, K. Mottaghy, R. Rossaint, and R. Kuhlen, "Effect of hirudin versus heparin on hemocompatibility of blood contacting biomaterials: an in vitro study," International Journal of Artificial Organs, vol. 28, no. 12, pp. 1272–1277, 2005.

15. C. M. Cripps, "Rapid method for the estimation of plasma haemoglobin levels," Journal of Clinical Pathology, vol. 21, no. 1, pp. 110–112, 1968.

16. Y. B. J. Aldenhoff, M. L. W. Knetsch, J. H. L. Hanssen, T. Lindhout, S. J. H. Wielders, and L. H. Koole, "Coils and tubes releasing heparin. Studies on a new vascular graft prototype," Biomaterials, vol. 25, no. 16, pp. 3125–3133, 2004.

17. Y. B. J. Aldenhoff, R. Blezer, T. Lindhout, and L. H. Koole, "Photo-immobilisation of dipyridamole (Persantin) at the surface of polyurethane biomaterials: reduction of in-vitro thrombogenicity," Biomaterials, vol. 18, no. 2, pp. 167–172, 1997.

18. T. W. Barrowcliffe, M. Cattaneo, G. M. Podda, et al., "New approaches for measuring coagulation," Haemophilia, vol. 12, supplement 3, pp. 76–81, 2006.

19. W. van Oeveren, J. Haan, P. Lagerman, and P. Schoen, "Comparison of coagulation activity tests in vitro for selected biomaterials," Artificial Organs, vol. 26, no. 6, pp. 506–511, 2002.

20. N. Weber, H. P. Wendel, and G. Ziemer, "Hemocompatibility of heparin-coated surfaces and the role of selective plasma protein adsorption," Biomaterials, vol. 23, no. 2, pp. 429–439, 2002.

21. G. M. Sreeram, A. D. Sharma, and T. F. Slaughter, "Platelet glycoprotein IIb/IIIa antagonists: perioperative implications," Journal of Cardiothoracic and Vascular Anesthesia, vol. 15, no. 2, pp. 237–240, 2001.

22. C. S. Rinder, J. L. Bonan, H. M. Rinder, J. Mathew, R. Hines, and B. R. Smith, "Cardiopulmonary bypass induces leukocyteplatelet adhesion," Blood, vol. 79, no. 5, pp. 1201–1205, 1992.

23. K. T. Lappegard, M. Fung, G. Bergseth, et al., "E ˚ ffect of complement inhibition and heparin coating on artificial surfaceinduced leukocyte and platelet activation," Annals of Thoracic Surgery, vol. 77, no. 3, pp. 932–941, 2004.

24. Y.-P. Wu, P. G. de Groot, and J. J. Sixma, "Shear stress-induced detachment of blood platelets from various surfaces," Arteriosclerosis, Thrombosis, and Vascular Biology, vol. 17, no. 11, pp. 3202–3207, 1997.

25. K. Kawahito, J. Mohara, Y. Misawa, and K. Fuse, "Platelet damage caused by the centrifugal pump: in vitro evaluation by measuring the release of α-granule packing proteins," Artifi- cial Organs, vol. 21, no. 10, pp. 1105–1109, 1997.

26. V. Kutay, T. Noyan, S. Ozcan, Y. Melek, H. Ekim, and C. Yakut, "Biocompatibility of heparin-coated cardiopulmonary bypass circuits in coronary patients with left ventricular dysfunction is superior to PMEA-coated circuits," Journal of Cardiac Surgery, vol. 21, no. 6, pp. 572–577, 2006.

27. R. A. Malinauskas, "Plasma hemoglobin measurement techniques for the in vitro evaluation of blood damage caused by medical devices," Artificial Organs, vol. 21, no. 12, pp. 1255– 1267, 1997.

28. R. Ohkawa, Y. Hirowatari, K. Nakamura, et al., "Platelet release of β-thromboglobulin and platelet factor 4 and serotonin in plasma samples," Clinical Biochemistry, vol. 38, no. 11, pp. 1023–1026, 2005.

29. K. T. Lappegard, M. Fung, G. Bergseth, J. Riesenfeld, and T. ˚ E. Mollnes, "Artificial surface-induced cytokine synthesis: effect of heparin coating and complement inhibition," Annals of Thoracic Surgery, vol. 78, no. 1, pp. 38–44, 2004.

30. A. E. Asberg and V. Videm, "Neutrophil dysfunction after bio- ˚ material contact in an in vitro model of cardiopulmonary bypass," European Journal of Cardio-Thoracic Surgery, vol. 30, no. 5, pp. 744–748, 2006.

31. A. E. Asberg and V. Videm, "Activation of neutrophil gran- ˚ ulocytes in an in vitro model of a cardiopulmonary bypass," Artificial Organs, vol. 29, no. 12, pp. 927–936, 2005.

32. J. Gong, R. Larsson, K. N. Ekdahl, T. E. Mollnes, U. Nilsson, and B. Nilsson, "Tubing loops as a model for cardiopulmonary bypass circuits: both the biomaterial and the blood-gas phase interfaces induce complement activation in an in vitro model," Journal of Clinical Immunology, vol. 16, no. 4, pp. 222–229, 1996.

33. J. Andersson, J. Sanchez, K. N. Ekdahl, G. Elgue, B. Nilsson, and R. Larsson, "Optimal heparin surface concentration and antithrombin binding capacity as evaluated with human nonanticoagulated blood in vitro," Journal of Biomedical Materials Research Part A, vol. 67, no. 2, pp. 458–466, 2003.

Chapter 2

STUDIES ON PROCESSING AND CHARACTERIZATION OF HYDROXYAPATITE BIOMATERIALS FROM DIFFERENT BIO WASTES

Sudip Mondal[1,2], Biswanath Mondal[1], Apurba Dey[2], and Sudit S. Mukhopadhyay[2]

[1]Centre for Advanced Material Processing, Central Mechanical Engineering Research Institute, Mahatma Gandhi Avenue, Durgapur-713209, India

[2]Department of Biotechnology, National Institute of Technology, Mahatma Gandhi Avenue Durgapur-713209, India

ABSTRACT

Development of suitable materials that acts as an interface between the implant and tissues in body system structurally, mechanically and bio functionally is important for the success of tissue engineering. This motivated materials scientists and biologists to find out suitable bioactive materials for the aforementioned purpose. There has been growing interest in developing bioactive synthetic ceramics that could closely mimic natural apatite characteristics. Hydroxyapatite (HAp) has been widely used as a biocompatible ceramic but mainly for contact with bone tissue, due to its resemblance to mineral bone. This study presents the synthesis and characterization of HAp materials from different sources like bovine bone and fish scales and their application in tissue engineering. The phase purity and crystallinity of different calcined HAp powder was determined by XRD and FTIR analysis. The Thermo Gravimetric and Differential Thermal Analysis were carried out to show the thermal stability of the HAp powder. The morphology of the powder was observed under Scanning Electron Microscopy (SEM). Cytotoxicity evaluation of the developed powder was carried out in RAW macrophage like cell line media for an incubation period of 72 hours. These results proved the biocompatibility of HAp powders obtained from different biosources for tissue engineering applications.

INTRODUCTION

Hydroxyapatite [$Ca_{10}(PO_4)_6(OH)_2$] has been acknowledged as a bone graft material in a range of medical and dental applications due to their similar chemical composition with natural bones. Generally, bone substitution materials such as autograft, allograft and xenograft are used to solve problems related to bone trauma and fractures. But, none of these materials provide a perfect replacement of the bone due to mechanical and biological instability and incompatibility. Recently, calcium phosphate bi o ceramics such as calcium phosphate, tri-calcium phosphate and HAp are identified as most suitable bone substitution materials to serve the demand. Unlike other calcium phosphates, HAp does not break under physiological conditions. In fact, it is thermodynamically stable at physiological pH and actively takes part in bone bonding. This property has been exploited for rapid bone repair after major trauma or surgery. HAp is derived from natural materials such as coral and fish bone (Jensen et al., 1996), fish scale (Mondal et al. 2010). Attempts have been taken to isolate fish scale derived HAp and use them as an alternate for synthetic HAp (Mondal et al. 2010). Generally, very high heat treatment (1250°C) is used for isolation of HAp from fish scale and this temperature gives a higher strength to HAp structure (Choi, Lee, Jeon, Byun, & Kim, 1999) and results an excellent biocompatible inorganic substance (Kim et al., 1998; Kim & Park, 2000; Kim, Park, & Kim, 2001). HAp and calcium phosphate based materials have attracted consider able interest in the field of Tissue Engineering because of similarities with the mineral fraction of natural bone and high biocompatibility with living tissues. It has good bio affinity, stimulates osteo conduction and is slowly replaced by the host bone after implantation. Application of the HAp biomaterial as a porous or granulated material useful in bone surgery or coating on metallic bio implants. A number of methods have been used for HAp powder synthesis such as solid state reaction, hydrothermal reaction, co-precipitation reaction, sol-gel synthesis, mechano-chemical synthesis etc. [1-5] . Natural structural HAp material from fish scale [6] and bovine bone not onl y provide an abundant source for novel bone and cartilage replacement but it also inspires investigations to develop biomimetic composites.

In this study HAp powder was synthesized from fish scales. Fish scales are mainly composed of collagen, connective tissue proteins, water and the remaining 41% to 84% [7] of other proteins. In course of evolution, scale formation process shows the same mechanism as in the formation of teeth and bone. This study shows that the biomimetic property may lead to the development of new biomaterials. There are several types of calcium phosphate salts, which are present in fish scales due to their extreme biological response in physiological environment. HAp powder was extracted by calcining the chemically treated fish scales at different temperatures. Extraction of HAp from bovine bone is biologically safe and economic, since it is easy to obtain. Bone is a unique composite, containing a collagenous hydrogel matrix consisting of about 33–43% apatite minerals, 32–44% organics, and 15–25% [8] water on a volumetric basis. HAp material manufactured from bovine bones has the advantage of inheriting some properties of the raw materials viz. its chemical composition and structure. The synthesized powder from these two different bio sources are ball milled for several hours and compacted. The Thermo Gravimetric- Differential Thermal Analysis, X - ray diffraction (XRD), Fourier Transform Infrared spectroscopy (FTIR) were employed to characterize the synthesized powder. The morphology of the derived HAp powder has also been studied by SEM. Many processing technologies have been employed to obtain porous ceramics for bone tissue engineering. In tissue repair application the macro pores and highly interconnected networks are required for in-growth of surrounding host tissues. The milled powder was mixed with surfactant and finally press injection method was applied to make small diameter fillers. As a first parameter of biocompatibility [9] the ability of the cells to attach to the material surface during the early period of cell/material interaction was used. Then the powders were screened *in vitro* for cytotoxic [10] effects on cultured RAW macrophage cells. Cell attachment [11] study was observed under inverted microscopic analysis. Cytotoxicity effects were analyzed by Trypan blue staining method.

EXPERIMENTAL PROCEDURE

Synthesis of Hydroxyapatite Powder from Fish Scale

Fish scales were collected from fresh water fish (*Labeo rohita*) and washed thoroughly in running tap water. The collected scales were initially de-proteinized through external washing with 1 (N) HCl (Merck, 35%) solution (2:1, v/w, water HCl /fish scale) for 24 hours at room temperature (25° ±2°C). Next, the de-proteinized fish scales were washed thoroughly several times with distilled water. Remaining proteins of fish scales were treated with 1(N) NaOH solution. The filtered fish scales were washed thoroughly with distilled water and dried at 60°C in hot air oven for several hours. Treated fish scales were calcined at different temperatures to synthesize HAp ceramics.

Synthesis of Hydroxyapatite Powder from Bovine Bone

Bovine bone were initially deproteinized externally with 1 (N) HCl (Merck, 35%) solution and finally 1(N) NaOH solution was added for removal of remaining proteins. The samples were then thoroughly washed with double distilled water and dried at 50-60°C at hot air oven. The dried samples were then calcined in air atmosphere for an hour at different temperatures viz. 1000°C, 1100°C and 1200°C to obtain HAp phase.

Preparation of Small Fillers

The synthesized powder was mixed with starch and milled for 48 hours in ball mill. Triton – X surfactant was added drop-wise with the powder to make a paste. Injection press method was employed to make small 2mm diameter and 4 mm long fillers with this paste. The small roshaped fillers were then dried at 80°C for several hours. Finally, the dried samples were sintered at 1100°C for two hours.

POWDER CHARACTERIZATIONS

The Thermo Gravimetric and Differential Thermal Analysis of HAp from treated fish scale and bovine bone was carried out using Thermal analyzer (Netzsch, STA 409) over a temperature range of 30°C-1250°C and heating rate of 10°C/min under air atmosphere. The crystalline phases of synthesized powders were identified by X- ray diffraction analysis (Shimadzu, XRD-6000, CuKα radiation). FTIR (Shimadzu) analysis of calcined powder at different temperatures were carried out to confirm the structural composition. The average particle sizes of powder samples were observed through SEM analysis. The optimized calcined HAp powder derived from fish scales were wet ball milled for several hours and compacted into cylindrical/square shapes. Cytotoxicity and cell attachment studies of synthesized HAp materials were also carried out in RAW macrophage like cell line media.

RESULTS AND DISCUSSION

TG DTA Analysis

The thermo gravimetric analysis (Fig.1.) of chemically treated fish scales were carried out between 35°C and 1250°C in air at a heating rate of 100C/min. In this analysis actual weight losses [12-13] are observed in three steps and the related temperature ranges are 30°C - 800°C. The first loss is due to the weakly entrapped water in the sample material, the second and third losses resulted from the decomposition and burning of organic components in the raw scales. As the washing treatment could not completely remove the organic compounds of the inner parts of scale structure, the large weight loss is resulted mainly from those organics. However, there was minor weight loss on heating up to 1250°C which indicates thermal stability of the sample in this range.

The thermo gravimetric analysis (Fi g.2.) of chemically treated bovine bone was carried out from room temperature to 1250°C in air atmosphere at a heating rate of 100C/min. In this analysis, actual weight losses were observed with rising temperature. The first loss is due to the removal of trapped water in the sample material, the second and third losses resulted from the decomposition and burning of organic components in the bovine bone constituents. However, minor weight loss was observed on heating up to 1250°C

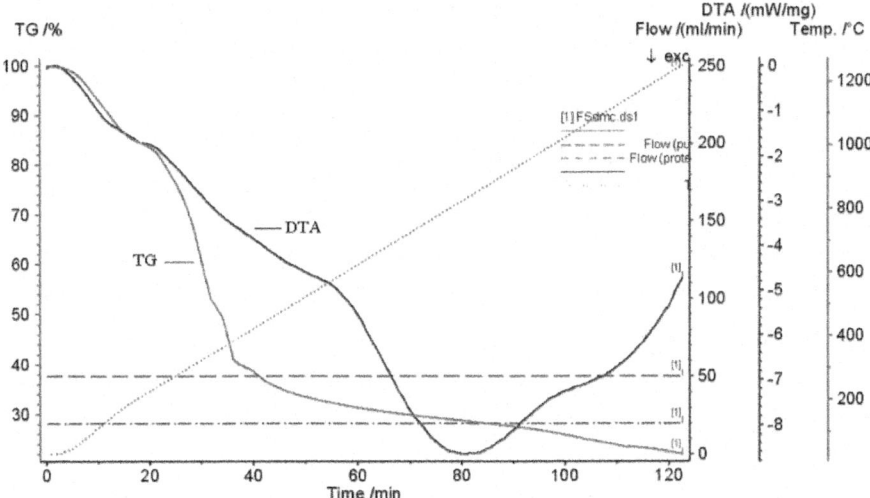

Figure 1. TG DTA of Fish scale.

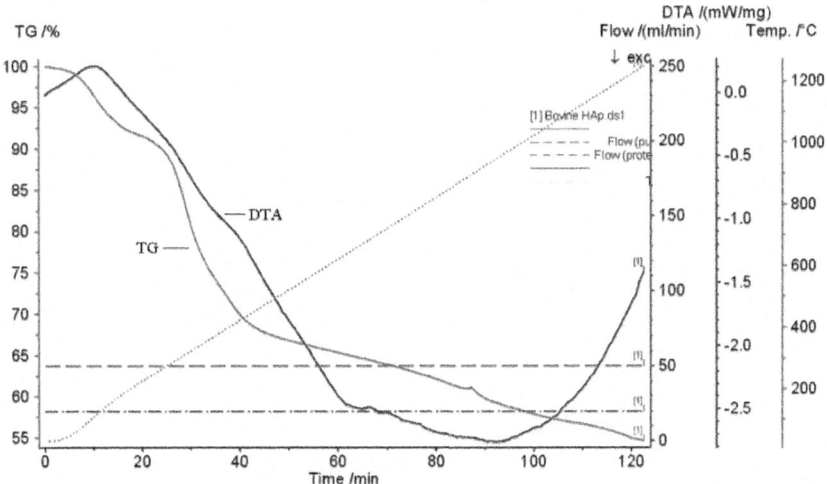

Figure 2. TG DTA of Bovine bone.

XRD Analysis

XRD patterns of synthesized HAp particles from fish scales and bovine bone are shown in Fig. 3 and 4 respectively. The crystalline phase analysis of the HAp powder from two different bio sources w er e carried out by x-ray diffraction studies. Identification of the phases was realized by comparing the experimental XRD pattern to standards complied by the International Centre for Diffraction Data (ICDD) using the cards 00-009-0432 for hexagonal HAp structure. Each pattern showed HAp as the only phase. Well-resolved characteristic peak of highest intensity for HAp was obtained at 2θ value of 31.77° corresponding to 211 plane. The phase formed was pure and matches well with standard pattern. The standard corresponding plane for HAp (viz. 100, 101, 200, 002, 211, 202, 301, 130, 131, 113, 203, 222, 132, 321, 004, 240, 241, 502, 323, 511) are well observed in case of both the synthesized powders. Sharp peak intensity and well resolved peaks in XRD patterns of the powders at high calcination temperature proves complete crystallization of the powder. The crystallite sizes of HAp particles were calculated using Scherer's equation

$$D = 0.9 \lambda / B \cos \theta$$

[Where, D represents mean grain size, B stands for full width at half maximum of the peak, λ is the diffraction wavelength (0.154059 nm) and θ is the diffraction angle

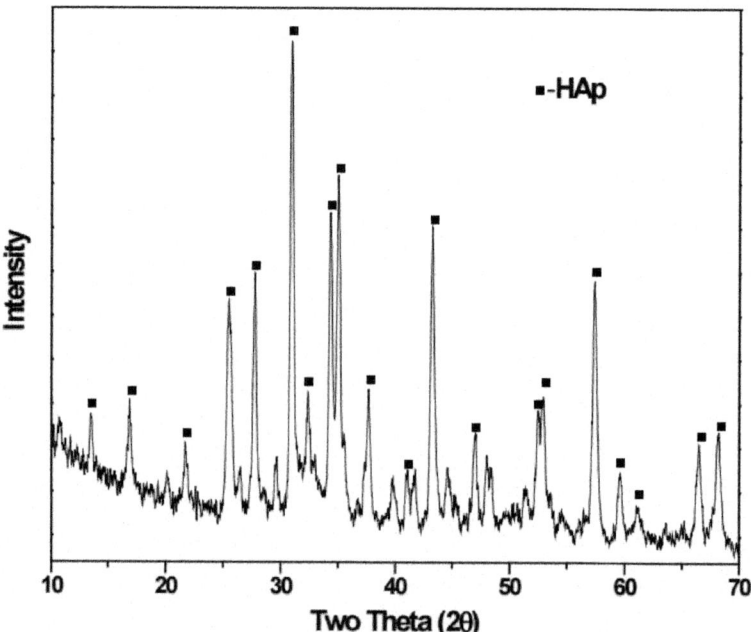

Figure 3. XR D Pattern of synthesized HA p powder from Fish scale.

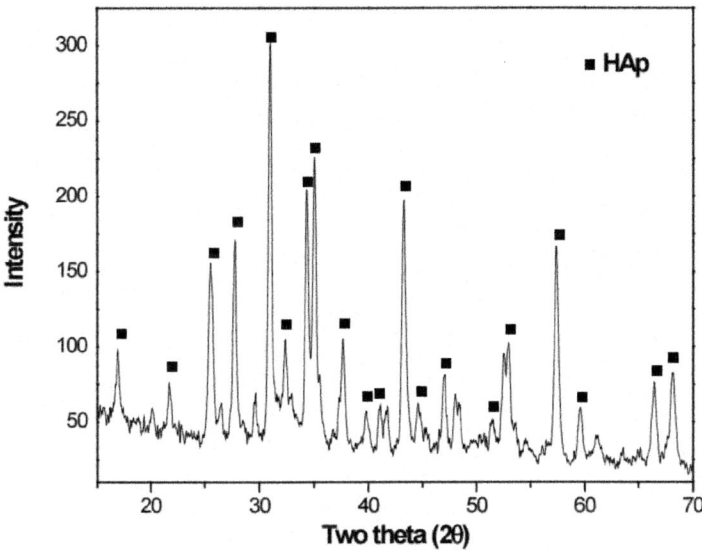

Figure. 4. XRD pattern of Hydroxyapatite powder from Bovine bone.

The Bragg reflection at (002) planes of HAp was considered to calculate the crystallite size. Crystallite size for HAp synthesized from fish scales and bovine bones are 69.6 nm, 77.62 nm respectively.

FTIR Analysis

Fourier transform infrared (FTIR) spectroscopy was employed to characterize the different functional groups of HAp Ca_{10} $(PO_4)_6(OH)_2$, (HAp) powder obtained from two bio sources. Figures 5 and 6 show the FTIR spectrum of synthesized HAp from fish scales and cow bone, respectively. The spectrum was recorded in the range of 4000–400 cm^{-1}. The representative FTIR spectrum shows all characteristic absorption peaks of HAp. The first indication for formation of HAp is in the form of a strong complex broad FTIR band centered at about 1000-1100 cm^{-1} due to asymmetric stretching mode of vibration for PO4 group [14]. The band at 576.30 cm^{-1} corresponds to n4 symmetric P-O stretching vibration of the PO4 group [15]. As a major peak of phosphate group, the n3 vibration peak could be identified in the region between 1100-960 cm^{-1} for all two powders which are due to P-O asymmetric stretching of PO 43- . The band at 2005-2079 cm^{-1} is due to overtone of 1040 cm^{-1} band. The presence of peak in the region 1400cm^{-1}- 1450 cm^{-1} was due to absorbed carbon dioxide. The crystalline powder generates two characteristic stretching modes of O-H bands at about 3497 cm^{-1} and 456c m^{-1} which are notice in all FTIR spectra of HAp.

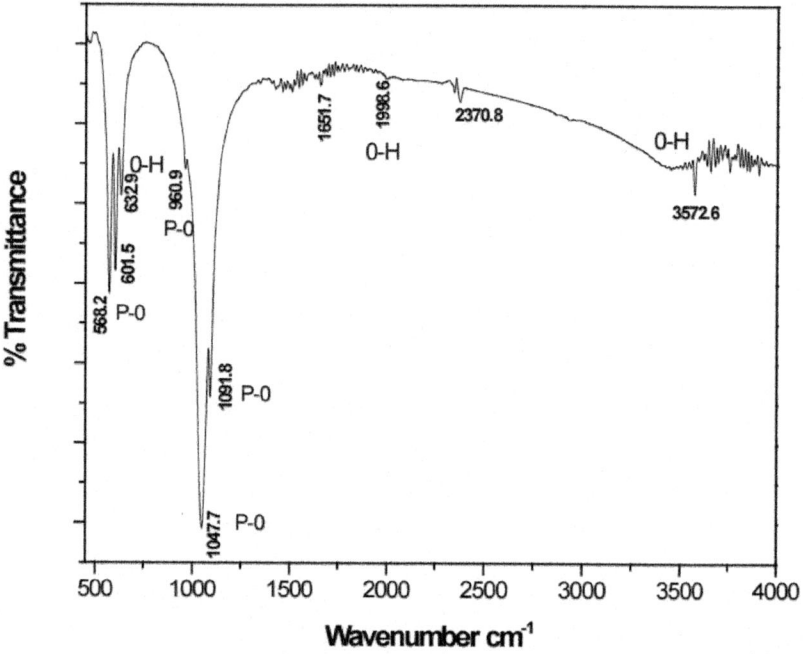

Figure 5. FTIR Spectrum of Hydroxyapatite powder from Fish scale.

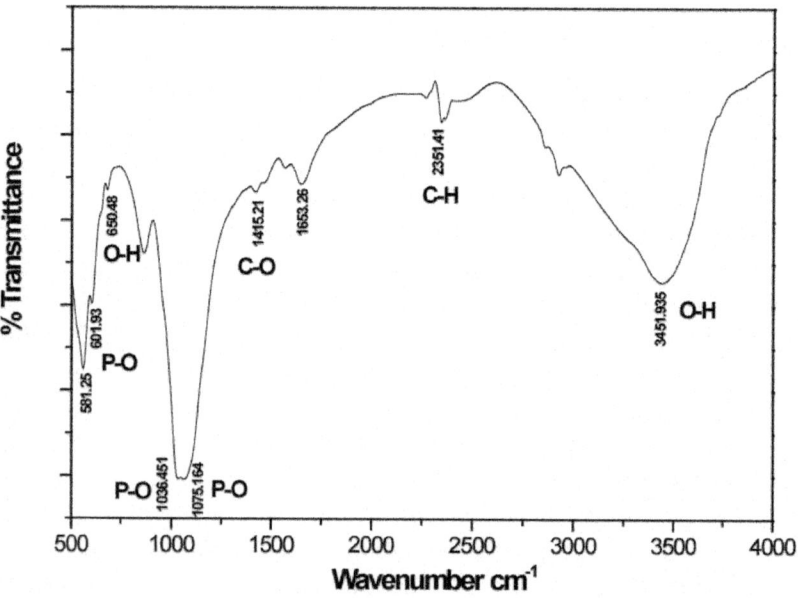

Figure 6. FTIR spectrum of Hydroxyapatite powder from Bovine bone.

SEM Analysis

The SEM micrographs of synthesized HAp powder (Fig. 7, 8) from fish scale and bovine bone sources were soft agglomerated ultra-fine HAp particles which break up easily during compaction due to high uniform pressure

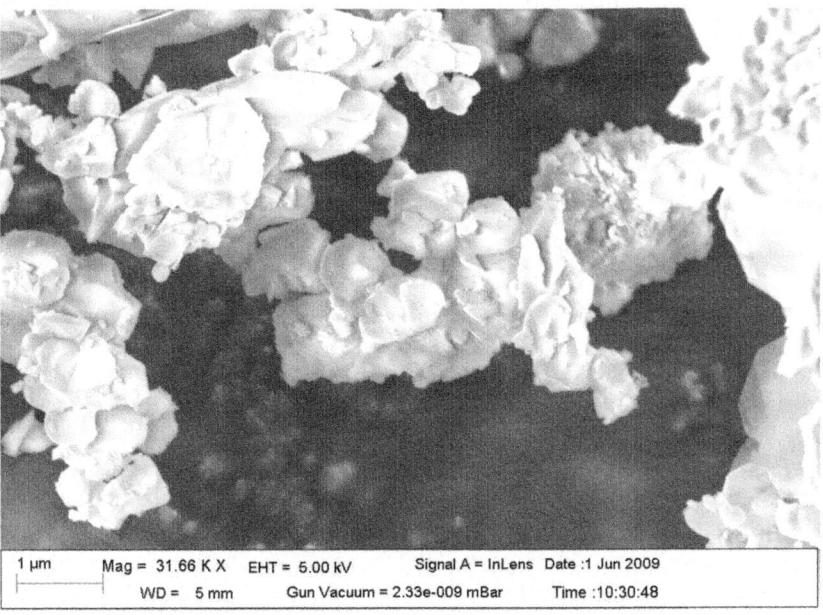

Figure 7. FE-SEM of HAp powder synthesized from Fish Scale

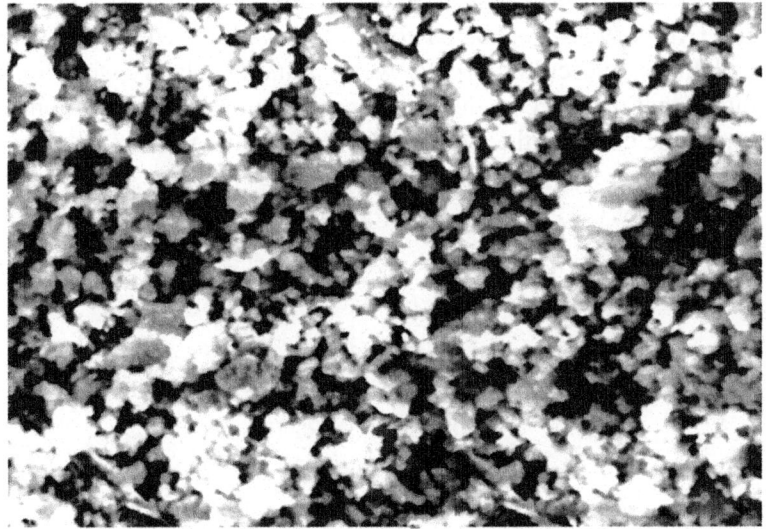

Figure 8. FE-SEM of HAp powder synthesized from Bovine Bone

Bio Fillers Made Up of Hap Powder

The synthesized powder was wet ball milled for several hours and by using surfactants like Triton-X small fillers were made for bio implants. These small fillers were then sintered at 1100° C temperature and prepared for *in vivo* bio implantation (Fig. 9 [a] and 9 [b]) and subsequent toxicity testing. The porosity of the sintered body in all the cases was around 10-15%

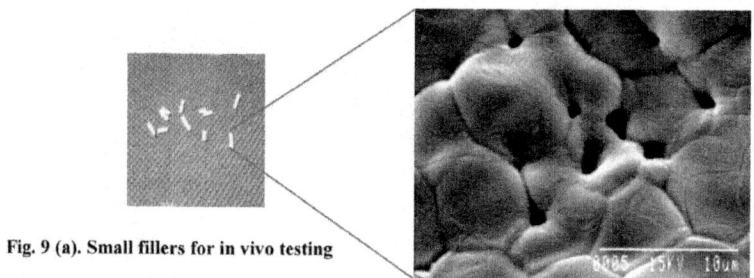

Fig. 9 (a). Small fillers for in vivo testing

Fig. 9 (b). SEM image of the small fillers

In vitro Analysis

HAp Powder samples as well as fillers and plates were utilized for further *in vitro* testing. First of all samples were sterilized by autoclaving at 16 lb /inch2 pressure for 20 minutes. Then the samples were placed into RPMI culture media. Here RAW cell lines were utilized for experimental purpose. Cell loads were given 10 5 cells/ 200 micro liter. After incubation in cell culture media samples are stained and observed under inverted microscopy. Fig. 10, 11 and 12 show HAp particles incubated for 72 hours along with macrophage like RAW cell lines. The cultured cells were stained with Trypan Blue and the result shows that there are no dead cells in the culture vessels. It confirms that there is no toxic effect of the synthesized HAp materials.

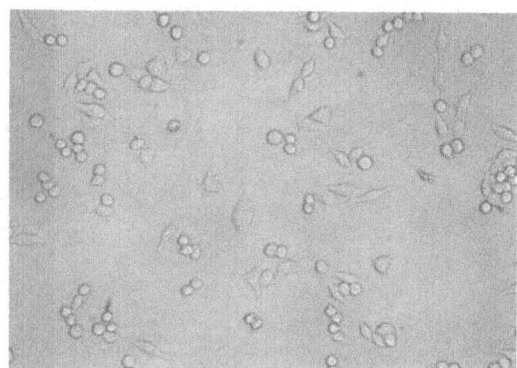

Figure 10. RAW cell line control media.

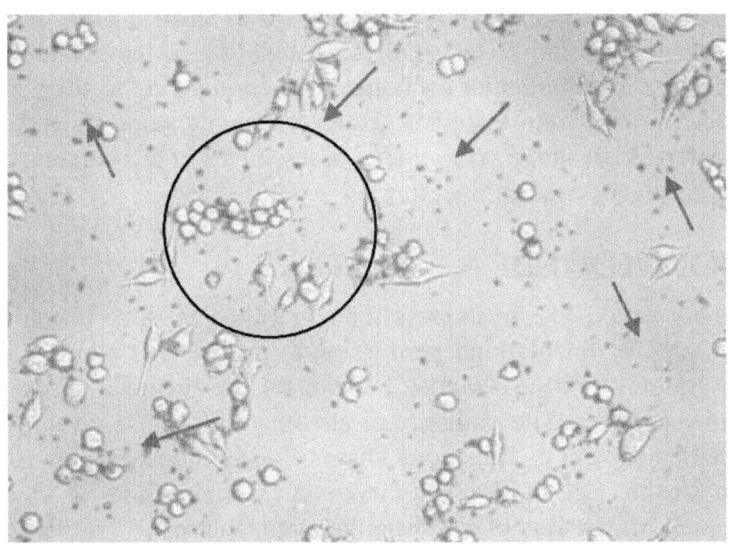

Figure 11. RAW cell line with Fish scale derived HAp particles (red arrow).

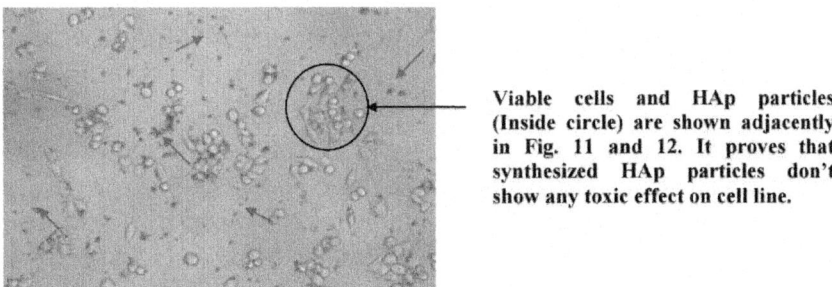

Viable cells and HAp particles (Inside circle) are shown adjacently in Fig. 11 and 12. It proves that synthesized HAp particles don't show any toxic effect on cell line.

Figure 12. RAW cell line with Bovine bone derived HAp particles (red arrow).

CONCLUSIONS

The present study reveals that HAp powder can be synthesized by thermal decomposition using fish scale and bovine bone in an eco-friendly manner. FTIR, X- ra y diffraction and EDX analysis indicated the phase purity and crystallinity of the HAp powder. TG-DTA analysis results showed the thermal stability of HAp powder derived from these two different biosources. The micro-structural stud y of comp acted powders show the presence of uniformly distributed very fine sub-micron particles. HAp ceramic fillers prepared from Injection press method are found to exhibit 30% porosity, which could be useful for biomedical applications such as fillers or scaffold. These small biocompatible osteo-conductive fillers appear to have a great potential for bone tissue engineering. The small biocompatible osteo-conductive fillers appear to have great potential for bone tissue engineering as the y showed no toxic effect on cell culture studies. More systematic studies are required for the characterization and *in vivo, in vitro* assessments of bio-ceramic composite scaffolds for bone tissue engineering

ACKNOWLEDGEME NT

The authors would like to express their gratitude to Prof. Gautam Biswas, Director, CMERI for his kind permission to present this paper. The authors are also grateful to CSIR, Govt. of India, for the financial support through networking projects. The authors are also thankful to Dr. Syamal Roy and all the staff members of Infectious Diseases & Immunology Division, IICB, Kolkata, for their cell culture and cytotoxicit y studies and Mr. P. Dhak, Mr. A. Paria and Mr. B. Das of IIT, Kharagpur for thermal, FE- SEM and XRD studies.

REFERENCES

1.   Mobasherpour, I., Heshajin, M. S., Kazemzadeh, A., M. Zakeri, M., 2007, "Synthesis of Nanocrystalline Hydroxyapatite by using Precipitation Method," J. Alloys Compd., Vol. 430, pp. 330-333.

2.   Parthiban, S.P., Elayaraja, K., Girija, E. K., Yokogawa, Y., Kesavamoorthy, R., Palanichamy, M., Asokan, K., and Narayana Kalkura, S., 2009, "Preparation of thermally stable nanocrystalline hydroxyapatite by hydrothermal method." J. Mater. Sc: Mater. Med., Vol. 20, pp. 77-83.

3.   Kim, W., Zhang, Q., and F. Saito., 2000, "Mechanochemical synthesis of hydroxyapatite from $Ca(OH)_2$-P_2O_5 and CaO-$Ca(OH)_2$-P_2O_5 mixtures." J. Mater. Sci., Vol. 35, pp. 5401-5405.

4.   Balamurugan, A., Kannan, S., and Rajeswari S., 2002, "Bioactive sol-gel hydroxyapatite surface for biomedical applications-in vitro study." Trends. Biomater. Artif. Organs, Vol. 16, pp. 18-20.

5.   Tadic D., and. Epple, M., 2003, "Mechanically stable implants of synthetic bone mineral by cold isostatic pressing.", Biomaterials, Vol. 24, pp. 4565-4571.

6.   Mondal, S., Mahata, S., Kundu, S., and Mondal, B., 2010, "Processing of natural resourced hydroxyapatite ceramics from fish scale." Adv. Appl. Ceram.: Struct. Funct. Bioceram., Vol. 109, pp. 234-239.

7.   [7]astry T.P., Sankar S., Mohan R., Rani S., Sundaraseelan T., 2008,

"Preparation and partial characterization of collagen sheet from fish (Lates calcarifer) scales" International Journal of Biological Macromolecules, Vol. 42, pp. 6-9.

8. Kalita, S.J., Bhardwaj, A., Bhatt, H.A., 2007, "Nanocrystalline calcium phosphate ceramics in biomedical engineering." Materials Science and Engineering: C, Vol. 27 Issue 3, pp. 441-449.

9. Liao, C. J., Lin, F. H., Chen, K. S., and J. S. Sun., J.S., 1999, "Thermal decomposition and reconstitution of hydroxyapatite in air atmosphere." Biomaterials, Vol. 20, pp. 1807–1813.

10. Roy, M., Krishna, B V., Bandyopadhya, A., Bose, S., 2011, "Compositionally graded hydroxyapatite/tricalcium phosphate coating on Ti by laser and induction plasma." Acta Biomaterialia, Vol. 7, pp. 866-873.

11. Stok, J. V. der, Lieshout, E. M. M. V., Massoudi, Y. E., Gerdine H. Van Kralingen, G. H. V., and Patka, P., 2011, "Bone substitutes in the Netherlands – A systematic literature review" Acta Biomaterialia., Vol. 7 , pp. 739-750.

12. Mortier, A., Lemaitre, J., and Rouxhet, P.G., 1989, "Temperature programmed characterization of synthetic calcium deficient hydroxyapatite." Thermochim. Acta,, Vol. 143, pp. 265-282.

13. Ozawa, M., Suzuki, S., 2002 "Microstructural Development of Natural Hydroxyapatite Originated from Fish-Bone Waste through Heat Treatment." J. Am. Ceram. Soc., Vol. 85, pp. 1315-1317.

14. Rocha, J. H. G., Lemos, A.F., Kannan, S., Agathopoulos, S., Ferreira, J. M. F., 2005, "Hydroxyapatite scaffolds hydrothermally grown from aragonitic cuttlefish bones", Journals of Materials Chemistry, Vol. 15, pp. 5007-5011.

15. Varma, H.K., and Babu, S., 2005. "Synthesis of Calcium Phosphate Bioceramics by Citrate Gel Pyrolysis Method." Ceram. Int., Vol. 31, pp. 109-114.

Chapter 3

BIODEGRADATION OF SILK BIOMATERIALS

Yang Cao[1] and Bochu Wang[1,2]

[1]College of Biological and Environmental Engineering, Jiangsu University of Science and Technology, Zhenjiang Jiangsu 212018, P.R. China

[2]College of Bioengineering, Chongqing University, Chongqing 400030, P.R. China

ABSTRACT

Silk fibroin from the silkworm, *Bombyx mori*, has excellent properties such as biocompatibility, biodegradation, non-toxicity, adsorption properties, etc. As a kind of ideal biomaterial, silk fibroin has been widely used since it was first utilized for sutures a long time ago. The degradation behavior of silk biomaterials is obviously important for medical applications. This article will focus on silk-based biomaterials and review the degradation behaviors of silk materials.

INTRODUCTION

What is a biomaterial? Biomaterial can be defined as "any substance (other than a drug) or combination of substances synthetic or natural in origin, which can be used any time, as a whole or as a part of a system which treats, augments, or replaces any tissue, organ or function of the body"[1]. Theoretically, any material, natural or man-made, can be a biomaterial as long as it serves the stated medical and surgical purposes. The development of biomaterials is not a new area. It encompasses elements of medicine, biology, physical, chemistry, tissue engineering and materials science. Nevertheless, the demand for biocompatible, biodegradable and bioresorbable materials has increased dramatically since the last decade. An ideal biomaterial is one that is non-immunogenic, biocompatible and biodegradable, which can be functionalized with bioactive proteins and chemicals. In particular, biodegradability is one of the essential properties of the biomaterials. Over the past decades, significant attention has been paid to the biodegradable biomaterials. Here are some of the important properties of biodegradable biomaterials [2]:

- The material should not evoke a sustained inflammatory or toxic response upon implantation *in vivo*.
- The material should have acceptable shelf life.
- The degradation time of the material should match the healing or regeneration process.
- The material should have appropriate mechanical properties for the indicated application, and any variation in mechanical properties with degradation should be compatible with the healing or regeneration process.
- The degradation products should be non-toxic, and easily metabolized and cleared from the body.
- The material should have appropriate permeability and processibility for the intended application.

Consequently, a wide variety of natural and synthetic biodegradable polymers have been investigated recently for medical and pharmaceutical applications. Natural biodegradable polymers like collagen, gelatin, chitosan and silk fibroin have promising advantages over synthetic polymers due to their favorable properties, including good biocompatibility, biodegradability and bioresorbability. Their physical and chemical properties can be easily modified to achieve desirable mechanical and degradation characteristics. Among these natural polymers, silk fibroin provides an important set of material options for biomaterials and scaffolds in biomedical applications because of its high tensile strength, controllable biodegradability, haemostatic properties, non-cytotoxicity, low antigenicity and noninflammatory characteristics [3–5].

Silk fibroin is a natural protein produced by the domestic silkworm, *Bombyx mori*. It can be used as a biomaterial in various forms [6], such as films [7–9], membranes [10], gels [11], sponges [12], powders [13], and scaffolds [14–16]. Applications include burn-wound dressings [17], enzyme immobilization matrices [18], nets [19], vascular prostheses and structural implants [20–21]. Silk has been commercially used as biomedical sutures since decades of years ago. Because of its special crystallization and orientation, as well as compact structure, natural fibroin is difficult to degrade. As a kind of FDA approved biomaterial, silk is defined by United States Pharmacopeia as non-degradable for its negligible tensile strength loss *in vivo*. However, according to the literature, silk is degradable but over longer time period. In general, silk is slowly absorbed *in vivo*. The rate of degradation depends on many factors. This article will focus on the silk-based biomaterials, and review the degradation behaviors of silk materials.

STRUCTURE AND PROPERTIES OF SILK BIOMATERIALS

The silk worm has been domesticated for thousands of years. The cocoon is wrapped in a continuous silk thread whose length can exceed 1 km [22]. Normally, native silk fiber consists of two types of self-assembled proteins: fibroin and sericin [23,24]. These two proteins both contain the same 18 amino acids such as glycine, alanine and serine in different amounts. The core fibroins are encased in a coat of sericin, a family of hydrophilic proteins which holds two fibroin fibers together [25–26]. There is a kind of proteins that non-covalently linked these proteins named P25, a 25 kDa glycoprotein [24,27]. The fibroin is a giant molecule comprising a crystalline portion of about two-thirds and an amorphous region of about one-third. The crystalline portion contains repetitive amino acids (-Gly-Ala-Gly-Ala-Gly-Ser-) along its sequence, forming an antiparallel β-sheet and leading to the stability and mechanical properties of the fiber [22,28–30].

Generally, the main secondary structures of fibroin are of the random-coil and amorphous type and the antiparallel β-sheet type, which is formed through hydrogen bonds between adjacent peptide chains [31]. The silk fibroins are characterized as natural block copolymers comprising hydrophobic blocks with short side-chain amino acids such as glycine and alanine, and hydrophilic blocks with larger side-chain amino acids, as well as charged amino acids [32]. The former blocks lead to β-sheets or crystals through hydrogen bonding [14]. The two main distinct structures in silk fibroin are silk I and silk II. The structure of silk I contains random-coil and amorphous regions. The silk II structural form of the silk fibroins has been characterized as an antiparallel β-sheet structure. The former structure is a water-soluble structure while the latter excludes water and is insoluble in several solvents including mild acid and alkaline conditions, and several chaotropes [33] (Table 1). In regenerated silk fibroins, the silk I structure easily converts to a β-sheet structure by chemical methods such as treatment with methanol [34–36].

Table 1. Structure of silk fibers.

Bombyx mori silk worm				
Silk fiber	Silk fibroin (72–81%)			Silk sericin (19–58%)
	H chain	L chain	P 25 glycoprotein	a glue-like protein
Molecular Weight	325 kDa	25 kDa	25 kDa	~300 kDa
Polarity	Hydrophobic			Hydrophilic
Structure	silk I(random-coil or unordered structure) silk II(crystalline structure) silk III (unstable structure)			non-crystalline structure
Function	the structure protein of fibers filament core protein			binds two fibroins together coating protein

Compared to other biomaterials, silk fibroins have excellent mechanical properties such as remarkable strength and toughness (Table 2). In the final molecular assembly of the proteins into silk fibers, the hydrophobic domains play an important role [35]. These domains take up a large portion of silk fibroin and are responsible for insolubility, the high strength of fibers and the thermal stability of the silk fibers which lead to the formation of β-sheet secondary structure [32]. It can be concluded that the materials properties of silk fibroins such as biodegradability and biocompatibility, are determined by their special molecular structure [35].

Table 2. Mechanical properties of biodegradable materials. Reprinted from [26] Biomaterials, 24 (2003), Gregory H. Altman, Frank Diaz, Caroline Jakuba, Tara Calabro, Rebecca L. Horan, Jingsong Chen, Helen Lu, John Richmond, David L. Kaplan, Silk-based biomaterials, Pages No.401–416, Copyright (2009), with permission from Elsevier.

Source of biomaterial	UTS (MPa)	Modulus (GPa)	Strain (%) at breakage	References
Bombyx mori silk (with sericin)	500	5–12	19	[37]
Bombyx mori silk (without sericin)	610–690	15–17	4–16	[37]
Bombyx mori silk	740	10	20	[38]
Collagen	0.9–7.4	0.0018–0.046	24–68	[39]
Cross-linked collagen	47–72	0.4–0.8	12–16	[39]
Polylactic acid	28–50	1.2–3.0	2–6	[40]

DEGRADATION BEHAVIORS OF SILK BIOMATERIALS

According to the US Pharmacopeia's definition, silk is classified as non-degradable. However, from the literature, it can be considered as a degradable material. The reason may be connected to the fact that silk degradation behavior is usually mediated by a foreign body response [26,41–43]. Different from synthetic materials, the degradable behavior of silk fibroins doesn't lead to an immunogenic response. Biodegradation is the breakdown of polymer materials into smaller compounds. The processes vary greatly, and the mechanisms are complex. Normally, the encompass physical, chemistry and biological factors. Depending on the mode of degradation, silk fibroins can be classified as enzymatically degradable polymers [44,45]. Enzymes play a significant role in the degradation of silk fibroins. Due to their enzymatic degradability, unique physic-chemical, mechanical and biological properties of silk fibroins have been extensively investigated. The enzymatic degradation of biomaterials is a two-step process. The first step is adsorption of the enzyme on the surface of the substrate through surface-binding domain and the second step is hydrolysis of the ester bond [45].

The Biodegradation Behavior of Silk Biomaterials with Sifferent Enzymes

As a protein, silk fibroin is susceptible to biological degradation by proteolytic enzymes such as chymotrypsin, actinase, and carboxylase [12,46–48]. Generally, the biodegradation behavior has two steps, as explained above. At first, silk biomaterials are adsorbed by different enzymes, which demands that the enzymes must find binding domains on the materials' surface. After that, silk biomaterials are digested by enzymes. The final wastes of silk fibroins are the corresponding amino acids, which are easily absorbed *in vivo*. That is one of advantages of silk biomaterials used in biomedical field.

The characteristics of silk biodegradation behaviors vary with different enzymes. Some literature has investigated the degradation behaviors of silk fibroins exposed to different proteolytic enzymes for various times. Chymotrypsin has been used to degrade amorphous regions of fibroins to obtain highly crystallizable fibroin protein [12]. When protease (Protease XIV) was compared with α-chymotrypsin, silk matrices incubated in the former enzyme significantly decreased in mass and UTS a week later, while, when in α-chymotrypsin, the UTS and mass of the silk matrices remained unchanged [49]. In another way, Li and his team [12] find α-chymotrypsin could degrade the dissolved fibroin proteins but not the fibroin sheet. In contrast, other enzymes (particularly protease XIV) extensively degraded the fibroin sheets demonstrating the potential of protease degradation of silk fibroin.

After biodegradation, significant changes have been reported according to the structure and molecular weight of silk fibroins. In *in vitro* studies of silk degradation behavior with proteolytic enzymes they will cleave the less-crystalline regions of the protein to peptides which are then capable of being phagocytosed for further metabolism by the cell [26,44]. In one study [10], protease E degraded the surface of silk fibroin membranes, especially the amorphous regions. Generally, degradation behavior varies from different silk materials forms with regard to enzymes. From other literature, when a silk fibroin sheet is immersed in various proteolytic enzyme solutions, the small amount of Silk II crystalline structure originally present in the sheet will disappear after degradation by protease XIV, and Silk I crystalline structure formed leading to an overall increase in crystallinity of the silk film over time. Collagenase IA is shown to degrade silk II as well, but to a lesser extent. α-Chymotrypsin is believed to degrade silk [44,50], however, it does not have an appreciable effect on the degradation of silk films [12,49].

In another way, biodegradation behavior has great effect on the final molecular weight after degradation. Upon incubation with proteolytic enzymes, silk films exhibit a noticeable decrease of sample weight and degree of polymerization to an extent which depended on the type of enzymes, on the enzyme-to-substrate ratio, and on the degradation time [44]. Focusing on three types of enzymes as examples, protease was more aggressive than α-chymotrypsin or collagenase. The average molecular weight of silk biomaterials after degradation follows the order protease XIV < collagenase IA < α-chymotrypsin [12].

From the literature, the changes in sample weight and degree of polymerization of silk fibers exposed to proteolytic attack are negligible. However, tensile properties are also significantly affected, as shown by the drop of strength and elongation as a function of the degradation time [44]. Silk can be proteolytically degraded and resorbed *in vivo* over a longer time period (typically within a year) [31,49]. *In vivo* studies, silks lose the majority of their tensile strength within one year, and fail to be recognized at the site within two years or even longer [25]. Great changes have happened to the morphology of silk fibroin, such as diameter, strength, and surface roughness. Enzymes, such as protease XXI, have been shown to degrade silk films and fibers altering surface roughness and strength over 17 days [42]. In order to know the biodegradation behavior of silk fibroin, several studies implanted silk materials under the skin of rats *in vivo*. After 6 weeks post-implantation, 55% of silk tensile strength and 16% of elastic modulus were found to be lost [51–52]. In another rat model, silk fibers lost 29% of tensile strength at 10 days, 73% at 30 days and 83% after 70 days [52]. Another study regarding molecular-weight distribution and amino acid composition indicates that part of silk fibroin materials is broken down into amino acids [12]. When immersed in collagenase IA, the weight of the fibroin sheets decreases as the degradation time increases. The percentage of free amino acids exceeded 50% of the total. Particularly, 70% of a silk fibroin sheet can be degraded in 15 days when exposed to protease XIV. Importantly the protease XIV does not only degrade silk fibroin, but also directly degraded the fibroin sheet into peptides and amino acids. This indicates that the biodegradation products of silk fibroin materials do less or even no harm to the human body.

Factors Influencing the Degradation Behavior of Silk Biomaterials

The degradation behavior of biomaterials is important in medical applications *in vivo*. The features of enzymes influence the biodegradable process for silk fibroins. For example, most proteolytic enzymes are better at degrading silk fibroins with low molecular weight and non-compact structures [53]. This indicates that the degradation behavior has a close relationship with the molecular weight and structure of silk biomaterials, so structure and molecular weight of polymers are two main factors influencing the biodegradation process. Low molecular weight and non-compact structure means that it is easy for enzymes to bind on the surface of silks as well as display hydrolysis behaviors.

As for silk fibroin porous sponges, their biodegradation behavior depends on the original preparation method and structural characteristics, such as processing condition, pore size, silk fibroin concentration, and host immune system elements during degradation [54]. It maybe has a close relationship with increased surface roughness or differences in content or distribution of crystallinity [34]. Thus it is possible to regulate the degradation behavior of silk fibroin by changing the crystallinity [10], pore size, porosity and molecular weight distribution of the silk fibroin. Wang's [54] research was conducted to systematically investigate the degradation behavior of silk fibroin three-dimensional scaffolds in both nude and Lewis rats. The study indicated that the *in vivo* behavior of the silk fibroin scaffolds can be predicted and thus can be controlled to match the diverse needs for the engineering and repairing of various tissues with specific functional requirements, repairing characteristics, and repairing rates.

It is generally accepted that the degradation of silk materials should match the function needs and ensure optimum mechanical and physiological integration of the device. Control over the rate is an important feature of function tissue design, for example the rate of scaffold degradation should match the rate of tissue growth [33]. Based on varieties studies on natural polymers, the rate and extent of degradation may be highly variable, depending on a series of factors related to structural and morphological features of the polymers, processing conditions, as well as characteristics of the biological environment at the location of implantation, and presence of different mechanical and chemical stresses [44]. Some researchers have indicated that variable rates of silk absorption *in vivo* are dependent on the animal model and tissue implantation site (Table 3) [26]. The degradability of silk fibroin also can be altered by processing conditions. Different processing conditions influence silk materials degradability significantly. As an enzymatically degraded biomaterial, the rate of silk degradation partly depends on the availability and concentration of the enzymes. Besides, chemical modification also affects the degradation behavior [33,45].

Table 3. Evidence of silk degradation *in vitro* and *in vivo*. Reprinted from [26] Biomaterials, 24 (2003), Gregory H. Altman, Frank Diaz, Caroline Jakuba, Tara Calabro, Rebecca L. Horan, Jingsong Chen, Helen Lu, John Richmond, David L. Kaplan, Silk-based biomaterials, Pages No.401–416, Copyright (2009), with permission from Elsevier.

Type of silk	In vivo/vitro	Mechanism	Degree and measure of degradation	References
Extracted fibroin film	*In vitro*	Proteolytic degradation	~10% weight loss 5 days following enzymatic digestion	[10]
Unknown/ assumed black raided	Rat/ subcutaneous	Unknown/ assumed foreign body response	55% loss in tensile strength 6 weeks *in vivo*	[51]
Black braided	Rat/ subcutaneous	Unknown/ assumed foreign body response	83% loss in tensile strength 10 weeks *in vivo*	[52]
Unknown/ assumed black raided	Rat/ abdominal wall muscle	Foreign body response (proteolytic degradation)	Fragmentation at 6 weeks; not detected at 24 weeks	[55]
Black braided	Rabbit/ cornea, sclera and ocular muscle	Foreign body response (proteolytic degradation)	Reduced number of filaments and diameter at 42 days; absorption at 90 days *in vivo*	[43]

Unknown/ assumed virgin silk	Rabbit/ abdominal wall muscle	Foreign body response (proteolytic degradation)	80% decrease in tensile strength at 12 weeks; 0% strength at 2 years; decrease in the number of fibers observed histologically; fragmentation following 4 weeks *in vivo*	[56]

Others

According to what has been discussed, protease cocktails and chymotrypsin are capable of enzymatically degrading silk [26]. Of interest, the silkworm, *Bombyx mori*, produces a protease inhibitor in the silk gland embedding it within the cocoon for protection against premature proteolytic degradation [57]. Generally, this 6kDa trypsin inhibitor is isolated from the water extract from silkworm cocoons, and protects the light chain of silk fibroin against tryptic degradation.

In addition to proteolytic enzymes, silk fibroins also can be degradated by other means, such as gamma radiation. Gamma radiation directly affects the decreasing tensile strength of the fibroin fibers. Due to the weakness of peptide bonding in fibroin's polypeptides, reduction of β-sheet structure in the silk fibroin, as well as the release of low-molecular-weight proteins in degradation products, the results of this study shows that the biodegradation of silk fibroin increases with increasing irradiation intensity [58].

CONCLUSIONS

Generally, biodegradability is one of the essential properties of the biomaterials. Over the past decades, significant attention has been paid to biodegradable biomaterials. Silk fibroins are obtained from the cocoons of mulberry silkworm *Bombyx mori*. Due to their high tensile strength, controllable biodegradability, haemostatic properties, non-cytotoxicity, low antigenicity and non-inflammatory characteristics, silk materials are increasingly used as biodegradable material.

Normally, silk fiber consists of two types of self-assembled proteins, fibroin and sericin. The fibroin is a major component of silk fiber serving as the core, while the sericin is a minor component serving as a coating protein. The former is comprised of highly organized β-sheet crystal regions and semi-crystalline regions responsible for silk's elasticity compared to fibers of similar tensile integrity [26]. Biodegradable materials are preferred candidates for developing therapeutic devices such as temporary prostheses, three-dimensional porous structures as scaffolds for tissue engineering and as controlled/sustained release drug delivery vehicles. The medical application demands biomaterial with special properties such as degradability. According to the US Pharmacopeia's definition, however, silk is classified as non-degradable. Although according to the literature, it can be considered as a degradable material, although over longer times. Depending on the mode of degradation, silk fibroins can be classified as enzymatically degradable polymers [45]. Enzymes play a significant role in the degradation of silk fibroins, especially proteolytic enzymes. The degradation behavior of biomaterials is important in the medical application *in vivo*. Control over the rate is an important feature of function tissue design, such as the rate of scaffold degradation matches the rate of tissue growth. Based on varieties studies on natural polymers, the rate and extent of degradation may be highly variable, depending on a series of factors related to structural and morphological features of the polymers, such as fibers, films, sponges, processing conditions, as well as characteristics of the biological environment at the location of implantation, and presence of different mechanical and chemical stresses [44]. Moreover, during the biodegradation, some other factors influence the silk biodegradation behavior, such as a protease inhibitor, produced by silk itself, and gamma radiation. Finally, a better understanding of the biodegradation behavior of silk fibers will provide greater insight into the appropriate silk biomaterials design for future medical appliaction.

REFERENCES

1. Von Recum, AF; LaBerge, M. Educational goals for biomaterials science and engineering: perspective view. *J. Appl. Biomater* 1995, *6*, 137–144.

2. Lloyd, AW. Interfacial bioengineering to enhance surface biocompatibility. *Med. Device Technol* 2002, *13*, 18–21.

3. Stitzel, J; Liu, J; Lee, SJ; Komura, M; Berrya, J; Sokerc, S; Limc, G; Dykec, MV; Richard, C; James, JY; *et al.* Controlled fabrication of a biological vascular substitute. *Biomaterials* 2006, *27*, 1088–1094.

4. Murugan, R; Ramakrishna, S. Development of nanocomposites for bone grafting. *Compos. Sci. Technol* 2005, *65*, 2385–2406.

5. Takasu, Y; Hiromi, Y; Kozo, T. Isolation of three main sericin components from the cocoon of the silkworm, Bombyx mori. *Biosci. Biotechnol. Biochem* 2002, *66*, 2715–2718.

6. Chitrangada, A; Boris, H; Subhas, CK. The effect of lactose-conjugated silk biomaterials on the development of fibrogenic fibroblasts. *Biomaterials* 2008, *29*, 4665–4675.

7. Minoura, N; Aiba, S; Higuchi, M; Gotoh, Y; Tsukada, M; Imai, Y. Attachment and growth of fibroblast cells on silk fibroin. *Biochem. Biophys. Res. Commun* 1995, *208*, 511–516.

8. Acharya, C; Ghosh, SK; Kundu, SC. Silk fibroin protein from mulberry and nonmulberry silkworms: cytotoxicity, biocompatibility and kinetics of L929 murine fibroblast adhesion. *J. Mater. Sci. Mater. Med* 2008, *19*, 2827–2836.

9. Kundu, J; Dewan, M; Ghoshal, S; Kundu, SC. Mulberry non-engineered silk gland protein vis-a-vis silk cocoon protein engineered by silkworms as biomaterial matrices. *J. Mater. Sci. Mater. Med* 2008, *19*, 2679–2689.

10. Minoura, N; Tsukada, M; Nagura, M. Physico-chemical properties of silk fibroin membrane as a biomaterial.*Biomaterials* 1990, *11*, 430–434.

11. Fini, M; Motta, A; Torricelli, P; Giavaresi, G; Aldini, NN; Tschon, M; Giardino, R; Migliaresi, C. The healing of confined critical size cancellous defects in the presence of silk fibroin hydrogel. *Biomaterials* 2005, *26*, 3527–3536.

12. Li, M; Ogiso, M; Minoura, N. Enzymatic degradation behavior of porous silk fibroin sheets. *Biomaterials* 2003, *24*, 357–365.

13. Hino, T; Tanimoto, M; Shimabayashi, S. Change in secondary structure of silk fibroin during preparation of its microspheres by spray-drying and exposure to humid atmosphere. *J. Colloid. Interface Sci* 2003, *266*, 68–73.

14. Wang, Y; Kim, HJ; Vunjak-Novakovic, G; Kaplan, DL. Stem cell-based tissue engineering with silk biomaterials.*Biomaterials* 2006, *27*, 6064–6082.

15. Mauney, JR; Nguyen, T; Gillen, K; Kirker-Head, C; Gimble, JM; Kaplan, DL. Engineering adipose-like tissue *in vitro*and *in vivo* utilizing human bone marrow and adipose-derived mesenchymal stem cells with silk fibroin 3D scaffolds.*Biomaterials* 2007, *28*, 5280–5290.

16. Uebersax, L; Hagenmuller, H; Hofmann, S; Gruenblatt, E; Müller, R; Vunjaknovakovic, G; Kaplan, DL; Merkle, HP; Meinel, L. Effect of scaffold design on bone morphology *in vitro*. *Tissue Eng* 2006, *12*, 3417–3429.

17. Santin, M; Motta, A; Freddi, G; Cannas, M. *In vitro* evaluation of the inflammatory potential of the silk fibroin. *J. Biomed. Mater. Res* 1999, *46*, 382–389.

18. Acharya, C; Kumar, V; Sen, R; Kundu, SC. Performance evaluation of a silk protein based matrix for the enzymatic conversion of tyrosine to

L-DOPA. *Biotech. J* 2008, *3*, 226–233.

19. Unger, RE; Peters, K; Wolf, M; Motta, A; Migliaresi, C; Kirkpatrick, CJ. Endothelialization of a non-woven silk fibroin net for use in tissue engineering: growth and gene regulation of human endothelial cells. *Biomaterials* 2004, *25*, 5137–5146.

20. Dalpra, I; Freddi, G; Minic, J; Chiarini, A; Armato, U. De novo engineering of reticular connective tissue *in vivo* by silk fibroin nonwoven materials. *Biomaterials* 2005, *26*, 1987–1999.

21. Meinel, L; Fajardo, R; Hofmann, S; Langer, R; Chen, J; Snyder, B; Vunjak-Novakovic, G; Kaplan, D. Silk implants for the healing of critical size bone defects. *Bone* 2005, *37*, 688–698.

22. Heslot, H. Arfificial fibrous proteins: A review. *Biochimic* 1998, *80*, 9–13.

23. Chitrangada, A; Sudip, KG; Kundu, SC. Silk fibroin film from non-mulberry tropical tasar silkworms: A novel substrate for *in vitro* fibroblast culture. *Acta Biomater* 2009, *5*, 429–437.

24. Zhou, CZ; Confalonieri, F; Medina, N; Zivanovic, Y; Esnault, C; Yang, T; Jacquet, M; Janin, J; Duguet, M; Perasso, R; *et al*. Fine organization of B. mori fibroin heavy chain gene. *Nucleic Acids Res* 2000, *28*, 2413–2419.

25. Inoue, S; Tanaka, K; Arisaka, F; Kimura, S; Ohtomo, K; Mizuno, Shigeki. Silk fibroin of B. mori is secreted, assembling a high molecular mass elementary unit consisting of H-chain, L-chain, and P25, with a 6:6:1 molar ratio. *J. Biol. Chem* 2000, *275*, 40517–40528.

26. Altman, GH; Diaz, F; Jakuba, C; Jakuba, Caroline; Calabro, T; Horan, RL; Chen, J; Lu, H; Richmond, J; Kaplan, DL. Silk-based biomaterials. *Biomaterials* 2003, *24*, 401–416.

27. Tanaka, K; Inoue, S; Mizuno, S. Hydrophobic interaction of P25, containing Asn-linked oligosaccharide chains, with the H–L complex of silk fibroin produced by B. mori. *Insect Biochem. Mol. Biol* 1999, *29*, 269–276.

28. He, SJ; Valluzzi, R; Gido, SP. Silk I structure in Bombyx mori silk foams. *Int. J. Biol. Macromol* 1999, *24*, 187–195.

29. Asakura, T; Yao, J; Yamane, T; Kosuke, U; Ulric, HS. Heterogeneous structure of silk fibers from Bombyx mori resolved by ^{13}C solid-state NMR spectroscopy. *J. Am. Chem. Soc* 2002, *124*, 8794–8795.

30. Kim, UJ; Park, J; Kim, HJ; Wada, M; Kaplan, DL. Three dimensional aqueous-derived biomaterial scaffolds from silk fibroin. *Biomaterials* 2005, *26*, 2775–2785.

31. Tsuboi, Y; Ikejiri, T; Shiga, S; Yamada, K; Itaya, A. Light can transform

the secondary structure of silk protein. *Appl. Phys. A* 2001, *73*, 637–640.

32. Bini, E; Knight, DP; Kaplan, DL. Mapping domain structures in silks from insects and spiders related to protein assembly. *J. Mol. Biol* 2004, *35*, 27–40.

33. Vepari, C; Kaplan, DL. Silk as a biomaterial. *Prog. Polym. Sci* 2007, *32*, 991–1007.

34. Valluzzi, R; Gido, SP; Zhang, W; Muller, WS; Kaplan, DL. Trigonal crystal structure of bombyx mori silk incorporating a threefold helical chain conformation found at the air-water interface. *Macromolecules* 1996, *29*, 8606–8614.

35. Huang, J; Foo, CWP; Kaplan, DL. Biosynthesis and applications of silk-like and collagen-like proteins. *Polym. Rev*2007, *47*, 29–62.

36. Huemmerich, D; Slotta, U; Scheibel, T. Processing and modification of films made from recombinant spider silk proteins. *Appl Phys A – Mat Sci Process* 2006, *82*, 219–22.

37. Perez-Rigueiro, J; Viney, C; Llorca, J; Elices, M. Mechanical properties of single-brin silkworm silk. *J. Appl. Polym. Sci*2000, *75*, 1270–1277.

38. Cunniff, P; Fossey, S; Auerbach, M; Song, JW; Kaplan, DL; Adams, WW; Eby, RK; Mahoney, D; Vezie, DL. Mechanical and thermal properties of dragline silk from the spider N. clavipes. *Polym. Adv. Technol* 1994, *5*, 401–410.

39. Pins, G; Christiansen, D; Patel, R; Silver, FH. Self-assembly of collagen fibers: Influence of fibrillar alignment and decorin on mechanical properties. *Biophys. J* 1997, *73*, 2164–2172.

40. Engelberg, I; Kohn, J. Physicomechanical properties of degradable polymers used in medical applications: a comparative study. *Biomaterials* 1991, *12*, 292–304.

41. Rossitch, E, Jr; Bullard, DE; Oakes, WJ. Delayed foreign-body reaction to silk sutures in pediatric neurosurgical patients. *Childs Nerv. Syst* 1987, *3*, 375–378.

42. Soong, HK; Kenyon, KR. Adverse reactions to virgin silk sutures in cataract surgery. *Ophthalmol* 1984, *91*, 479–483.

43. Salthouse, TN; Matlaga, BF; Wykoff, MH. Comparative tissue response to six suture materials in rabbit cornea, sclera, and ocular muscle. *Am. J. Ophthalmol* 1977, *84*, 224–233.

44. Arai, T; Freddi, G; Innocenti, R; Tsukada, M. Biodegradation of Bombyx mori silk fibroin fibers and films. *J. Appl. Polym. Sci* 2004, *91*, 2383–2390.

45. Naira, LS; Laurencina, CT. Biodegradable polymers as biomaterials. *Prog. Polym. Sci* 2007, *32*, 762–798.

46. Chen, K; Iura, K; Aizawa, R; Hirabayashi, K. The digestion of silk fibroin by rat. *J. Seric. Sci. Jpn* 1991, *60*, 402–403.

47. Chen, K; Umeda, Y; Hirabayashi, K. Enzymatic hydrolysis of silk fibroin. *J. Seric. Sci. Jpn* 1996, *65*, 131–133.

48. Chen, G; Arai, M; Hirabayashi, K. Isolation of tyrosine from silk fibroin by enzyme hydrolysis. *J. Seric. Sci. Jpn* 1996, *65*, 182–184.

49. Horan, RL; Antle, K; Collette, AL; Wang, Y; Huang, J; Moreau, JE; Volloch, V; Kaplan, DL; Altman, GH. *In vitro* degradation of silk fibroin. *Biomaterials* 2005, *26*, 3385–3393.

50. Tsukada, M. Effect of α-chymotrypsin on the structure of silk fibroin. *J. Seric. Sci. Jpn* 1986, *55*, 120–126.

51. Greenwald, D; Shumway, S; Albear, P; Gottlieb, L. Mechanical comparison of 10 suture materials before and after *in vivo* incubation. *J. Surg. Res* 1994, *56*, 372–377.

52. Bucknall, TE; Teare, L; Ellis, H. The choice of a suture to close abdominal incisions. *Eur. Surg. Res* 1983, *15*, 59–66.

53. Zou, B; Wu, DZ. Analysis of structure and properties of biodegradable regenerated silk fibroin fibers. *J. Mater. Sci* 2006, *41*, 3357–3361.

54. Wang, YZ; Rudym, DD; Walsh, A; Abrahamsen, L; Kim, HJ; Kim, HS; Kirker-Head, C; Kaplan, DL. *In vivo* degradation of three-dimensional silk fibroin scaffolds. *Biomaterials* 2008, *29*, 3415–3428.

55. Lam, KH; Nijenhuis, AJ; Bartels, H; Postema, AR; Jonkman, MF; Pennings, AJ; Nieuwenhuis, P. Reinforced poly(L-Lactic Acid) fibers as suture material. *J. Appl. Biomater* 1995, *6*, 191–197.

56. Postlethwait, RW. Tissue reaction to surgical sutures. In *Repair and regeneration*; Dumphy, JE, van Winkle, W, Eds.; McGraw-Hill: New York, USA, 1969; pp. 263–285.

57. Kurioka, A; Yamazaki, M; Hirano, H. Primary structure and possible functions of a trypsin inhibitor of Bombyx mori. *Eur. J. Biochem* 1999, *259*, 120–126.

58. Kojthung, A; Meesilpa, P; Sudatis, B; Treeratanapiboon, L; Udomsangpetch, R; Oonkhanond, B. Effects of gamma radiation on biodegradation of Bombyx mori silk fibroin. *Int. biodeter. biodegr* 2008, *62*, 487–490.

Chapter 4

BIOENGINEERING FUNCTIONAL COPOLYMERS. XVII. INTERACTION OF ORGANOBORON AMIDE-ESTER BRANCHED DERIVATIVES OF POLY(ACRYLIC ACID) WITH CANCER CELLS

Mustafa Türk[1], Gülten Kahraman[2], Sevda A. Khalilova[3], Zakir M. O. Rzayev[4*], Serpil Oguztüzün[1]

[1]Department of Biology, Faculty of Arts and Sciences, Kırıkkale University, Yahşihan, Turkey

[2]Sarayköy Nuclear Research and Training Center, Turkish Atomic Energy Authority, Ankara, Turkey

[3]Scientific Research Institute of Medicinal Prophylaxis, Ministry of Public Health, Baku, Azerbaijan

[4]Institute of Science & Engineering, Division of Nanoscience and Nanomedicine, Hacettepe University, Ankara, Turkey.

ABSTRACT

Novel bioengineering functional organoboron polymers were synthesized by 1) amidolysis of poly(acrcylic acid) (PAA) with 2-aminoethyldiphenyl borinate (2-AEPB), 2) esterification of organoboron PAA polymer (PAA-B) with a-hydroxy-w-methoxypoly(ethylene oxide) (PEO) as a compatibilizer and 3) conjugation of organoboron PEO branches (PAA-B-PEO) with folic acid (FA) as a targeting agent. Structure and composition of the synthesized polymers were characterized by FTIR-ATR and ^{1}H (^{13}C) NMR spectroscopy, chemical and physical analysis methods. Antitumor activity of organoboron functional polymer and its complex with FA (PAA-B-PEO-F) against cancer and normal cells were evaluated by using different biochemical methods such as cytotoxicity, statistical, apoptotic and necrotic cell indexes, double staining and caspase-3 immune staining, light and fluorescence inverted microscope analyses. It was found that citotoxicity and apoptotic/necrotic effects of polymers significantly depend on the structure and composition of studied polymers, and increase the following raw: PAA << PAA-B < PAA-B-PEO < PAA-B-PEO-F. Among them, PAA-B-PEO-F complex at 400 mg *

mL^{-1} concentration as a therapeutic drug exhibits minimal toxicity toward the normal cells, but influential for HeLa cancer cells.

INTRODUCTION

Many natural polymers such as polylysine, polyarginine, dextran derivatives, heparin and chitosan, and synthetic bioengineering polymers such as poly(acrylic acid) (PAA), copolymers of maleic anhydride, have now been reported to have direct or indirect antitumor activity via stimulation of the immune system [1-3]. In recent years, the PAA and its copolymers have been often used as carriers in drug release systems, because of their multifunctional nature, unique properties and good biocompatibility [4,5]. Dimitrov et al. [5] studied the biopharmaceutical characterization of hydrogels based on crosslinked PAA and showed that this studied systems provide retarded drug release and appear to be potential candidates for use in the pharmaceutical practice. PAA is grafted to the poly(ethylene glycol) hydro-gel by photo-induced graft polymerization. Due to carboxyl functionality of PAA, collagen and cell adhesion protein, they could be covalently immobilized on to the poly(ethylene glycol) hydrogel [6]. Most of the hydrogels utilized as adhesives for dermatological patches were composed using PAA and its salts as matrix polymers. The ionic interactions between the carboxyl groups of the polymer and polyvalent cations such as calcium, copper, and aluminum cause the formation of the chemical crosslinking used to increase their mechanical strengths [7]. Acrylate-based polymers, containing carboxylic groups, exhibit a swelling behaviour depending on pH and ionic strength of solution [8,9]. Argentiere et al. [10] investigated PAA nanogels as pH-sensitive carriers for biomedical applications. They prepared PAA–biopolymer nanogels by loading and release of an oligothiophene fluorophore and its albumin conjugate onto the PAA macromolecules. On the other hand, several synthetic boron-containing compounds exhibiting important biological properties were investigated as potential therapeutics [11,12]. The mild electrophilic nature of the boronic acid moiety has led to its use at the 'warhead' site of enzyme inhibitors, particularly for inhibiting proteases. For this purposes, several researchers developed some α-aminoboronic acid derivatives [11,13]. One such compound, the novel proteasome inhibitor bortezomib (Velcade) has been recently approved for clinical use as an anticancer agent for the treatment of myeloma [14]. Ban et al. [15] synthesized a series of o-carboranyl phenoxy derivatives as potent inducers for the activation of the 20S proteasome and as chemical probes for the investigation of proteasome-dependent degradation pathways. Other types of bioactive boron-containing compounds have been investigation as therapeutic agents. These include certain boron analogues of biomolecules

[16], diazaborine as an antibacterial and antimalarial agent [17], various antibacterial oxazaborolidines [18], the antibacterial diphenyl borinic esters to inhibit bacterial cell wall growth [19], the antifungal agent benzoxaborole (AN2690) [20], and an oestrogen receptor modulator containing a B–N bond [21]. Some organoboron compounds, including boronic acids and its functional derivatives, and carboranes, were also investigated as agents for boron-neutron capture therapy (BCNT) for the treatment of brain tumors [12,22, 23].

The goal of this work is synthesis and characterization of novel organoboron amide-ester derivatives by amidolysis of PAA with 2-aminoethyldiphenyl borinate (2-AEPB) and their a,ω-hydroxy-methoxypoly(ethylene oxide) (PEO) macrobranched derivative by grafting of synthesized organoboron polymer with PEO to improve the biocompatibility and degree of conjugation with cancer biomacromolecules.

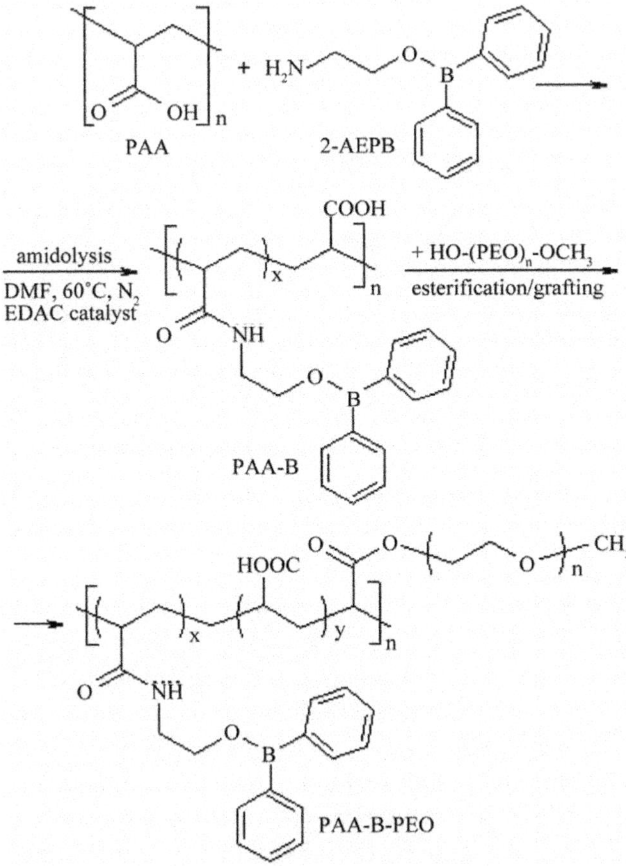

Scheme 1. Synthetic partway of the organoboron amideester-carboxyl functionalized polymers via amidolysis and esterification/grafting reactions.

An important aspect of this work is comparative investigations of the interactions of these novel functionalized organoboron polymers with HeLa (human cervix carcinoma cell) cancer cells and L929 Fibroblast normal cells, and evaluation of their antitumor activity (cytotoxicity, apoptotic and necrotic effects) using various biochemical methods such as hematoxylen/eosin and immune cytochemical staining, light and fluorescence inverted microscopy analyses.

Synthetic partway of the side-chain amide-, esterand carboxyl-functionalized organoboron polymers can be represented as follows (Scheme 1).

EXPERIMENTAL

Materials

PAA (BDH) was used as 25% aqueous solution with M_w 230.000 g/mol and density 1.09 g/ml. 2-Aminoethyl diphenylborinate (2-AEPB) (Sigma-Aldrich, Germany) was purified by recrystallization from anhydrous ethanol: m.p. 193.5°C (by DSC); FTIR-ATR spectra of 2-AEPB, cm^{-1}: 3284 (vs) and 3220 (s) N-H stretching in NH_2, 3066 (vs)-2870(s) C-H stretching, 1611(vs) NH_2 bending and C=C stretching in phenyl groups, 1491(m) and 1334 (m) B-O band, 1432 (vs) fairly strong, sharp band due to benzene ring vibration in phenyl-boronic acid linkage, 1263-1154 (s) fairly strong, sharp bands due to C-N stretching in C-NH_2, 1061(vs) N-H bending in NH_2 and 750-710(s) sharp bands due to boron-phenyl linkage; ^1H NMR spectra (δ, ppm) in CHCl$_3$-d$_1$: CH$_2$-O 1.49, CH$_2$-NH$_2$ 2.96, and 7.38-7.40 (1H), 7.19-7.24 (2H) and 7.13-7.16 (2H) for protons of p-, oand m-positions in benzene ring, respectively.

a-Hydroxy-ω-methoxy-PEO (M_n 2000 g · mol^{-1}) (Fluka). ^1H NMR spectra (δ, ppm) in CHCl$_3$-d$_1$: CH$_2$-O3.75-3.45, OH end group 2.61 and O-CH$_3$ end group 2.16.

N-Ethyl-N-(3-dimethylaminopropyl)carbodiimide hydrochloride (EDAC) as a catalyst and folic acid (FA) as a targeting agent were supported from Aldrich-Sigma (Germany). All solvents and reagents were of analytical grade and used without purification HeLa (human cervix carcinoma cell) cancer cells and L929 Fibroblast cells were obtained from the tissue culture collection of the SAP Institute (Ankara, Turkey). Cell culture flasks and other plastic material were purchased from Corning (NY, USA). The growth medium, which is Dulbecco Modified Medium (DMEM) without L-glutamine supplemented fetal calf serum (FCS), and Trypsin-EDTA were purchased from Biological Industries (Kibbutz Beit Haemek, Israel). The primary antibody, caspase-3 was purchased from Lab Vision (Germany).

Synthesis of 2-Amidoethyldiphenylborinate-poly(Acrylic Acid)

Amidolysis of PAA with 2-AEPB using various [PAA]/[2-AEPB] mole ratios was carried out in N,N'-dimethylformamide (DMF) at 60°C with EDAC catalyst under the nitrogen atmosphere using a standard Pyrex-glass reactor supplied by a mixer, temperature control unit and condenser. Reaction conditions: [2-AEPB] = 0.066 mol · L^{-1}, mole ratios of [PAA]/ [2-AEPB] = 1: 1, 3: 1, 5: 1 and EDAC = 1.0 wt %. Appropriate quantities of PAA, 2-AEPB, DMF and EDAC were placed in a reactor and the reaction mixture was flushed with dried nitrogen gas for at least 2 min, then sealed and placed in a thermo stated silicon oil bath at 60°C to intensive mixing for 5 h. The organoboron amide polymer was isolated from reaction mixture by precipitation with diethyl ether and dried under vacuum. Synthesized organoboron polymer has the following average parameters: T$_g$ (by DSC) 190.6°C, [h]$_{in}$ in deionized water at 25°C 2.72 dL · g^{-1}; FTIR-ATR spectra of PAA-g-2-AEPB (KBr pellet), cm^{-1}: 1702 (m) C=O stretching (amide I band), 1642 (w) and 1542 (m) N-H deformation (amide II band), 1446(m) and 1407(w) C-N stretching (amide III band); ^{1}H NMR spectra (in DMSO-d$_6$ at 25°C) δ ppm: protons of phenyl groups 7.9, 2H from CH$_2$ in -CH$_2$-CO-NHfragment 7.3, 2H from B-O-CH$_2$ group 3.6, 2H from NH-CH$_2$ group 3.0 and 2H from backbone -CH-CH- 3.3, 2.2 and 1.2-1.7; ^{13}C NMR spectra (δ ppm): C=O of PAA unit/amide linkage 177, CH= in phenyl groups 162-158, backbone CH$_2$ and CH128-127 and 57, NH-CH$_2$ 41-42, CH$_2$-O 31-36.

Synthesis of PEO Branched Organboron Copolymer

The esterification (grafting) of organoboron amide of PAA, containing 19.24 mol % of organoboron groups, with PEO (M$_n$ 2000 g · mol^{-1}) at organoboron polymer/PEO feed molar ratio 1: 0.01 was carried out in DMF at 60°C for 1 h. PEO branched polymer was isolated from reaction mixture by precipitation with diethyl ether and dried 40°C under vacuum. Prepared PEO ester of organoboron polymer has the following average characteristics: T$_g$ 175.8°C (by DSC); [h]$_{in}$ in deionized water at 25°C 0.9 dL · g^{-1}; ^{1}H NMR spectra (in DMSO-d$_6$ at 25°C) δ ppm: protons of phenyl groups 7.8, CH$_2$ in CH$_2$-CO-NHamide group 7.2, 2H in B-O-CH$_2$ 3.5, CH$_2$CH$_2$ in PEO branch 3.35, 3H in OCH$_3$end group 3.1 and 2H in NH-CH$_2$ 2.9; ^{13}C NMR spectra (δ ppm): C=O in –COOH 176, CH= in phenyl groups 162, backbone CH$_2$ and CH 128 and 127, respectively, O-CH$_2$ in PEO 69, end OCH$_3$group of PEO 57, NH-CH$_2$ 41-42, and CH$_2$-O-B 31-36.

Characterization

Fourier transform infrared (FTIR-ATR) spectra were recorded with FTIR Nicolet 8700 spectrometer in the 3700 - 600 cm^{-1} range. ^{1}H and ^{13}C NMR spectra were performed on a Bruker Avance (300 MHz) spectrometer with DMSO-d$_6$ as a solvent at 25°C. Thermo gravimetric (TGA) and differential scanning calorimetric (DSC) analyses were performed in a TGA-DTA (Perkin Elmer TG/DTA6300) and a DSC2010 Thermal Analyzers, respectively, under nitrogen atmosphere at a heating rate of 10°C/min. The intrinsic viscosity [h]$_{in}$ values of the organoboron polymers were determined in deionized water at 25°C ± 0.1°C in the concentration range 0.003 - 0.06 g · dL^{-1} using an Ubbelohde viscometer.

Analyses of cytotoxicity, apoptotic and necrotic cells with double staining and immune cytochemical stains of the synthesized novel organoboron functional polymers were performed according to the modified methods using in our recent published work [25,26]. For cytotoxicity experiments, HeLa and L 929 Fibroblast cells (50 × 10^3 cells per well) were placed in DMEM by using 24-well plates. Different amounts of pristine PPA and organoboron polymers (PAA-B, PPA-PEO-B and PAA-PEO-B-F) (about 0-650 mg · mL^{-1} in aqueous solutions) were put into wells containing cells, respectively. The plates were kept in the CO$_2$ incubator (37°C in 5% CO$_2$) for 24 h; the medium was replaced with fresh medium, and incubated at the same conditions for 24 h. Following of this incubation, HeLa cells were harvested with trypsin–EDTA, and then were dyed with trypan blue. The number of living and dead cells were counted with a haemacytometer (C.A. Hausse & Son Phluila, USA), using light microscope at ×200 magnification. Analysis of apoptotic and necrotic cells with double staining were performed to quantify the number of apoptotic cells in culture on basis of scoring of apoptotic cell nuclei. HeLa and L929 fibroblast cells (20 × 10^3 cells per well) were placed in DMEM by using 24-well plates. After treating with different amount functional oligomers (about 0 - 650 mg · mL^{-1} in aqueous solutions) for 24 hours period, both attached and detached cells were collected, then washed with PBS and stained with Hoechst dye 33342 (2 mg · mL^{-1}), propodium iodide (PI) (1.0 mg · mL^{-1}) and DNAse free-RNAse (100 mg · mL^{-1}) for 15 min at room temperature. After that 10 - 50 mL of cell suspension was smeared on slide and cover slip for examination by fluorescence microscopy. The nuclei of normal cells were stained light blue but apoptotic cells were stained dark blue by the Hoechst dye.

The apoptotic cells were identified by their nuclear morphology as a nuclear fragmentation or chromatin condensation. Necrotic cells were staining red by PI. Necrotic cells lacking plasma membrane integrity and PI dye cross cell membrane, but PI dye don't cross non necrotic cell membrane. The number of apoptotic and necrotic cells in 10 randomly chosen microscopic fields were counted and the result expressed as a ratio of apoptotic and necrotic to normal cells. The number of apoptotic and necrotic cells were determined by light and fluorescence inverted microscope (Leica, Germany). The cell images were also recorded using the both above mentions microscopes with DAPI and FITC filters, respectively. For immunocytochemical stains, about 2 ml HeLa (20×10^3 cells per well), treated with functional oligomers (about 0 - 650 mg · mL^{-1} in aqueous solutions) suspension was centrifuged for 5 min in a Hettich centrifuge. Cytospin preparations were fixed in 70 % ethanol for immunocytochemistry.

For an indirect immunocytochemical procedure, cytology specimens were treated with 3% H_2O_2 for 10 min, taken to water, and then rinsed in PBS (pH 7.4) for 5 min. Nonspecific protein binding was blocked on specimen by incubating with blocking solution for 10 min. The primary antibody, caspase-3 (Lab Vision) used at 1:300 dilution, incubated for 1 h at room temperature. Specimens were washed with PBS buffer (pH 7.4) and incubated in biotinylated secondary antibody solution for 10 min. Diaminobenzidine (Dako) served as the chromagen and Mayer's hematoxylin as the counter stain. For the negative control the primary antibody was omitted in one of the slides.

The immunocytochemical staining results were controlled independent and blindly by observers without the knowledge of treatment. The immunoreactivity of the caspase-3 antibody is confined to the cytoplasm of apoptotic cells. We counted the number of caspase-3-positive cytoplasmic staining cells in all fields found at ×400 final magnification. For each image, three randomly selected microscopic fields were observed, and at least of 100 cells/field were evaluated.

RESULTS AND DISCUSSION

Structure of Organoboron Polymers

The structures of synthesized organoboron polymers and their PEO branches were confirmed by FTIR-ATR and ^1H (^{13}C) NMR analysis. Comparative analysis of FTIR-ATR spectra (**Figure 1**) of 2-AEPB, PAA and its organoboron derivative indicates that the characteristic bands of acid C=O groups disappearance in the spectra of PAA-B-1 polymer prepared from 1:1 molar feed ratio of PAA: 2-AEPB.

The formation of amide bound in this organoboron polymer is confirmed by the appearance of new bands such as 1702 (amide-I band), 1642 and 1542 (amide-II band), 1446 cm^{-1} and 1407 (amide-III band). Simultaneously a very broad band between 3500 and 2500 cm^{-1} appearances in spectra due to increase hydrogen bonded fragments in organoboron polymer (PAA-B-1). As the intensities of amide bands significantly decrease in spectra of PAA-B-2 and PAA-B-3 polymers prepared from PAA/ 2-AEPB mixtures enchasing with PAA (PAA>> 2-AEPB), the intensities of free acid group bands increase.

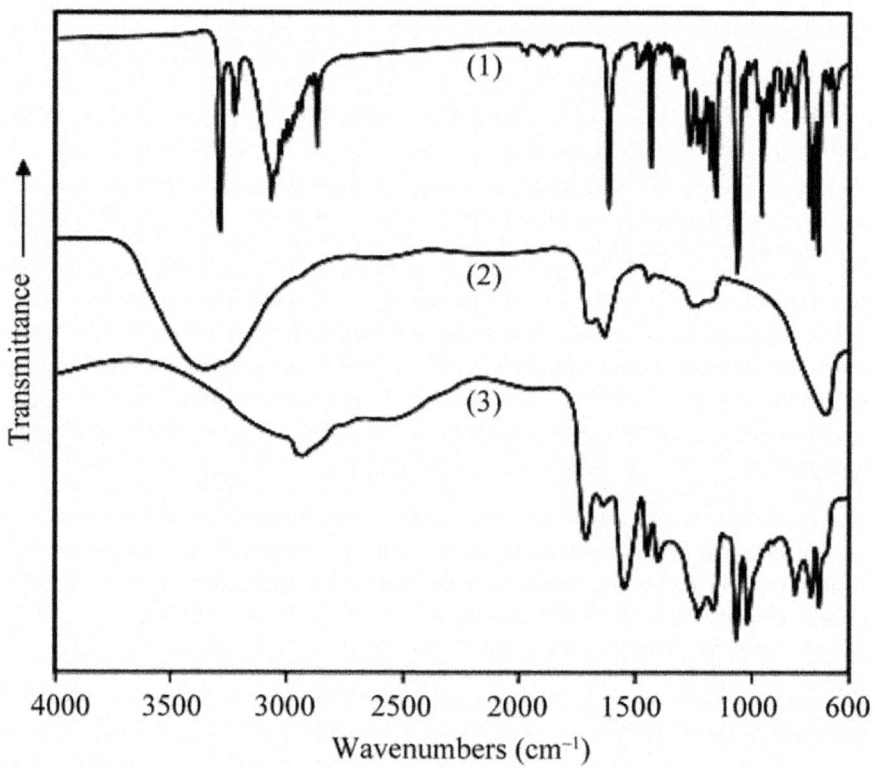

Figure 1. FTIR spectra: (1) 2-AEPB, (2) PAA and (3) PAAg-2-AEPB-1 organoboron amide polymer.

Similar effect has been observed from comparative analysis of the ^{1}H and ^{13}C NMR spectra of A-B-2and its PEO branch (PAA-B-PEO). The results of this analysis are illustrated in Figures 2 and 3. The formation of H-bonded amide linkages is confirmed by a presence of characteristic broad peaks at 7.3 and 177 ppm in the ^{1}H and ^{13}C NMR spectra of PAA-B-2, respectively (**Figure 2**). In addition, the presence of characteristic proton peaks of organoboron linkages such as quarter phenyl peak at 7.9 ppm, triplet B-O-CH$_2$ peak at 3.6 ppm andquarter NH-CH$_2$ peak at 3.0 ppm (**Figure 2**(a)) also confirmed that 2-AEPB is covalently bound to anhydride units. In the ^{13}C NMR spectra of PAA-B-2 polymer (**Figure 2**(b)), the characteristic carbon resonances (162, 158, 41, 42, 31 and 36 ppm) from organoboron fragment are also observed.

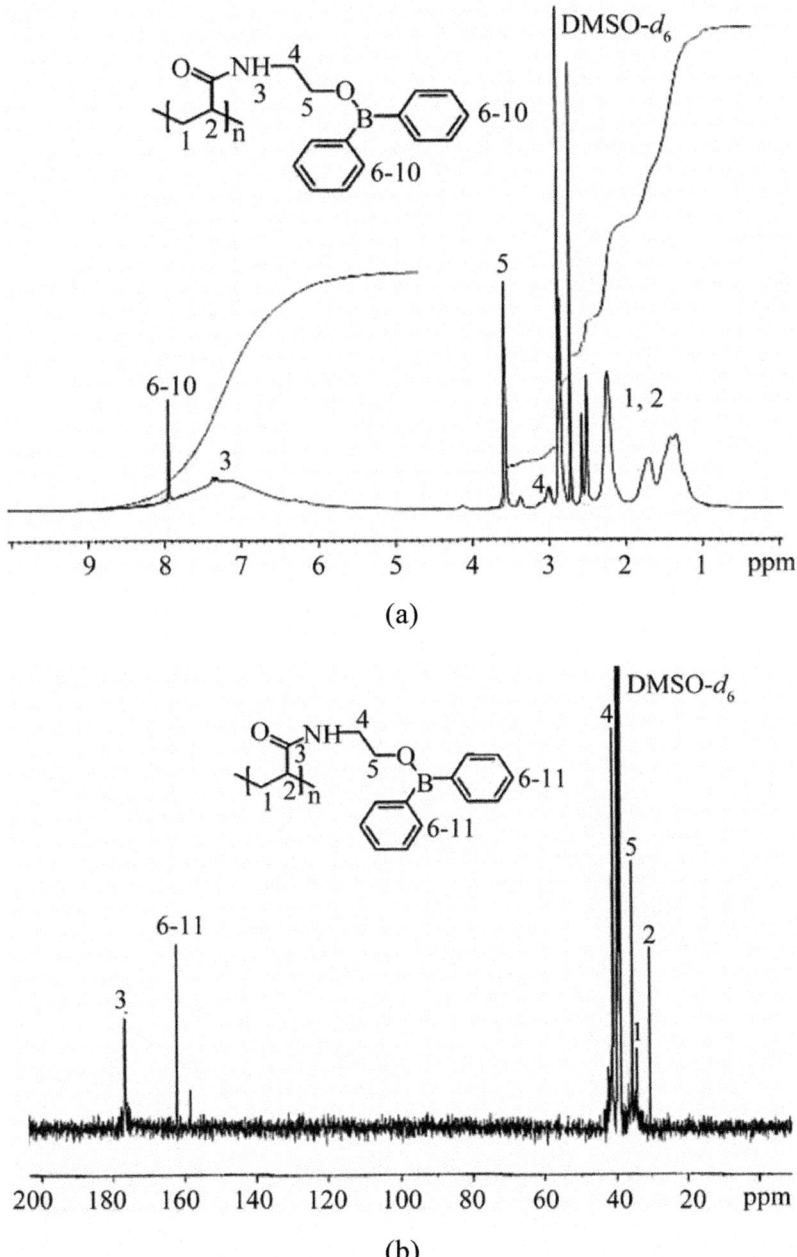

Figure 2. (a) ¹H NMR and (b)¹³C NMR spectra of organoboron polymer (PAA-B) in DMSO-d₆.

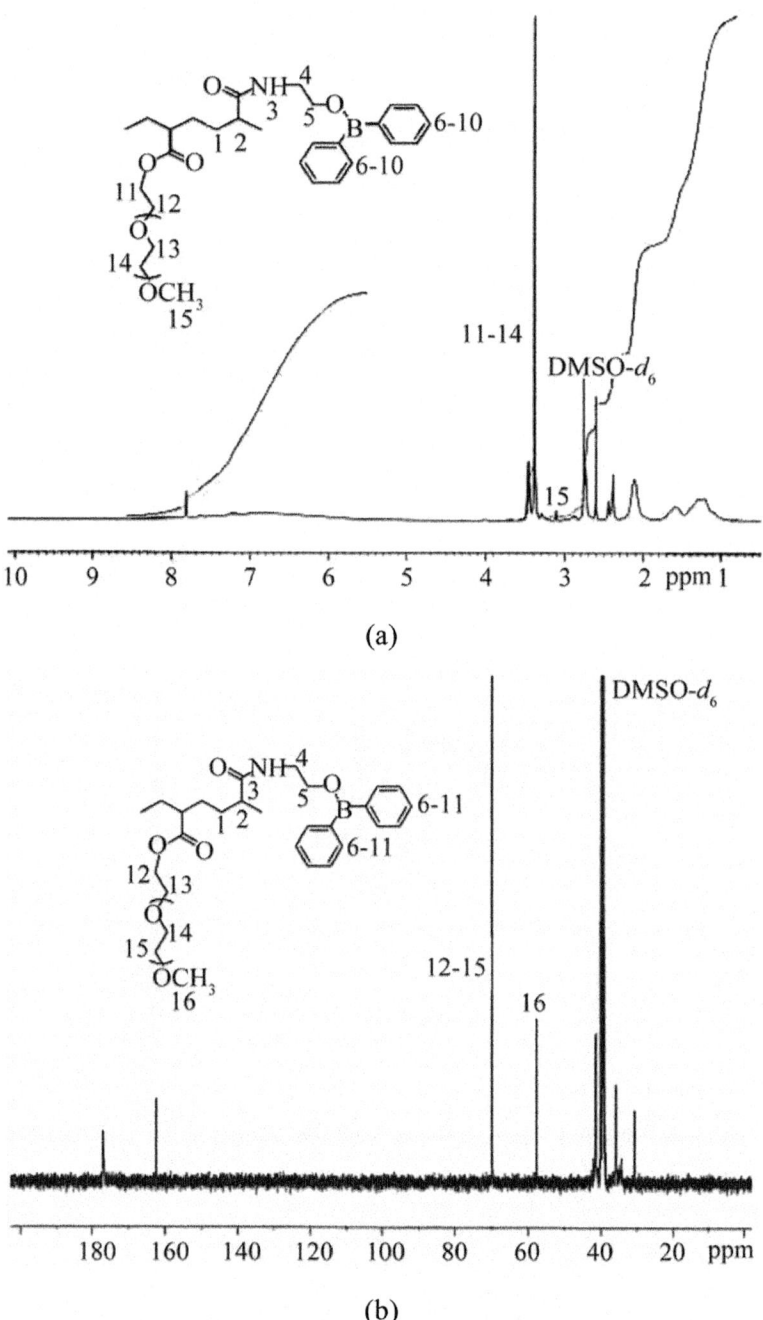

Figure 3. (a) ^{1}H NMR and (b) ^{13}C NMR spectra of PAA-gAEPB-2-g-PEO in DMSO-d[6].

^{1}H (^{13}C) NMR spectra of PEO grafted organoboron PAA polymer (PAA-B-PEO) were illustrated in **Figure 3**. The observed proton signals from of side-chain PEO branches at 3.4 and 3.1 ppm for (CH$_2$-CH$_2$-O)$_n$ units (**Figure 3**(a)) and carbon atom resonances (69 ppm for O-CH$_2$ and 57 ppm for OCH$_3$ end group) (**Figure 3**(b)) may be served an additional fact to confirm the formation of side-chain macrobranched PEO linkages.

Functional Polymer Composition–Property Relationship

The results of intrinsic viscosity measurements from the plots of h$_{sp}$/c (specific viscosity) vs. c (polymer concentration in deionized water) for the organoboron PAA and PEO derivatives having different compositions are illustrated in **Figure 4**.

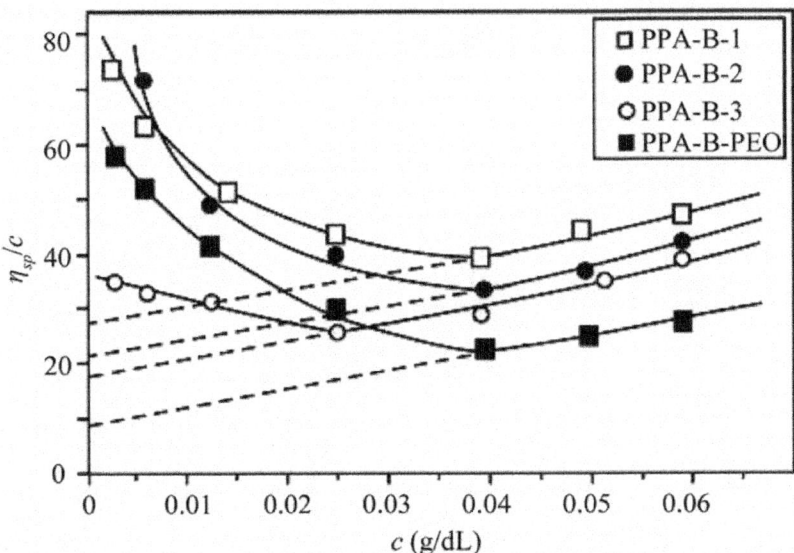

Figure 4. The plots of η$_{sp}$/c (specific viscoity) versus c (polymer concentrations in deionized water) for the determination of intrinsic viscosity and evaluation of polymer composition-viscosity relationships (dilution effect and polyelectrolyte behaviour): –□– PPA-B-1, –·– PPA-B-2, –o– PAA-B-3 and –■– PAA-B-PEO.

Table 1. Some characteristic parameters of organoboron amide (PAA-B) and PEO branched (PAA-B-PEO) derivatives of PAA.

Functional polymers	B content (%)	$[\eta]_{in} (dL \cdot g^{-1})$ in water at 25°C	T_g (°C)
PAA-B-1	3.64	2.75	190.6
PAA-B-2	2.45	2.16	185.0
PAA-B-3	1.85	1.74	181.2
PAA-B-2-PEO	2.16	0.85	175.8

A visible decrease of h_{in} value with increasing the organoboron fragment in PAA polymer was observed (**Table 1**). Unlike the PEO branched derivative the organoboron polymers exhibit typical polyelectrolyte behavior, i.e., increase in viscosity with a dilution of polymer water solution, which can be explained by specific behavior of complexed macromolecules and their conformational changes resulting in the expansion of polymer coil in the dilution solution. Similar effect was observed for the other carboxyl-containing polymers [27,28].

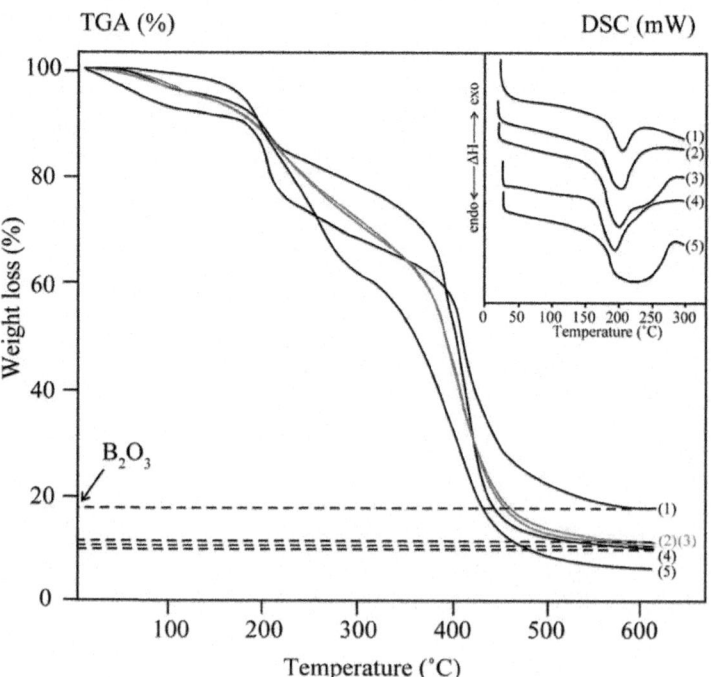

Figure 5. DSC and TGA curves of functional organoboron polymers: (1) PAA-B-1, (2) PAA-B-2, (3) PAA-B-3, (4) PAA-B-PEO and (5) pristine PAA. Heating rate 10°C / min under a nitrogen atmosphere.

Thermal behavior and phase transitons of synthesized organoboron polymers were investigated by differential scanning calorimetric (DSC) and thermal gravimetrical analysis (TGA) methods. The obtained results were summarized in **Figure 5**. It was found that PAA and its organoboron and PEO branched derivatives exhibit amorphous structure with characteristically broad endo-peaks, which are associated with the glass-transition temperatures (T_g), significantly depend on the composition and content of organoboron linkages in the functional polymers. The higher values of T_g are observed for the polymers containing relatively high organoboron linkages.

Therefore, rigid H-bonded structure provides high T_g in the organoboron polymers (curves 1-3). The results of TGA analyses (**Figure 5**) indicate that the organoboron polymer and PEO branched derivative of PAA show higher thermal stability which increases with increasing degree of grafted organoboron linkage in the polymer. The observed two step degradation of the PAA and its functionalized derivatives indicates occurrence of some macromolecular reactions. TGA analyses also allow us to determine the content of boron in studied functionalized polymers, results of which are summarized in **Table 1**.

Cytotoxicity

The obtained cytotoxicity results of the pristine PAA and its organoboron amide (PAA-B) and organoboron amide-ester (PAA-B-PEO) branches, and PAA-BPEO/ folic acid complex (PAA-B-PEO-F) on cancer cells using a trypan blue staining were illustrated in **Figure 6**. As seen from plots of concentration of polymers versus percent of cell viability, the toxicity of pristine PAA against cancer and normal cells decreased with an increasing in polymer concentration from 100 to 200mg $\cdot$ mL^{-1}for 24 h incubation at 37°C. If polymer concentration was higher than 20 mg $\cdot$ mL^{-1}, its toxicity increased, especially higher toxicity exhibits for 24 h incubation. The toxicity of PAA-B (organoboron amide polymer) was more significant than other polymer systems.

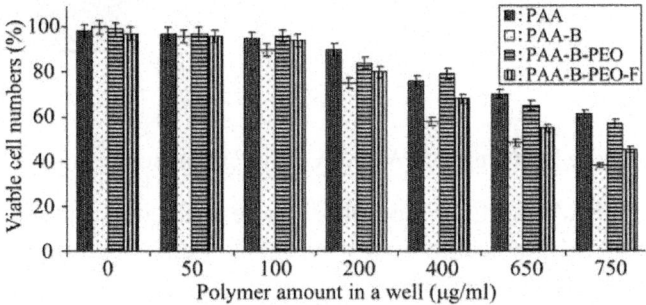

Figure 6. In vitro cytotoxicity of pristine PAA and functionalized organoboron.polymers with different amounts at 24 h incubation. Results are presented as means ± SEM.

Figure 6 shows that the number of viable cells is above 80% for normal and cancer cells after incubation of the cells with PAA-B at concentrations around 100 - 200 mg · mL^{-1} for 24 h incubating time in cell culture media. The number of viable cells was over 50 % or normal cells in the range of 400 - 650 mg · mL^{-1} concentration. However, the toxicity of cancer cells was increased beginning from 400 mg · mL^{-1}.

The PAA-B and PAA-B-PEO-F polymers had higher toxicity for cancer cells (55% alive cells) than normal cells (68% alive cells) in 650 mg · mL^{-1} concentration of polymer...FA complex. It was observed that the cytotoxicity of PAA-B-PEO decreases as compared with organoboron polymers, which can be explained by compatibilizing effect of PEO branched linkages. The cytotoxicity of PEO containing polymer was lower than those without PEO at 400 - 650 mg · mL^{-1} concentration (**Figure 6**). To improve the targeting of polymer macromolecules to cancer cells, folic acid (FA) was inserted to the structure through complex-formation.

The formation of organoboron polymer...FA complex through interaction of amide or carboxylic groups with pseudo-aromatic amine of FA and its conjugation with HeLa cells may be schematically represented as follows (Scheme 2).

When the polymer...FA complex was incubated, the toxicity of the HeLa cells was higher than that of the normal cells, because cancer cells had more FA receptors than normal cells.

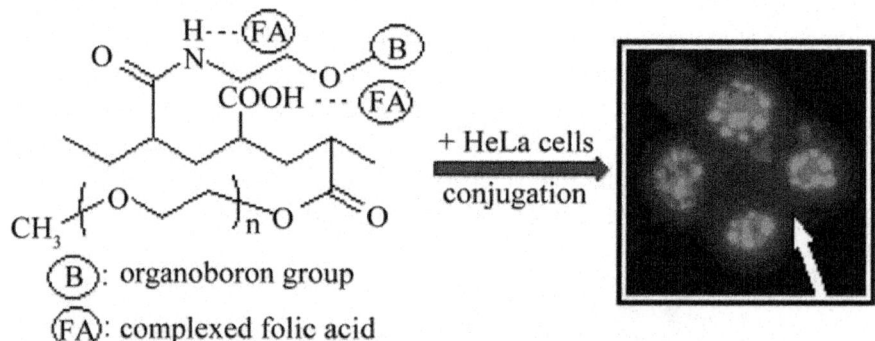

Scheme 2. Proposed structure of PAA...FA complex and conjugation with HeLa cells.

Therefore PAA-B-PEO-F complex can be utilized as a therapeutic drug at 200 - 400 mg · mL^{-1} concentration, where its toxicity was minimal for normal cells, but influential for cancer cells.

Double Staining and Capase 3 Immune Staining Results

Apoptotic index was obtained by both double staining and caspase 3 immune staining methods. The results were presented in **Table 2**. If the cells treated by PAA-B at 400 - 650 mg $\cdot$ mL^{-1} concentration, the number of apoptotic cells was not high. While PPA-B-PEO-F complex at 400 mg $\cdot$ mL^{-1} concentration exhibits the highest apoptotic ratios on cancer cells. In addition, the number of apoptotic cells was high as well for the organoboron polymer/folic acid complex at 400 mg $\cdot$ mL^{-1} concentration (**Table 2**). The results of light and fluorescent microscope investigation of the interaction of organoboron polymers with cancer cells were illustrated in **Figure 7**. The cytoplasm's of apoptotic cells treated with complex were stained brown (**Figure 7(b)**) but, the cytoplasm of non apoptotic cells were not stained brown (**Figure 7(a)**). According to double staining results, apoptotic cells' nucleus stained bright blue and compartmentalized **Figure 7(d)**), but non-apoptotic cells' nuclei stained lifeless blue (**Figure 7(c)**). When the PEO-containing branched polymers applied, the number of apoptotic cells was decreased. However, the number of apoptotic cells was increased as 7 % when they treated by PAA-PEO-BF complex in 400 mg $\cdot$ mL^{-1} concentration. Apoptotic index for Fibroblast cells was 18 % at 400 mg $\cdot$ mL^{-1} concentration of PAA-PEO-B-F. Moreover, there was no significant change on apoptotic index (18%) of Fibroblast cell targeting by folic acid. Apoptotic indexes in cancer and normal cells was estimated of caspase-3 and double staining result. The important observations can be summarized as follows: we checked for apoptosis or necrosis with double staining (Hoechst 33342 and PI) and caspase 3 immune staining. It was observed that both the cytotoxicity and necrotic indexes of synthesized functional organoboron polymers show approximately same values.

Table 2. The comparative analysis of apoptotic and necrotic HeLa cells index for (I) PAA, and its (II) organoboron amide (PAA-B), (III) PEO branched (PAA-B-PEO) and (IV) FA complexed (PAA-B-PEO-F) derivatives at 24 h incubation. Results are presented as means ± SEM.

[Polymer] ($\mu g \cdot mL^{-1}$)	Apoptotic index (%)				Necrotic index (%)			
	I	II	III	IV	I	II	III	IV
0	1 ± 1	1 ± 1	1 ± 1	1 ± 1	1 ± 1	1 ± 1	1 ± 1	1 ± 1
100	5 ± 1	10 ± 2	12 ± 2	16 ± 1	2 ± 1	8 ± 2	2 ± 1	7 ± 1
200	2 ± 2	16 ± 2	15 ± 1	20 ± 1	10 ± 2	25 ± 3	7 ± 1	18 ± 2
400	5 ± 1	21 ± 1	18 ± 2	5 ± 2	24 ± 2	46 ± 3	20 ± 1	30 ± 3
600	6 ± 1	6 ± 1	15 ± 2	20 ± 1	34 ± 2	53 ± 3	33 ± 2	45 ± 2

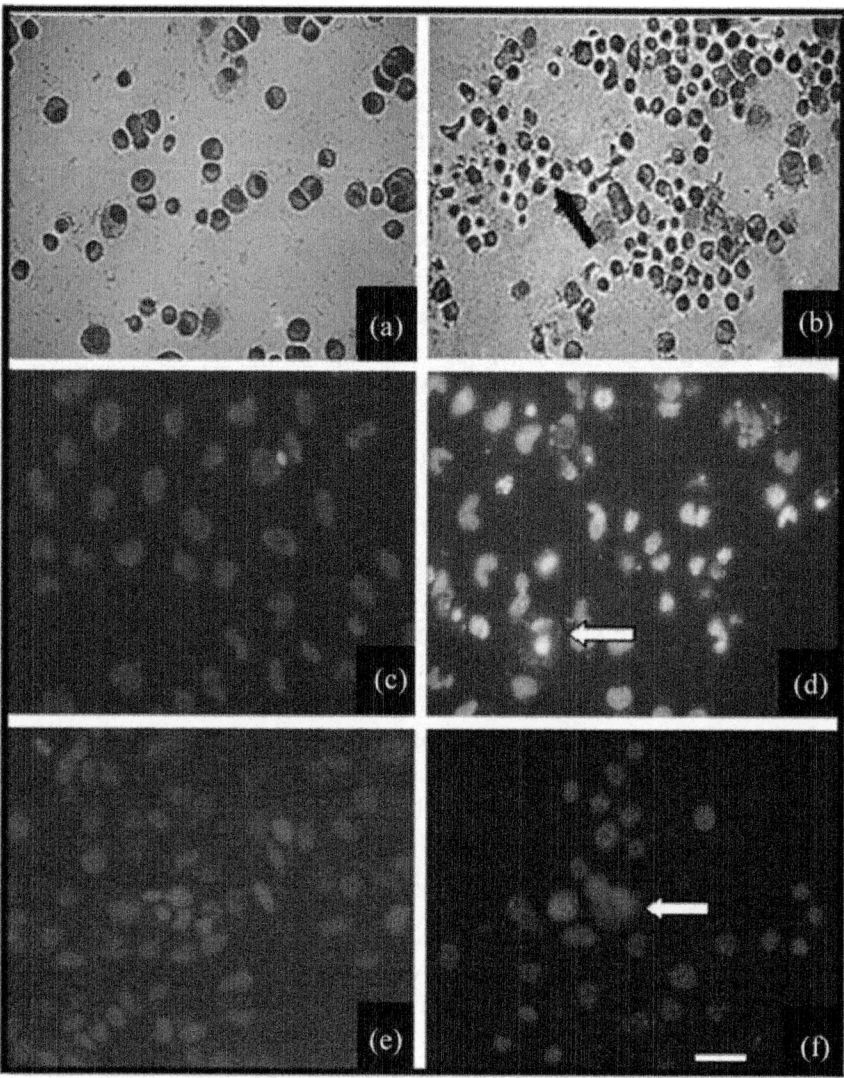

Figure 7. Light microscope images of (a) virgin (non-apoptotic) HeLa cells as a control group (stained with caspas-3 immune staining kit), and (b) 400 mg · mL⁻¹ concentration of organoboron polymer (PolyAC-B-2-PEO-F)/HeLa cells conjugate (stained with caspas-3 immune staining kit); (c) Fluorescent microscope image of nucleus of untreated HeLa cells (stained with Hoechst 33342 dye) as a control, (d) nucleus of HeLa cells (stained with Hoechst 33342); (e) Fluorescent microscope image of nucleus of untreated HeLa cells (stained with PI dye) as a control; (f) nucleus of HeLa cells (stained with PI dye); Photos (c) and (d) taken under DAPI filter, photos (e) and (f) taken under FITC filter. Figure (a) and (b) were recorded with ×200 magnification. Figure (d), (e) and (f) were recorded with ×400 magnification. Scale bar is 20 μm.

The polymers with lower concentrations ($100\text{-}200$ mg $\cdot$ mL^{-1}) decrease in necrosis stained with PI dye. While the necrotic indexes of normal and cancer cells increase at relatively higher concentration (400 mg $\cdot$ mL^{-1}) of polymers, especially PAA-B (**Table 2** and Figures 7(e) and (f)). However, when the polymer containing PEO was incubated to cancer cells, the necrotic index was decreased in cancer and normal cells.

Fluorescent microscope image of nucleus of untreated HeLa cells (stained with PI dye) as a control was presented in **Figure 7**(e), where formation of green spots indicates the nucleus of non-necrotic cells. Cancer cells exposed to polymer...FA complex became highly PI-positive. This observed fact indicated that the cells were undergoing to necrosis. HeLa and Fibroblast cells incorporated with PPA-B polymer provide a lysing the cellmembrane (necrosis) and relatively higher necrotic indexes 53% and 43% for the cancer and normal cells, respectively. When both the cells treated with PAAPEO-B-F copolymer, necrotic indexes decrease for HeLa (49%) and Fibroblast cells (41%).

CONCLUSIONS

This work presents the synthesis and characterization of organoboron, PEO branched and FA complexed derivatives of PPA and investigation of their antitumor activity (cytotoxicity, apoptotic and necrotic effects) toward HeLa and Fibroblast cells by using a combination of various biochemical, statistical and microscopy methods. It was observed that antitumor activity significantly depends on the structure, amount of ionizable free carboxylic groups, organoboron linkages and complexed fragments in the functionalized polymers, and changes in the following row: PAA << (PAA-B)s < PPA-B-PEO < PAA-B-PEO-F. Among them, PAA-B-PEO-F copolymer system showed promising antitumor activity against cancer cells through apoptosis and necrosis induced caspase-3-dependent partway. Apoptotic indexes in cancer and normal cells were estimated of caspase-3 immune staining and double staining (Hoechst 33342 and PI) results. These observations are confirmed the realization of apoptosis and necrosis processes in the interaction of functionalized polymers with normal and cancer cells. Apoptotic index of cancer cells were obtained higher than normal cells. Especially, apoptotic effect of FA containing copolymer was increased compared with non-targeted copolymers. HeLa and Fibroblast cells incorporated with organobron polymer provide a lysing the cell-membrane (necrosis) and relatively higher necrotic indexes 53% and 43% for the cancer and normal cells, respectively. It was found that interactions of both the cells with PPA-PEO-B-F copolymer were decreased the necrotic indexes for HeLa (45%) and Fibroblast cells (41%). Utilization of this novel organoboron polymer as precursors in boron neutron capture therapy (BNCT) will be a subject for our future investigations.

ACKNOWLEDGEMENTS

The supports of this work by the TAEK (Turkish Atomic Energy Authority) and TÜBİTAK (Turkish Scientific and Technology Research Council) through TAEK-A3.H2.P2.01 and TBAG-2386 projects, respectively, are gratefully acknowledged.

REFERENCES

1. L. Seymour, "Synthetic Polymers with Intrinsic AntiCancer Activity," Journal of Bioactive and Compatible Polymers, Vol. 6, No. 2, 1991, pp. 178-216.doi:10.1177/088391159100600205

2. J. Liao and R. M. Ottenbrite, "Controlled Drug Delivery: Challenges and Strategies," ACS, Washington DC, 1997.

3. S. Akhtar, "Non-Viral Cancer Gene Therapy: Beyond Delivery," Gene Therapy, Vol. 13, No. 5, 2006, pp. 739- 740. doi:10.1038/sj.gt.3302692

4. M. Dittgen, M. Durrani and K. Lehmann, "Acrylic Polymers. A Review of Pharmaceutical Applications," S. T. P. Pharma Science, Vol. 7, No. 6, 1997, pp. 403-437.

5. M. Dimitrov, M. Lambovi, S. Shenkov, V. Dosseva and V. Y. Baranovski, "Hydrogels Based on the Chemically Crosslinked Polyacrylic Acid: Biopharmaceutical Characterization," Acta Pharmaceutica, Vol. 53, No. 1, 2003, pp. 25-31.

6. W. Lee, T. G. Lee and W.-G. Koh, "Grafting of Poly- (Acrylic Acid) on the Poly(Ethylene Glycol) Hydrogel Using Surface-Initiated Photopolymerization for Covalent Immobilization of Collagen," Industrial & Engineering Chemistry Research, Vol. 13, No. 7, 2007, pp. 1195- 1200.

7. Y. Onuki, M. Nishikawa, M. Morishita and K. Takayama, "Development of Photocrosslinked Polyacrylic Acid Hydrogel as an Adhesive for Dermotological Patches: Involvement of Formulation Factors in Physical Properties and Pharmacological Effects," International Journal of Pharmacology, Vol. 349, No. 1-2, 2008, pp. 47-52.doi:10.1016/j. ijpharm.2007.07.021

8. B. R. Saunders, H. M. Crowther and B. Vincent, "Poly- [(methyl methacrylate)-co-(methacrylic acid)] Microgel particles: Swelling Control Using pH, Cononsolvency, and Osmotic Deswelling," Macromolecules,

Vol. 30, No. 3, 1997, pp. 482-487.doi:10.1021/ma961277f

9. T. Sawai, S. Yamazaki, Y. Ikariyama and M. Aizawa, "pH-Responsive Swelling of the Ultrafine Microsphere," Macromolecules, Vol. 24, No. 8, 1991, pp. 2117-2118.doi:10.1021/ma00008a067

10. S. Argentiere, L. Blasi, G. Ciccarella, G. Barbarella, R. Cingolani and G. Gigli, "Synthesis of Poly(Acrylic Acid) Nanogels and Application in Loading and Release of on Oligothiophene Fluorophore and Its Bovine Albumin Conjugate," Macromolecular Symposia, Vol. 281, No. 1, 2009, pp. 69-76. doi:10.1002/masy.200950709

11. N. A. Petasis, "Expanding Roles for Organoboron Compounds–Versatile and Valuable Molecules for Synthetic, BIOLOGICal and Medicinal Chemistry," Australian Journal of Chemistry, Vol. 60, No. 11, 2007, pp. 795-798. doi:10.1071/CH07360

12. W. Yang, S. Gao and B. Wang, "Boronic Acid Compounds as Potential Pharmaceutical Agents," Medicinal Research Reviews, Vol. 23, 2003, pp. 346-368.doi:10.1002/med.10043

13. V. M. Dembitsky and M. Srebnik, "Synthesis and Biological Activity of a-Aminoboronic Acid, Aminocarboranes and Their Derivatives," Tetrahedron, Vol. 59, No. 5, 2003, pp. 579-593. doi:10.1016/S0040-4020(02)01618-6

14. P. G. Richardson, C. Mitsiades, T. Hideshima and K. C. Anderson, "Bortezomib: Proteasome Inhibition as an Effective Anticancer Therapy," Annual Review of Medicine, Vol. 57, 2006, pp. 33-47. doi:10.1146/annurev.med.57.042905.122625

15. H. S. Ban, H. Minegishi, K. Shimizu, M. Maruyama, Y. Yasui and H. Nakamura, "Discovery of Carboranes as Inducers of 20S Proteasome Activity," Chemistry & Medicinal Chemistry, Vol. 5, No. 8, 2010, pp. 1236-1241. doi:10.1002/cmdc.201000112

16. C. Morin, "The Chemistry of Boron Analogues of Bio Molecules," Tetrahedron, Vol. 50, No. 44, 1994, pp. 12521-12569. doi:10.1016/S0040-4020(01)89389-3

17. C. Baldock, G.-J. de Boer, J. B. Rafferty, A. R. Stuitje and D. W. Rice, "Mechanism of Action of Diazaborines," Biochemical Pharmacology, Vol. 55, No. 10, 1998, pp. 1541- 1549.

18. A. Jabbour, D. Steinberg, V. M. Dembitsky, A. Moussaieff, B. Zaks and M. Srebnik, "Synthesis and Evaluation of Oxazaborolidines for Antibacterial Activity against Streptococcus Mutants," Journal of Medicinal Chemistry, Vol. 47, No. 10, 2004, pp. 2409-2410. doi:10.1021/jm049899b

19. S. J. Benkovic, S. J. Baker, M. R. K. Alley, Y.-H. Woo, Y.-K. Zhang, T. Akama, W. Mao, J. Baboval, P. T. Ravi Rajagopalan, W. Wall, L. S. Kahng, A.Tavassoli and L. Shapiro, "Identitication of Borinic Esters as Inhibitors of Bacterial Cell Growth and Bacterial Methyltransferases, CcrM and MenH," Journal of Medicinal Chemistry, Vol. 48, No. 23, 2005, pp. 7468-7476. doi:10.1021/jm050676a

20. S. J. Baker, Y.-K. Zhang, T. Akama, A. Lau, H. Zhou, V. Hernandez, W. Mao, M. R. K. Alley, V. Sanders and J. J. Plattner, "Discovery of a New Boron-Containing Antifungal Agent," Fluoro-1,3-dihydro-1-hydroxy-2,1-benzoxa-borole (AN2690), for the potential treatment of onychomycosis," Journal of Medicinal Chemistry, Vol. 49, No. 15, 2006, pp. 4447-4450. doi:10.1021/jm0603724

21. H. B. Zhou, K. W. Nettles, J. B. Bruning, Y. Kim, A. Joachimiak, S. Sharma, K. E. Carlson, F. Stossi, B. S. Katzenellenbogen, G. L. Greene and J. A. Katzenellenbogen, "Elemental Isomerism: A Boron-Nitrogen Surrogate for a Carbon-Carbon Double Bond Increases the Chemical Diversity of Estrogen Receptor Ligands," Chemistry & Biology, Vol. 14, No. 5, 2007, pp. 659-669. doi:10.1016/j.chembiol.2007.04.009

22. J. F. Valliant, K. J. Guenther, A. S. King, P. Morel, P. Schaffer, O. O. Sogbein and K. A. Stephenson, "The Medical Chemistry of Carborones," Coordination Chemistry Reviews, Vol. 232, No. 1-2, 2002, pp. 173-230. doi:10.1016/S0010-8545(02)00087-5

23. W. Chen, S. C. Mehta and D. R. Lu, "Selective Boron Drug Delivery to Brain Tumors for Boron Neutron Capture Therapy," Advanced Drug Delivery Reviews, Vol. 26, No. 2-3, 1997, pp. 231-247. doi:10.1016/S0169-409X(97)00037-9

24. F. Shosseler, F. Ilmain and S. J. Candau, "Structure and Properties of Partially Neutralized Poly(Acrylic Acid) Gels," Macromolecules, Vol. 24, No. 1, 1991, pp. 225- 234.doi:10.1021/ma00001a035

25. M. Türk, Z. M. O. Rzayev and S. A. Khalilova, "Bioengineering Functional Copolymers. XIV. Synthesis and Interaction of Poly(N-isopropyl Acrylamide-co-2,3-dihydro-2H-pyran-alt-maleic Anhydride)s with SCLC Cancer Cells," Bioorganic & Medicinal Chemistry, Vol. 18, No. 22, 2010, pp. 7975-7984. doi:10.1016/j.bmc.2010.09.031

26. Türk, Z. M. O. Rzayev and G. Kurucu, "Bioengineering Functional Copolymers. XII. Interaction of Boron-Containing and PEO Branched Derivatives of Poly(MA-alt-MVE) with HeLa Cells," Health, Vol. 2, No. 1, 2010, pp. 51-61. doi:10.4236/health.2010.21009

27. T. Shimisu and A. Minakata, "Effect of Divalent Cations on the Volume of a Maleic Acid Copolymer Gel Examined by Incorporating Lysozyme," European Polymer Journal, Vol. 38, No. 6, 2002, pp. 1113-1120. doi:10.1016/S0014-3057(01)00283-X

28. O. Nobumichi and S. Shintaro, "Conformational Characterization of a Maleic Acid Copolymer with an Inflexible Side Chain," Journal of Macromolecular Science: Pure and Applied Chemistry, Vol. 27, No. 7, 1990, pp. 861-873. doi:10.1080/10601329008544810

Chapter 5

GENERATION AND CHARACTERIZATION OF NOVEL MAGNETIC FIELD-RESPONSIVE BIOMATERIALS

Modesto T. Lopez-Lopez[1], Giuseppe Scionti[2], Ana C. Oliveira[2], Juan D. G. Duran[1], Antonio Campos[2], Miguel Alaminos[2], Ismael A. Rodriguez[2,3]

[1]Department of Applied Physics, Faculty of Sciences, University of Granada, Granada, Spain, and Instituto de Investigación Biosanitaria ibs.GRANADA, Granada, Spain

[2]Department of Histology, Faculty of Medicine, University of Granada, Granada, Spain, and Instituto de Investigación Biosanitaria ibs.GRANADA, Granada, Spain

[3]Department of Histology, School of Dentistry, National University of Cordoba, Cordoba, Argentina

ABSTRACT

We report the preparation of novel magnetic field-responsive tissue substitutes based on biocompatible multi-domain magnetic particles dispersed in a fibrin–agarose biopolymer scaffold. We characterized our biomaterials with several experimental techniques. First we analyzed their microstructure and found that it was strongly affected by the presence of magnetic particles, especially when a magnetic field was applied at the start of polymer gelation. In these samples we observed parallel stripes consisting of closely packed fibers, separated by more isotropic net-like spaces. We then studied the viability of oral mucosa fibroblasts in the magnetic scaffolds and found no significant differences compared to positive control samples. Finally, we analyzed the magnetic and mechanical properties of the tissue substitutes. Differences in microstructural patterns of the tissue substitutes correlated with their macroscopic mechanical properties. We also found that the mechanical properties of our magnetic tissue substitutes could be reversibly tuned by noncontact magnetic forces. This unique advantage with respect to other biomaterials could be used to match the mechanical properties of the tissue substitutes to those of potential target tissues in tissue engineering applications.

INTRODUCTION

Biomaterials intended for applications in regenerative medicine must imitate the histological structure of natural tissues. They should thus meet a number of requirements, including biocompatibility [1–4]. Various scaffold materials have been tested, including both naturally-derived and synthetic polymers. Although natural materials provide a physiological environment for cell adhesion and proliferation, they have several disadvantages, such as their suboptimal mechanical properties [5–8]. Synthetic materials are extensively used because of their easy molding characteristics, relatively easy production and their ability to control dissolution and degradation [9]. The main drawback of synthetic materials is that they do not have natural sites for cell adhesion [10].

One alternative to choosing between natural or synthetic materials is to use them in combination [11]. For example, several authors have very recently used magnetic nanoparticles in combination with polymers to prepare innovative magnetic scaffolds for tissue substitutes [12–29]. These magnetic scaffolds have several advantages. First, the ferromagnetic behavior of the magnetic scaffolds allows visualization and in-vivo follow-up by magnetic resonance imaging [28]. Second, in-vitro studies indicate that magnetic nanoparticles in the scaffolds do not compromise cell adhesion, proliferation or differentiation [12,13,25]. Furthermore, the main advantage of novel magnetic scaffolds is that they acquire a magnetic moment when an external magnetic field is applied, i.e. they act as magnets, attracting functionalized magnetic nanoparticles injected close to them [13,21,28]. This represents a promising strategy to guide and accumulate growth factors, drugs and cells previously attached to the injected magnetic nanoparticles.

To the best of our knowledge, all magnetic scaffolds described to date are based on the use of magnetic particles measuring on the order of 10 nm in diameter. Magnetic particles of this size are single-domain in terms of their magnetic behavior. Moreover, because of their small size the magnetic energy of interaction between particles is weak compared to the energy of Brownian motion [30]. As a result, even for strong applied magnetic fields, Brownian motion dominates over the magnetic forces, and the mechanical properties of the scaffolds cannot be controlled by noncontact magnetic forces. The situation is radically different for magnetic particles larger than approximately 50–100 nm. Particles of this size are multi-domain in terms of their magnetic behavior. This means that there is no magnetic interaction between them prior to the application of a magnetic field. In addition, because of their relatively large size, Brownian motion is negligible compared to magnetic interaction in the presence of moderate magnetic fields [30], which makes it theoretically possible to control, via noncontact magnetic forces, the mechanical properties of biomaterials that contain the particles.

The main aim of the present study was to generate magnetic biomaterials whose mechanical properties can be controlled by noncontact magnetic forces. To this end we used a mixture of fibrin and agarose as a polymer matrix. We chose this combination because fibrin is a natural polymer used frequently in tissue engineering. The main drawback of fibrin hydrogels lies in their suboptimal biomechanical properties, which fortunately can be enhanced by combining them with agarose [31]. We previously showed that these fibrin–agarose biomaterials have better biomechanical and structural properties than fibrin alone [31–33]. In addition, we recently demonstrated that the biomechanical properties of fibrin–agarose hydrogels reproduce the properties of several native soft human tissues [31]. Fibrin–agarose biomaterials have been used successfully to generate bioengineered substitutes of several human tissues such as the cornea, oral mucosa, skin and peripheral nerves, and were shown to be effective in vivo [32–34]. In the present study we demonstrate that the incorporation of magnetic particles gives rise to bioengineered oral mucosa tissue substitutes with a tunable, reversible mechanical response. In tissue engineering applications this versatility should make it possible to adjust the mechanical properties of the artificial tissue substitutes with precision, in order to match the properties of the target tissue at the site of implantation.

MATERIALS AND METHODS

Ethics Statement

This study was approved by the Ethics Committee of the University of Granada, Granada, Spain. Each tissue donor signed an informed consent form for this study.

Establishment of Primary Cultures of Oral Mucosa Fibroblasts

Ten normal human oral mucosa biopsies with an average volume of 8 mm^3 were obtained from healthy donors at the School of Dental Sciences of the University of Granada. To obtain primary cultures of human oral mucosa fibroblasts, tissues were enzymatically de-epithelized and the lamina propria was digested in a mixture of Dulbecco's Modified Eagle's Medium (DMEM) and 2 mg/mL *Clostridium histolyticum* collagenase I (Gibco BRL Life Technologies, Karlsruhe, Germany). Detached fibroblasts were collected by centrifugation and expanded in culture fiasks containing DMEM supplemented with 10% fetal calf serum (FCS) and 1% antibiotic–antimycotic solution (final concentration 100 U/mL penicillin G, 0.10 mg/mL streptomycin and 0.25 μg/ mL amphotericin B) (all from Sigma-Aldrich, Steinheim, Germany). Cells were incubated at 37°C in 5% carbon dioxide under standard culture conditions. The medium was changed every 3 days, and the cells were subcultured in a solution of 0.5 g/L trypsin and 0.2 g/L EDTA at 37°C for 10 min. For all experiments we used cells from the first 3 passages of these human oral mucosa fibroblast cell cultures.

Preparation of the Biomaterials (Three-dimensional Tissue Substitutes)

For the magnetic phase we used MagP-OH particles (Nanomyp, Granada, Spain). According to the manufacturer, MagP-OH particles consist of biocompatible nanoparticles with a mean diameter of 115 nm, comprising a single magnetic core of magnetite (γ-Fe_3O_4) coated by a polymer layer of methyl methacrylate-co-hydroxyl ethyl methacrylate-co-ethylene glycol dimethacrylate. MagP-OH particles were supplied as an aqueous suspension stabilized with surfactants, and were treated before use with 5 washing cycles (centrifugation at 15000 g for 30 min, supernatant discarded, ultrapure water added, particles redispersed) to remove the surfactant. We then replaced the water carrier with 70% ethanol and left the nanoparticles in this solution for 12 h for sterilization. Finally the ethanol was removed, and the nanoparticles were suspended in DMEM.

For the continuous matrix we used a mixture of fibrin and agarose as the biopolymer. The target tissue was human oral mucosa, thus, seeding with human oral mucosa fibroblasts was required. To prepare the magnetic tissue substitutes we used a variation of a previous method for fibrin–agarose nonmagnetic scaffolds [32]. Briefly, we used 3.8 mL human plasma obtained from blood donors (provided by the Granada Biobank of the Andalusian Regional Government), to which we added 1,000,000 oral mucosa fibroblasts resuspended in 0.625 mL DMEM, together with 75 μL of a solution of tranexamic acid at a concentration of 0.1 g/mL. The final concentration of tranexamic acid in the biomaterial was 1.5 mg/mL. This acid is an anti-fibrinolytic agent that prevents degradation of the scaffold. We then added the appropriate amounts of a concentrated suspension of MagP-OH particles in DMEM to a final concentration of approximately 2 mL of particles per 100 mL of mixture. Subsequently, 0.25 mL of a mixture of type VII agarose (a polysaccharide polymer material with a molecular weight of approx. 120,000 g/mol, supplied by Sigma-Aldrich Química SA, Madrid, Spain) in phosphate-buffered saline (PBS) (0.02 g/mL concentration) was added to the mixture to a final agarose concentration of 0.1%. Then 0.25 mL of 2% $CaCl_2$ was added to the mixture to activate the fibrin polymerization process. The final volume of the mixture was 5 mL, which contained 200,000 cells per mL of mixture. This cell density is on the same order of magnitude as (or higher than) the number of cells validated for fibrin–agarose gels in previous studies [32–34].

The mixtures were seeded on petri dishes and kept at 37°C for 2 h until gelation was complete. We applied a vertical magnetic field to the mixtures during the first 5 min of gelation with a coil connected to a DC power supply. We subjected different samples to different field strengths ranging from 0 to 48 kA/m in intensity (0, 16, 32 or 48 kA/m). After 2 h we added to the gels (tissue substitutes) DMEM medium supplemented with 10 vol% FCS and 1 vol% antibiotic–antimycotic solution, and incubated the cultures for 24 h at 37°C in the culture dishes.

For comparison we also prepared nonmagnetic tissue substitutes (control samples) with the same procedure as described above, except for the addition of magnetic particles. We also subjected these samples to applied magnetic fields of different intensity during gelation (0, 16, 32 or 48 kA/m) in order to analyze the effect of the magnetic field on the biological constituents in the tissue substitutes. To analyze the effect of the magnetic MagP-OH particles on the substitute properties more precisely, we also prepared a nanoparticle control sample (Ctrl-NP) which contained nonmagnetic polymer particles. These particles (PolymP-C, NanoMyP) were uniformly spherical and similar in diameter (approximately 130 nm) to MagP-OH particles, but lacked magnetic properties. Their chemical composition was similar to the polymer layer constituting the shell of MagP-OH, since they are made from the same polymers with OH functionalization. We prepared Ctrl-NP tissue substitutes with the same procedure as described above for magnetic tissue substitutes, but with PolymP-C particles instead of MagP-OH particles. Prior to use we sterilized the PolymP-C particles by immersion for 12 h in 70% ethanol, followed by ethanol removal and dispersion in DMEM.

In all, we prepared oral mucosa substitutes with 9 different protocols (Table 1). The density of all substitutes was approximately 1.1 g/mL.

Table 1. Summary of the different oral mucosa substitutes prepared for this study.

Magnetic field strength during gelation (kA/m)	Approx. concentration of particles (volume %)	Type of particles	Sample name
0	0	—	Ctrl-MF0
0	2	MagP-OH [a]	M-MF0
0	2	PolymP-C [b]	Ctrl-NP
16	0	—	Ctrl-MF16
16	2	MagP-OH [a]	M-MF16
32	0	—	Ctrl-MF32
32	2	MagP-OH [a]	M-MF32
48	0	—	Ctrl-MF48
48	2	MagP-OH [a]	M-MF48

[a] Magnetite (core)/polymer (shell) MagP-OH particles (Nanomyp).
[b] Nonmagnetic polymer PolymP-C particles (Nanomyp).

doi:10.1371/journal.pone.0133878.t001

Structural Analysis

After 24 h of cell culture, we fixed the oral mucosa tissue substitutes in formalin, embedded them in paraffin, and cut them in 5-μm-thick sections. After deparaffination and hematoxylin–eosin staining, we analyzed structural features in the biomaterial sections by light microscopy. For scanning electron microscopy (SEM), samples were fixed in 2.5% glutaraldehyde and postfixed in 1% osmium tetroxide for 90 min. After fixation, the samples were dehydrated in increasing concentrations of acetone (30%, 50%, 70%, 95% and 100%), critical point-dried, mounted on aluminum stubs and sputter-coated with gold according to routine procedures.

Cell Viability Analysis

We evaluated cell viability by measuring intracellular esterase activity, and by examining the integrity of the plasma and nuclear membranes with a fluorescence-based method using the Live/Dead commercial kit (Life Technologies, Carlsbad, CA, USA). This method uses calcein-AM, which is metabolically modified by living cells to a green pigment, and ethidium homodimer-1, which stains the nuclei of dead cells red. We obtained aliquots of 3 mm in diameter of all biomaterial samples after 24 h of cell culture, discarded the supernatants and washed the aliquots with PBS, then cut them into very thin films, incubated them with the Live/Dead solution for 15 min as indicated by the manufacturer, and washed them with PBS. We then observed the samples by fluorescence microscopy and processed the images with ImageJ software to quantify the number of live (green) and dead cells (red).

We also evaluated cell death as nuclear membrane integrity by quantifying the DNA released to the culture medium. We obtained supernatants of each sample and diluted 10-μL aliquots in distilled water free of nuclease (Ambion-Life Technologies, Austin, TX, USA). The DNA in the medium was quantified spectrophotometrically (SmartSpec Plus, Bio-Rad, Hercules, CA, USA) at wavelengths in the range of 260–280 nm.

The mean values ± standard deviations of 8 independent experiments are reported here for each experimental group and each analysis. The Kruskal–Wallis test was used to identify statistical differences among study groups, and the Mann–Whitney test was used to identify significant differences between two groups. Values of p less than 0.05 were considered statistically significant in two-tailed tests.

Magnetic Properties

We measured the magnetization (M) of dry MagP-OH particles at 37°C as a function of the magnetic field strength (H) in a Squid Quantum Design MPMS XL magnetometer. In addition, we obtained the magnetization curve of soaked tissue substitutes 24 h after cell culture. The magnetization curves reported here correspond to the mean of 3 independent measurements.

Mechanical Properties

We characterized the mechanical properties of the tissue substitutes (summarized in Table 1) with a Haake MARS III (Thermo Fisher Scientific, Waltham, MA, USA) controlled stress rheometer at 37°C. The measuring system geometry was a 3.5 cm diameter parallel plate set with rough surfaces to avoid wall slip.

We obtained measurements as follows. First we placed the sample in the rheometer measuring system and squeezed it by lowering the rotating plate until a normal force of 5 N was reached. The rheometer gap at which this force was seen varied slightly depending on the sample, but was in all cases approximately 300 μm. We obtained measurements both in the absence and presence of a magnetic field. For this purpose we used a coil connected to a DC power supply, with the axis of the coil aligned with the axis of the parallel plate measuring system. For measurements obtained during magnetic field application, we applied the magnetic field from 1 min before measurement was started until the measurement was recorded. We used two types of rheological test: oscillatory shear at a fixed frequency, and steady-state shear strain ramps, as described below.

Oscillatory Shear in Fixed Frequency–Variable Amplitude Sweeps

For these tests, we subjected the samples to sinusoidal shear strains at a fixed frequency (1 Hz) and increasing amplitude (logarithmically spaced in the 0.05–1.0 range), and measured the corresponding oscillatory shear stresses. Each frequency–amplitude pair was maintained during 5 oscillatory cycles, although we only used data for the last 3 cycles to rule out transients. These measurements were used to calculate the elastic modulus G' as a function of shear strain.

Steady State Shear Strain Ramps

In these tests the samples were subjected to a constant shear strain for 10 s and the resulting shear stress was measured. Measurements were repeated at increasing (linearly spaced) shear strain values until the nonlinear regime was reached.

We carried out each type of measurement for 3 different aliquots of each sample. For each aliquot we carried out at least 3 repetitions to record a minimum of 9 values per data point. First we recorded measurements at $H = 0$ kA/m, then at $H = 9$ kA/m, $H = 17$ kA/m, and $H = 26$ kA/m. Then we returned to $H = 0$ kA/m and repeated this cycle at least twice for each aliquot. The results obtained for each sample and experimental condition showed no statistically significant differences.

RESULTS AND DISCUSSION

Structural Analysis

Macroscopically, the magnetic tissue substitutes (M-MF0, M-MF16, M-MF32, M-MF48) were similar in appearance to nonmagnetic tissue substitutes (Ctrl-MF0, Ctrl-MF16, Ctrl-MF32, Ctrl-MF48, Ctrl-NP), although the former were darker than control tissue substitutes without particles (Ctrl-MF0 to Ctrl-MF48), which were whitish and semitransparent, and control tissue substitutes with nonmagnetic particles (Ctrl-NP), which were bright white.

For the control group without particles gelled in the absence of an applied magnetic field (Ctrl-MF0), microscopic analysis showed normally-shaped fusiform and star-shaped cells (Fig 1A). The cells were distributed throughout the fibrin–agarose matrix in a normal, net-like appearance. There were no cell–cell contacts, but cell–matrix contacts were evident, as expected in a connective tissue substitute. Cells in the control groups without particles gelled in the presence of an applied magnetic field were similar in appearance (not shown). In samples containing particles, we found that in the magnetic tissue substitute gelled in the absence of an applied magnetic field (M-MF0), as well as the control tissue substitute with nonmagnetic polymer particles (Ctrl-NP), the particles were distributed randomly in an isotropic, homogeneous pattern (Fig 1B and 1C). In contrast, magnetic samples gelled in the presence of a magnetic field (M-MF16, M-MF32, and M-MF48) presented a microscopic pattern consisting of filament-like structures aligned in the same direction, regardless of the intensity of the applied field (Fig 1D).

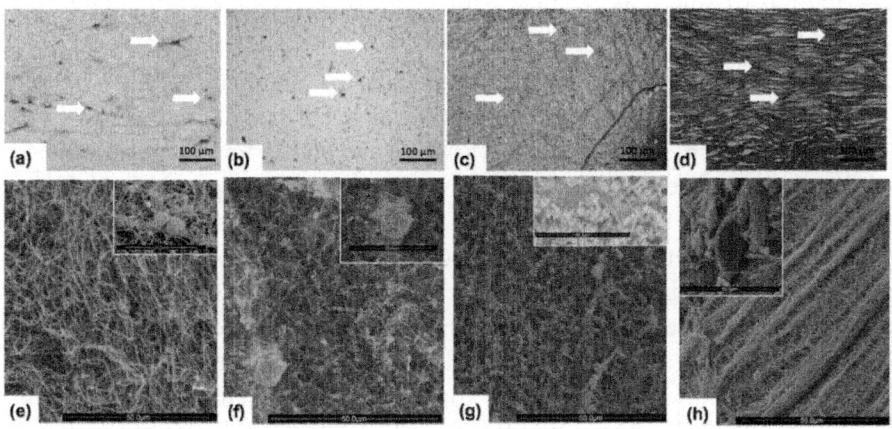

Figure 1. Microscopic images of tissue substitutes. 1a-1d: Light microscopy. 1e-1h: Scanning electron micrographs with individual cells shown in the insets. 1a and 1e: control (nonmagnetic) samples gelled in the absence of a magnetic field (Ctrl-MF0). 1b and 1f: control (nonmagnetic) samples with nonmagnetic polymer particles (Ctrl-NP). 1c and 1g: magnetic samples gelled in the absence of a magnetic field (M-MF0). 1d and 1h: magnetic samples gelled during application of a magnetic field (32 kA/m in 1d, and 48 kA/m in 1h). A few of the cells are marked with arrows in Fig 1a to 1d. Scale bars: Fig 1a-1d, 100 μm; Fig 1e-1h, 50 μm including insets, except for insets in Fig 1e and 1f, 20 μm.

Scanning electron micrographs showed that control samples without particles (Ctrl-MF0 to Ctrl-MF48) presented an isotropic, homogeneous network of randomly aligned fibrin fibers (see Ctrl-MF0, Fig 1E). Application of a magnetic field during gelation in these control samples did not lead to significant changes in their microscopic morphology. Samples Ctrl-MF16 to Ctrl-MF48 (not shown) were similar in appearance to Ctrl-MF0. The presence of magnetic or nonmagnetic nanoparticles induced changes in the fibrillar pattern even in the absence of a magnetic field during gelation. Although the tissue substitutes retained their homogeneous morphology, some particles and particle aggregates were homogeneously distributed throughout the fibrin network, disrupting its mesoscopic ordering (Fig 1F and 1G). When a magnetic field was applied during gelation in magnetic samples, the fibrin network presented an anisotropic pattern (with one direction predominating) characterized by thick stripes containing closely packed fibrin fibers aligned and braided in the direction of the stripes, and isotropic net-like spaces between the stripes, with fewer fibers (Fig 1H, M-MF48). The stronger the field applied during gelation, the more evident the thick stripes. At the highest field strength (sample M-MF48) these stripes were 3.2 ± 1.3 μm in diameter. The aligned distribution of fibers associated with the formation of stripes might induce contact guidance of cells.

The reasons for the striped appearance of magnetic tissue substitutes gelled during exposure to a magnetic field merit consideration. To prepare samples M-MF16, M-MF32 and M-MF48 we applied a magnetic field from the beginning of gelation for 5 min. Application of a magnetic field to multi-domain magnetic particles (such as MagP-OH nanoparticles) induces the appearance of a net magnetic moment aligned with the field direction in each particle (i.e., polarization of the particle). This results in magnetostatic forces of attraction between particles, and when particles are free to move (i.e., when they are dispersed in a liquid-like carrier), they migrate and aggregate into chain-like structures aligned with the field direction, in order to minimize the energy of the system [30]. Since the speed of particle polarization and migration is on the order of milliseconds [30], it is reasonable to assume that fibrin gelation in samples M-MF16, M-MF32 and M-MF48 took place, from the first few seconds, in the presence of MagP-OH particle structures distributed throughout the biomaterial and oriented in the direction of the applied field. Our hypothesis for the formation of the thick fibrin stripes we observed is that these chain-like particle structures acted as condensation fibers for the braid of biopolymer fibers, so that only some residual fibers gelled outside the stripes, giving rise to the microscopic pattern seen in samples M-MF16, M-MF32 and M-MF48 (Fig 1H). This hypothesis is also supported by the fact that no MagP-OH nanoparticles were observed in Fig 1H, from which we infer that all the particles were trapped in the fibrin stripes.

In this connection, we note that according to Tampieri et al. [23], in scaffolds made of magnetic particles and hydroxyapatite–collagen composites, the magnetic phase acts as a cross-linking agent for the collagen. Furthermore, Panseri et al. [21] showed that the fibril network in scaffolds made of magnetic particles and hydroxyapatite–collagen composites was influenced by the preparation method. When the particles were already dispersed in the solution before polymer gelation started (as in the engineered biomaterials described here), the magnetic phase was completely amalgamated and homogeneously distributed throughout the fibril network. On the other hand, when the magnetic scaffold was obtained by soaking a previously prepared nonmagnetic scaffold in a ferrofluid, the nanoparticles were simply adsorbed onto the surface of the collagen fibers. Thanikaivelan et al. [35] found that the collagen fibers were considerably stabilized when superparamagnetic Fe_2O_3 nanoparticles suspended in a liquid carrier were used upon application of a magnetic field of approximately 2,000 Oe (approximately 160 kA/m).

Cell Viability Analysis

Representative fluorescence microscopy images from the viability assays are shown in Fig 2. From these images we obtained the number of viable cells, which remained above 90% in all experimental groups, with no significant differences (p>0.05) among groups (Fig 2).

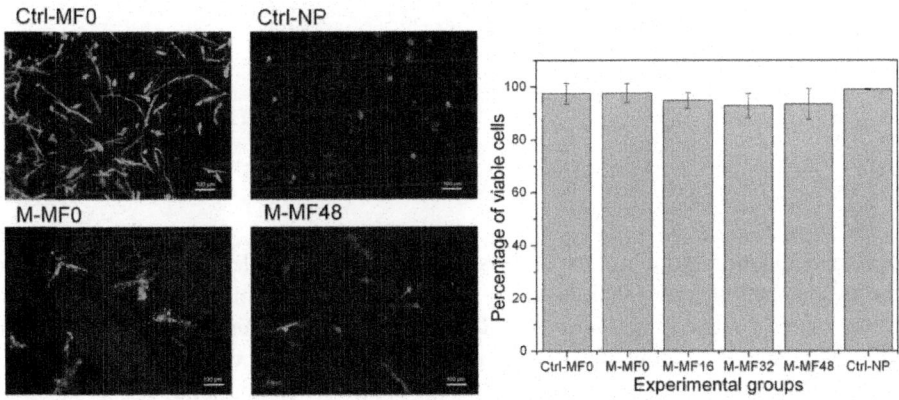

Figure 2. Cell viability tests. Fluorescence microscopy images (scale bar: 100 μm) representative of each experimental group. Live cells are stained green, and dead cells red. The graph shows the mean values ± standard deviations for live cells from 8 independent experiments for each experimental group. Ctrl-MF0: control (nonmagnetic) tissue substitute without particles, gelled in the absence of a magnetic field; Ctrl-NP: control (nonmagnetic) tissue substitute with nonmagnetic polymer particles; M-MF0: magnetic tissue substitute gelled in the absence of a magnetic field; M-MF16, M-MF32 and M-MF48: magnetic tissue substitutes gelled during application of a 16 kA m^{-1}, 32 kA m^{-1} or 48 kA m^{-1} field, respectively.

Similarly, we observed no significant difference (p>0.05) in the amount of free DNA among the different experimental groups (Fig 3).

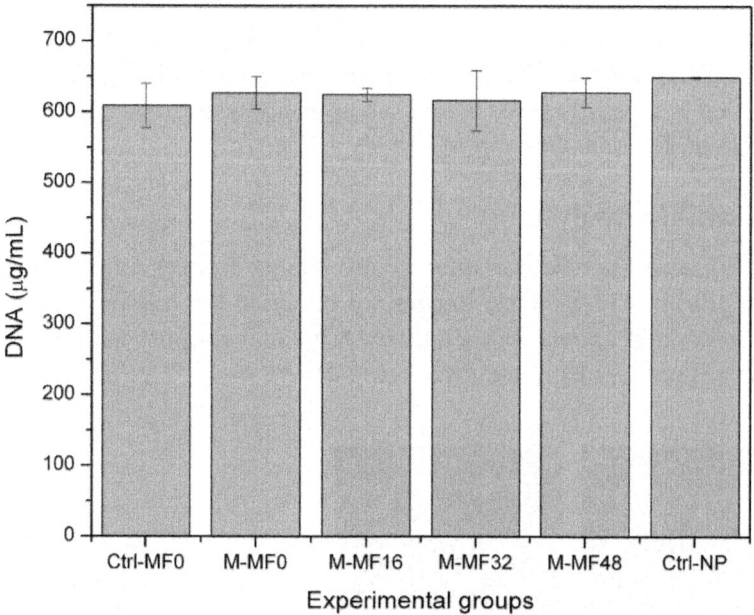

Figure 3. Quantification of DNA release. Integrity of the nuclear membrane was studied by quantifying the DNA released in the culture medium. The graph shows the mean values ± standard deviations of 8 independent experiments for each experimental group. Ctrl-MF0: control (nonmagnetic) tissue substitute without particles, gelled in the absence of a magnetic field; Ctrl-NP: control (nonmagnetic) tissue substitute with nonmagnetic polymer particles; M-MF0: magnetic tissue substitute gelled in the absence of a magnetic field; M-MF16, M-MF32 and M-MF48: magnetic tissue substitutes gelled during application of a 16 kA m^{-1}, 32 kA m^{-1} or 48 kA m^{-1} field, respectively.

According to results in Figs 2 and 3, cell viability was high in both magnetic and the nonmagnetic control tissue substitutes. We interpret this to mean that magnetic and nonmagnetic nanoparticles did not alter cell viability, and that magnetic tissue substitutes are likely to be safe for use in vivo, in agreement with previous results [12,13].

Magnetic Properties

The magnetization curve of MagP-OH particles (not shown) displayed typical soft ferromagnetic features, with a saturation magnetization of 161 ± 7 kA/m, obtained by fitting the experimental data to the Fröhlich–Kennely law [36]. Similarly, magnetic tissue substitutes showed soft ferromagnetic features, although with much lower saturation magnetization values (Fig 4).

Differences in the saturation magnetization values between different magnetic tissue substitutes were most likely due mainly to their different MagP-OH particle content. In fact, the concentration of MagP-OH particles in the tissue substitutes can be estimated by comparing their saturation magnetization (obtained by fitting the experimental data to the Fröhlich–Kennely law) to the saturation magnetization of MagP-OH powder, on the basis of the mixing law [37]. From the best fits to the mixing law, we obtained the following values for MagP-OH particle volume concentration (ϕ), M-MF0: 2.9 ± 0.3 vol%; M-MF16: 2.5 ± 0.3 vol%; M-MF32: 1.66 ± 0.16 vol%; M-MF48: 2.22 ± 0.22 vol%. Note that as expected, nonmagnetic control tissue substitutes did not show any ferromagnetic behavior.

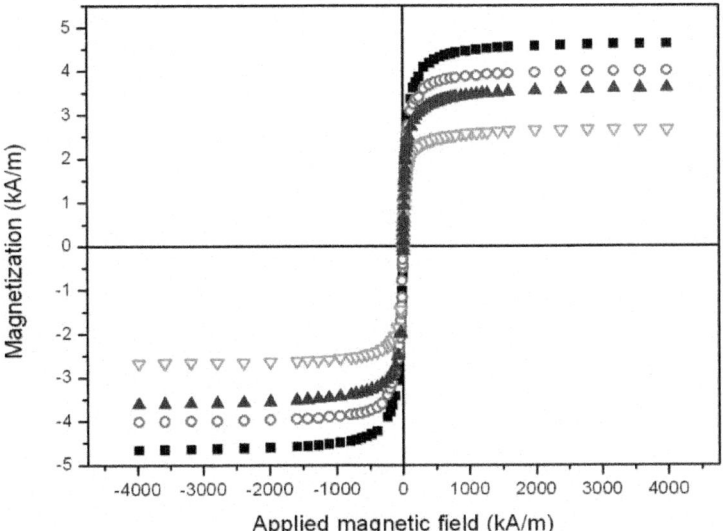

Figure 4. Magnetization curves of magnetic tissue substitutes. Filled squares: tissue substitute gelled in the absence of a magnetic field (M-MF0); open circles: tissue substitute gelled during application of a 16 kA m^{-1} field (M-MF16); open triangles: tissue substitute gelled during application of a 32 kA m^{-1} field (M-MF32); filled triangles: tissue substitute gelled during application of a 48 kA m^{-1}field (M-MF48). Values for saturation magnetization (kA/m) were obtained according to the Fröhlich–Kennely law [36]: M-MF0: 4.7 ± 0.3; M-MF16: 4.04 ± 0.24; M-MF32: 2.67 ± 0.15; M-MF48: 3.57 ± 0.20.

Mechanical Properties

In the absence of a magnetic field, we observed much higher values for elastic modulus G′ (up to 4 times as high) and shear stress (up to 5 times as high for a given value of shear strain) in the oral mucosa tissue substitutes that contained either magnetic or nonmagnetic particles compared to tissue substitutes without particles (Fig 5).

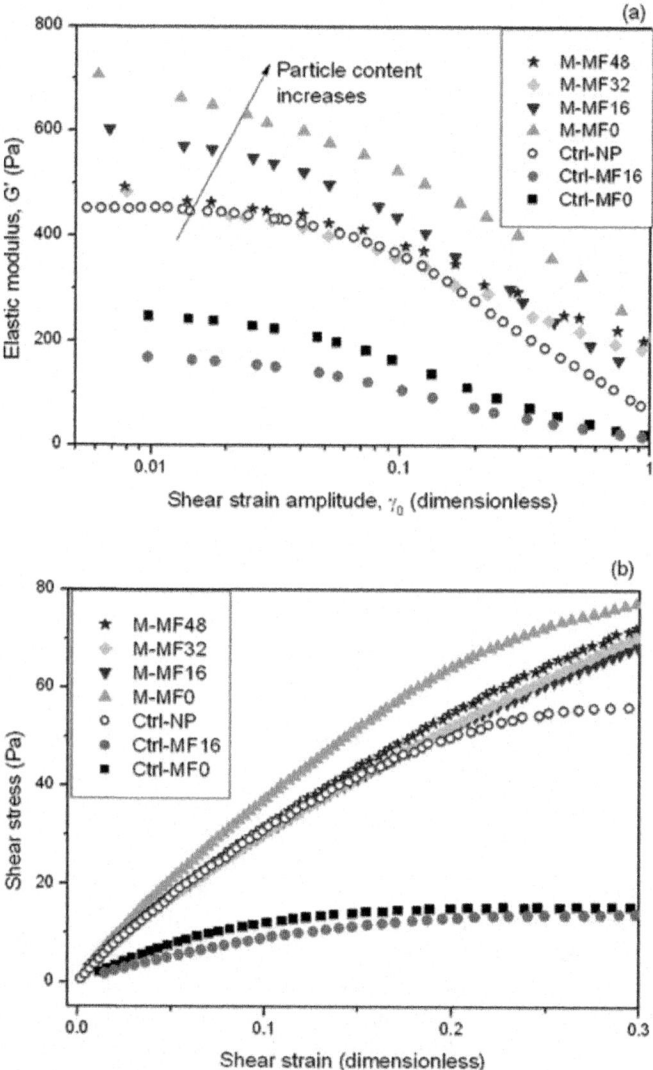

Figure 5. Mechanical properties of tissue substitutes in the absence of a magnetic field. (a) Elastic modulus as a function of the amplitude of shear strain in oscillatory tests at an oscillation frequency of 1 Hz. (b) Shear stress as a function of shear strain obtained under steady-state conditions. Experimental groups: Ctrl-MF0 and Ctrl-MF16: control (nonmagnetic) tissue substitute without particles, gelled in the absence of a magnetic field or during application of a 16 kA m⁻¹ field, respectively; Ctrl-NP: control (nonmagnetic) tissue substitute with nonmagnetic polymer particles; M-MF0: magnetic

tissue substitute gelled in the absence of a magnetic field; M-MF16, M-MF32 and M-MF48: magnetic tissue substitutes gelled during application of a 16 kA m^{-1}, 32 kA m^{-1} or 48 kA m^{-1} field, respectively.

The differences between the values for nonmagnetic control tissue substitutes without particles were small. On the other hand, tissue substitutes containing particles differed in G′ by as much as 40%, whereas shear stress was approximately similar in all samples with the exception of magnetic samples gelled in the absence of an applied field (M-MF0), and nonmagnetic control samples containing polymer particles (Ctrl-NP) at the highest strain values. Regarding the correlation between G′ and shear strain amplitude, we found that in all cases G′ showed an initial pseudoplateau at low amplitude, followed by a decrease at medium and high amplitudes. The initial pseudoplateau determines the so-called viscoelastic linear region (VLR) and the rest of the curve is referred to as the nonlinear viscoelastic region. Usually, the value of G′ pertaining to the VLR is considered an indicator of the strength of the material: the higher the G′, the stronger the material. With respect to the shape of the curves of shear stress vs. shear strain, we observed an initial linear portion at low strain values, where stress was proportional to strain. The proportionality constant is known as the shear modulus, G. At higher values of shear strain linearity was lost, and stress increased more slowly. Apart from the higher values of G for samples containing either magnetic or nonmagnetic particles compared to nonmagnetic control samples without particles (up to 3 times as high), we note that linearity was maintained up to much higher strain values in the former samples, especially magnetic tissue substitutes gelled during field application, compared to the nonmagnetic samples (Fig 5B). Note that G is also usually considered a measure of the strength of a material.

With respect to the differences in G′ among different magnetic samples, to analyze the effect of the concentration of magnetic particles on this value, we calculated the increase in G′ with respect to the average value in control tissue substitutes without particles (G′control) and normalized these values to the volume fraction of magnetic particles, ϕMagP–OH, and G′control:

$$\frac{G' - G'_{control}}{\phi_{MagP-OH} \cdot G'_{control}} \cdot$$

$$(1)$$

The normalized G′ values approximately overlapped in a single master curve, as shown in Fig 6.

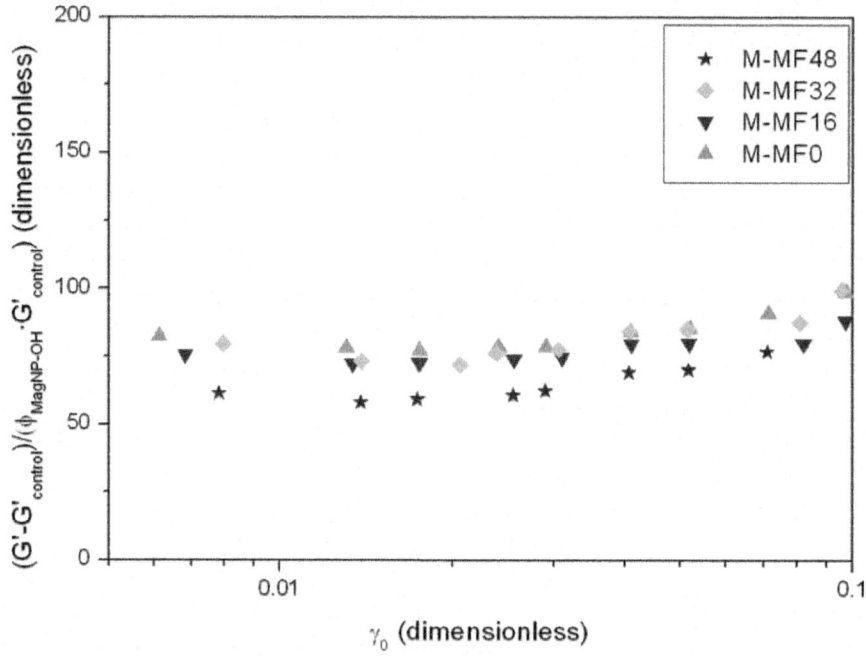

Figure 6. Normalized elastic modulus of magnetic tissue substitutes plotted as a function of shear strain amplitude. The elastic modulus, G′, of different magnetic tissue substitutes was normalized to account for the increase with respect to the elastic modulus of control (nonmagnetic) tissue substitutes without particles (Ctrl-MF0 to Ctrl-MF48), $G'_{control}$, per unit volume concentration of magnetic particles, $_{MagP-OH}$. Experimental groups: M-MF0: magnetic tissue substitute gelled in the absence of a magnetic field; M-MF16, M-MF32 and M-MF48: magnetic tissue substitutes gelled during application of a 16 kA m⁻¹, 32 kA m⁻¹ or 48 kA m⁻¹ field, respectively.

From the initial linear portion of the curves in Fig 5B we obtained the shear modulus (G) of the samples as the slope of the curves. As per our procedure for elastic modulus, we analyzed the effect of magnetic nanoparticles by defining a normalized shear modulus:

$$\frac{G - G_{control}}{\phi_{MagP-OH} \cdot G_{control}} \cdot$$

(2)

Normalized shear modulus data are shown in Table 2. Although normalized shear modulus values differed among samples, they overlapped when experimental error was taken into account.

Table 2. Normalized shear modulus (Eq 2) of different magnetic tissue substitutes. $G_{control} = 101 \pm 10$ Pa represents the mean value for control samples without particles (Ctrl-MF0 to Ctrl-MF48). Uncertainties were estimated according to theory of error propagation.

Sample name[a]	M-MF0	M-MF16	M-MF32	M-MF48
Normalized shear modulus: (dimensionless)	81 ± 21	49 ± 16	74 ± 22	58 ± 17

[a] Experimental groups: M-MF0: magnetic tissue substitute gelled in the absence of a magnetic field; M-MF16, M-MF32 and M-MF48: magnetic tissue substitutes gelled during application of a 16 kA m^{-1}, 32 kA m^{-1} or 48 kA m^{-1} field, respectively.

doi:10.1371/journal.pone.0133878.t002

The results in Fig 6 and Table 2 indicate that the higher G' and G in magnetic tissue substitutes than control samples without particles (Ctrl-MF0 to Ctrl-MF48) were approximately proportional to the volume concentration of magnetic particles. This result is consistent with the predictions of the classical theory of mechanics of composite materials for a continuous matrix with spherical inclusions [38]. Note that the higher G' and G in control samples with nonmagnetic polymer particles (Ctrl-NP) compared to control samples without particles (Ctrl-MF0 to Ctrl-MF48) are assumed to be governed by the same theory. In particular, in the special case where the spherical inclusions are completely rigid and under dilute conditions, and the matrix material is incompressible, the classical theory of mechanics of composite materials predicts [38]:

$$G = (1 + 2.5\phi)G_c \Rightarrow \frac{G - G_c}{\phi G_c} = 2.5$$

(3)

where G_c is the shear modulus of the continuous matrix. The quotient in Eq (3) has the same structure as the normalized shear modulus defined by Eq (2), where $G_{control}$ is replaced by G_c. The value of 2.5 in Eq (3) can thus be interpreted as the theoretical value predicted by the classical theory of mechanics of composite materials for the normalized shear modulus. It is therefore informative to compare this theoretical value of 2.5 against the experimental normalized shear modulus (Table 2). As observed, the normalized shear modulus of magnetic tissue substitutes was much higher than 2.5, which can be taken as evidence of the much stronger structure of the continuous matrix of magnetic tissue substitutes compared to control tissue substitutes without particles. In fact, Eq (3) can be used to calculate the shear modulus of the continuous matrix of magnetic tissue substitutes (Table 3).

Table 3. Shear modulus of the continuous matrix of magnetic tissue substitutes, as calculated with Eq (3). Note the mean value of the shear modulus in control samples without particles (Ctrl-MF0 to Ctrl-MF48), $G_{control} = 101 \pm 10$ Pa. Uncertainties were estimated according to the theory of error propagation.

Sample name[a]	M-MF0	M-MF16	M-MF32	M-MF48
Shear modulus of continuous matrix (Pa)	315 ± 4	211 ± 3	217 ± 3	218 ± 3

[a] Experimental groups: M-MF0: magnetic tissue substitute gelled in the absence of a magnetic field; M-MF16, M-MF32 and M-MF48: magnetic tissue substitutes gelled during application of a 16 kA m^{-1}, 32 kA m^{-1} or 48 kA m^{-1} field, respectively.

doi:10.1371/journal.pone.0133878.t003

As shown in Table 3, there was a twofold increase in the shear modulus of the continuous matrix in magnetic tissue substitutes gelled during exposure to a magnetic field, compared to control tissue substitutes without particles. In magnetic tissue substitutes gelled without a magnetic field, the shear modulus of the continuous matrix was even higher, with a threefold increase compared to control tissue substitutes. These enhancements in the mechanical properties of the continuous matrix when magnetic particles were included in the formulation of the engineered tissue substitutes may be due to the changes in the microscopic pattern of the fibrin network induced by the magnetic particles. The same argument would apply for the enhanced mechanical properties of control tissue substitutes containing nonmagnetic polymer particles (Ctrl-NP) compared to control tissue substitutes without particles (Ctrl-MF0 to Ctrl-MF48). These microstructural changes were evident in samples that were gelled during exposure to a magnetic field (M-MF16, M-M32, M-MF48), with thick stripes containing closely packed fibrin fibers aligned in the same direction, as discussed above. Changes in the microscopic pattern of the continuous matrix were not so intense in magnetic tissue substitutes gelled without application of a magnetic field (M-MF0) or in control tissue substitutes containing nonmagnetic polymer particles (Ctrl-NP); in both cases the likely reason for the enhanced mechanical properties is bonding and amalgamation of the fibers to the homogeneously distributed nanoparticles.

With regard to the influence of magnetic field intensity during the rheological measurements, we observed–as expected–no effect in nonmagnetic control tissue substitutes. In M-MF0 tissue substitutes, there was little difference in the values of G′ (not shown). For these samples the effect on shear stress (results not shown) was larger, with a clear tendency of shear stress to increase with strength of the field applied. For M-MF16, M-MF32 and M-MF48 tissue substitutes, the magnetic field applied during rheological measurements had a notable effect on both G′ and shear stress values, as illustrated in Fig 7. We note that as described in the Material and Methods section, each point in this figure is the average of at least 9 measurements, including at least 3 successive cycles of increasing the magnetic field from 0 kA/m to 26 kA/m and then decreasing it again to 0 kA/m. Since we found no statistically significant differences among values for the same sample and field strength, we infer that the changes in mechanical properties after application of a magnetic field are reversible.

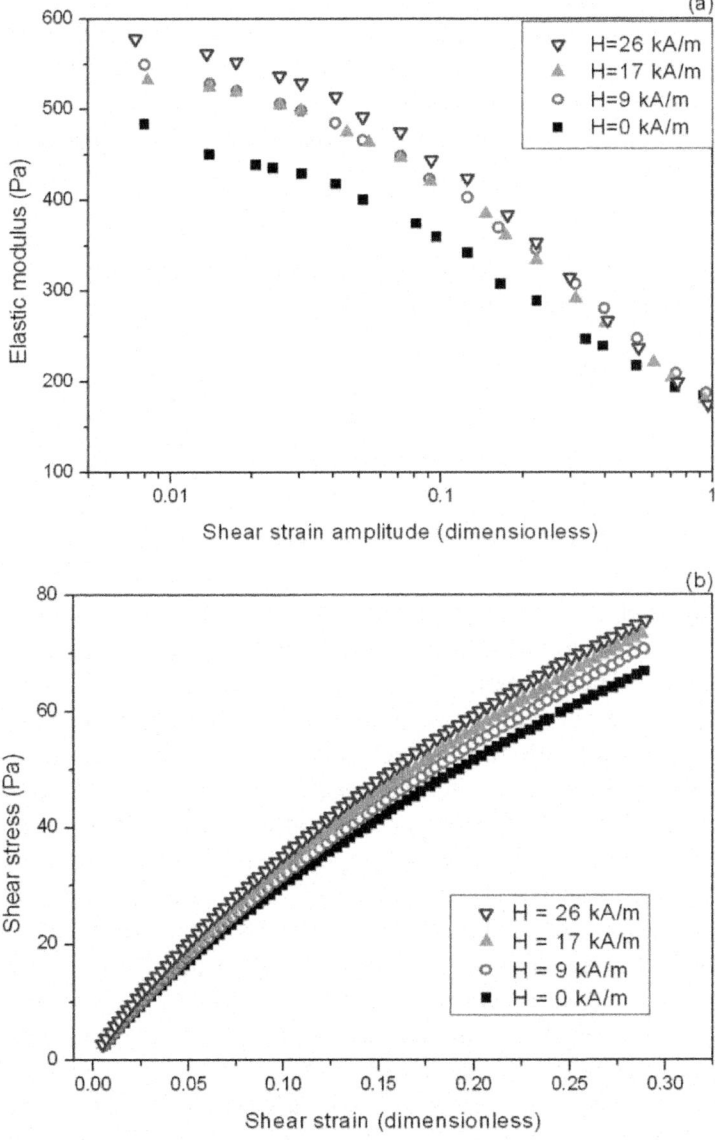

Figure7. Effect of a magnetic field on the mechanical properties of magnetic tissue substitutes. Sample M-MF32 is a magnetic tissue substitute gelled during application of a 32 kA m⁻¹ field. The effect of a magnetic field applied during measurement on the mechanical properties of the tissue substitute is shown as (a) the elastic modulus as a function of shear strain amplitude, and (b) the initial portion of the shear stress vs. shear strain curves. The intensities (H) of the magnetic field applied are shown.

As observed, the shape of the G′-vs.-amplitude curves remained similar as the intensity of the magnetic field increased, despite the fact that G′ increased in average terms together with the strength of the magnetic field. The same was true for the shear stress-vs.-shear strain curves. From the linear portion of these curves we obtained the values of shear modulus, and observed a clear tendency for G to increase with the strength of the magnetic field applied in all magnetic tissue substitutes (Table 4).

Table 4. Effect of the magnetic field applied during measurement on the shear modulus (Pa) of magnetic tissue substitutes. Data in this table correspond to the best linear fit including experimental uncertainties.

Magnetic field strength (kA/m)	Sample M-F0 [a]	Sample M-MF16 [a]	Sample M-MF32 [a]	Sample M-MF48 [a]
0	338 ± 3	224 ± 3	225.8 ± 2.2	230 ± 3
9	363 ± 3	237 ± 3	243.6 ± 2.1	237 ± 3
17	369 ± 4	246 ± 3	239.6 ± 1.9	252 ± 3
26	370 ± 4	253 ± 3	245.0 ± 1.9	254 ± 3

[a] Experimental groups: M-MF0: magnetic tissue substitute gelled in the absence of a magnetic field; M-MF16, M-MF32 and M-MF48: magnetic tissue substitutes gelled during application of a 16 kA m^{-1}, 32 kA m^{-1} or 48 kA m^{-1} field, respectively.

doi:10.1371/journal.pone.0133878.t004

We note that the increases in characteristic mechanical parameters (shear modulus, elastic modulus, Young modulus, etc.) in samples exposed to increasingly strong magnetic fields is typical of dispersions of multi-domain magnetic particles in a polymer matrix [30]. This phenomenon is known as the magnetorheological (MR) effect, and we refer to these systems as MR gels and MR elastomers. In fact, the magnitude of the increases we observed in shear modulus and elastic modulus with increasingly intense magnetic fields in magnetic tissue substitutes agrees well with previous research on MR elastomers. For example, Jolly et al. [39] found a maximum increase in shear modulus of 30% upon application of a magnetic field in an MR elastomer consisting of 10 vol% iron particles dispersed in a silicone-based polymer matrix. More recently, Ge et al. [40] reported a 43% increase in an MR elastomer consisting of approximately 7 vol% iron particles dispersed in natural rubber. The enhancements reported here were weaker most probably because of the lower concentration of magnetic particles in the polymer matrix and the weaker magnetic properties of magnetite (the main constituent of MagP-OH nanoparticles) compared to iron. Note, for example, that shear modulus increased by 10% in our magnetic tissue substitutes exposed to a 26 kA/m field compared to no exposure to a magnetic field during measurement, and elastic modulus showed a slightly large increase.

Finally, it is worth noting that both the magnetic and nonmagnetic tissue substitutes reported here had values of G and G′ on the same order of magnitude as those obtained in previous studies of fibrin–agarose scaffolds and oral mucosa tissue substitutes [31,33,41]. Moreover, G and G' values were within the range of values reported for native human soft tissues (G ≈ 5–2500 Pa, G' ≈ 10–5000 Pa) [31].

CONCLUSIONS

We report a straightforward, versatile method for the preparation of a new type of tissue-engineered biomaterial characterized by the inclusion of multi-domain magnetic particles in a biopolymer matrix. Cell viability analyses of oral mucosa fibroblasts showed no significant differences in comparison to control (nonmagnetic) tissue substitutes of proven applicability in tissue regeneration. Thanks to their magnetic behavior, these novel tissue substitutes could be visualized and followed for in vivo applications by magnetic resonance imaging, and also act as magnets, attracting functionalized magnetic nanoparticles injected close to them. Although these advantages are also shared by other magnetic scaffolds described previously, a unique feature of our magnetic tissue substitutes is that their mechanical properties can be tuned in a controlled, reversible manner by noncontact magnetic force fields. Furthermore, we found that in the off state (absence of an applied field) the strength of our engineered magnetic tissue substitutes is also affected by the concentration of particles and other technical details, such as the application of a magnetic field during gelation. This versatility could be exploited in clinical applications to match the mechanical properties of tissue substitutes to those of natural target tissues. Several other potential advantages can be envisaged for our magnetic tissue substitutes, such as their adhesion by magnetic attraction in tissue replacements, which would reduce the need for surgical sutures in (for example) treatments for gingival recession. To conclude, we foresee that other similar field-responsive biological tissue substitutes will be generated in the near future, as applied research contributes to the development of a broad range of promising novel applications for smart magnetic biomaterials.

ACKNOWLEDGMENTS

We thank Nanomyp (Granada, Spain) for supplying the particles used in this work, and K. Shashok for improving the use of English in the manuscript.

AUTHOR CONTRIBUTIONS

Conceived and designed the experiments: MTLL JDGD AC MA IAR. Performed the experiments: MTLL GS ACO IAR. Analyzed the data: MTLL GS MA IAR. Contributed reagents/materials/analysis tools: MTLL JDGD AC MA. Wrote the paper: MTLL GS ACO IAR.

REFERENCES

1. Baddour JA, Sousounis K, Tsonis PA. Organ repair and regeneration: an overview. Birth Defects Res Part C-Embryo Today-Rev. 2012; 96: 1–29. doi: 10.1002/bdrc.21006

2. Van Vlierberghe S, Dubruel P, Schacht E. Biopolymer-based hydrogels as scaffolds for tissue engineering applications: a review. Biomacromolecules. 2011; 12: 1387–1408. doi: 10.1021/bm200083n. pmid:21388145

3. Dhandayuthapani B, Yoshida Y, Maekawa T, Kumar DS. Polymeric Scaffolds in Tissue Engineering Application: A Review. Int J Polym Sci. 2011; 2011: 290602. doi: 10.1155/2011/290602

4. Gunatillake PA, Adhikari R. Biodegradable synthetic polymers for tissue engineering. Eur Cells Mater. 2003; 5: 1–16.

5. Ochi M, Uchio Y, Tobita M, Kuriwaka M. Current concepts in tissue engineering technique for repair of cartilage defect. Artif Organs. 2001; 25: 172–179. pmid:11284883 doi: 10.1046/j.1525-1594.2001.025003172.x

6. Pabbruwe MB, Esfandiari E, Kafienah W, Tarlton JF, Hollander AP. Induction of cartilage integration by a chondrocyte/collagen-scaffold implant. Biomaterials. 2009; 30: 4277–4286. doi: 10.1016/j. biomaterials.2009.02.052. pmid:19539365

7. Ng KW, Wang CCB, Mauck RL, Kelly TAN, Chahine NO, Costa KD, et al. A layered agarose approach to fabricate depth-dependent inhomogeneity in chondrocyte-seeded constructs. J Orthop Res. 2005; 23: 134–141. pmid:15607885 doi: 10.1016/j.orthres.2004.05.015

8. Lee SH, Shin H. Matrices and scaffolds for delivery of bioactive molecules in bone and cartilage tissue engineering. Adv Drug Deliv Rev. 2007; 59: 339–359. pmid:17499384 doi: 10.1016/j.addr.2007.03.016

9. Capito RM, Spector M. Scaffold-based articular cartilage repair. IEEE Eng Med Biol Mag. 2003; 22: 42–50. pmid:14699935 doi: 10.1109/ memb.2003.1256271

10. Getgood A, Brooks R, Fortier L, Rushton N. Articular cartilage tissue engineering: today's research, tomorrow's practice? J Bone Joint Surg Br. 2009; 91: 565–576. doi: 10.1302/0301-620X.91B5.21832. pmid:19407287

11. Kon E, Delcogliano M, Filardo G, Pressato D, Busacca M, Grigolo B, et al. A novel nano-composite multi-layered biomaterial for treatment of osteochondral lesions: technique note and an early stability pilot clinical trial. Injury-Int J Care Inj. 2010; 41: 693–701. doi: 10.1016/j.

injury.2009.11.014

12. Bañobre-López M, Piñeiro-Redondo Y, De Santis R, Gloria A, Ambrosio L, Tampieri A, et al. Poly(caprolactone) based magnetic scaffolds for bone tissue engineering. J Appl Phys. 2011, 109, 07B313. doi: 10.1063/1.3561149

13. Bock N, Riminucci A, Dionigi C, Russo A, Tampieri A, Landi E, et al. A novel route in bone tissue engineering: magnetic biomimetic scaffolds. Acta Biomater. 2010; 6: 786–796. doi: 10.1016/j.actbio.2009.09.017. pmid:19788946

14. Das B, Mandal M, Upadhyay A, Chattopadhyay P, Karak N. Bio-based hyperbranched polyurethane/Fe3O4 nanocomposites: smart antibacterial biomaterials for biomedical devices and implants. Biomed Mater. 2013; 8: 035003. doi: 10.1088/1748-6041/8/3/035003. pmid:23532037

15. De Santis R, Gloria A, Russo T, D'Amora U, Zeppetelli S, Dionigi C, et al. A basic approach toward the development of nanocomposite magnetic scaffolds for advanced bone tissue engineering. J Appl Polym Sci. 2011; 122: 3599–3605. doi: 10.1002/app.34771

16. Gloria A, Russo R, D'Amora U, Zeppetelli S, D'Alessandro T, Sandri M, et al. Magnetic poly(epsilon-caprolactone)/iron-doped hydroxyapatite nanocomposite substrates for advanced bone tissue engineering. J R Soc Interface. 2013; 10: 20120833. doi: 10.1098/rsif.2012.0833. pmid:23303218

17. Hu SH, Liu TY, Tsai CH, Chen SY. Preparation and characterization of magnetic ferroscaffolds for tissue engineering. J Magn Magn Mater. 2007; 310: 2871–2873. doi: 10.1016/j.jmmm.2006.11.081

18. Hu H, Jiang W, Lan F, Zeng X, Ma S, Wu Y, et al. Synergic effect of magnetic nanoparticles on the electrospun aligned superparamagnetic nanofibers as a potential tissue engineering scaffold. RSC Adv. 2013; 3: 879–886. doi: 10.1039/c2ra22726f

19. Lai K, Jiang W, Tang JZ, Wu Y, He B, Wang G, et al. Preparation and characterization of magnetic ferroscaffolds for tissue engineering. RSC Adv. 2012; 2: 13007–13017.

20. Li Y, Huang G, Zhang X, Li B, Chen Y, Lu T, et al. Magnetic Hydrogels and Their Potential Biomedical Applications. Adv Funct Mater. 2013; 23: 660–672. doi: 10.1002/adfm.201201708

21. Panseri S, Cunha C, D'Alessandro T, Sandri M, Giavaresi G, Marcacci M, et al. Intrinsically superparamagnetic Fe-hydroxyapatite nanoparticles positively influence osteoblast-like cell behaviour. J Nanobiotechnology. 2012; 10: 32. pmid:22828388 doi: 10.1186/1477-3155-10-32

22. Skaat H, Ziv-Polat O, Shahar A, Last D, Mardor Y, Margel S. Magnetic Scaffolds Enriched with Bioactive Nanoparticles for Tissue Engineering. Adv Healthc Mater. 2012; 1: 168–171. doi: 10.1002/adhm.201100056. pmid:23184719

23. Tampieri A, Landi E, Valentini F, Sandri M, D'Alessandro T, Dediu V, et al. A conceptually new type of bio-hybrid scaffold for bone regeneration. Nanotechnology. 2011; 22: 015104. doi: 10.1088/0957-4484/22/1/015104. pmid:21135464

24. Tampieri A, D'Alessandro T, Sandri M, Sprio S, Landi E, Bertinetti L, et al. Intrinsic magnetism and hyperthermia in bioactive Fe-doped hydroxyapatite. Acta Biomater. 2012; 8: 843–851. doi: 10.1016/j.actbio.2011.09.032. pmid:22005331

25. Zeng XB, Hu H, Xie LQ, Lan F, Jiang W, Wu Y, et al. Magnetic responsive hydroxyapatite composite scaffolds construction for bone defect reparation. Int J Nanomed. 2012; 7: 3365–3378. doi: 10.2147/ijn.s32264

26. Zeng XB, Hu H, Xie LQ, Lan F, Wu Y, Gu ZW. Magnetic responsive hydroxyapatite composite scaffolds construction for bone defect reparation. J Inorg Mater. 2013; 28: 79–84. doi: 10.2147/ijn.s32264

27. Zhu Y, Shang F, Li B, Dong Y, Liu Y, Lohe MR, et al. Magnetic mesoporous bioactive glass scaffolds: preparation, physicochemistry and biological properties. J Mater Chem B. 2013; 1: 1279–1288. doi: 10.1039/c2tb00262k

28. Ziv-Polat O, Skaat H, Shahar A, Margel S. Novel magnetic fibrin hydrogel scaffolds containing thrombin and growth factors conjugated iron oxide nanoparticles for tissue engineering. Int J Nanomed. 2012; 7: 1259–1274. doi: 10.2147/ijn.s26533

29. Singh RK, Patel KD, Lee JH, Lee EJ, Kim JH, Kim TH, et al. Potential of magnetic nanofiber scaffolds with mechanical and biological properties applicable for bone regeneration. PLOS ONE. 2014; 9: e91584. doi: 10.1371/journal.pone.0091584. pmid:24705279

30. Bossis G, Volkova O, Lacis S, Meunier A. Magnetorheology: Fluids, Structures and Rheology. Lect Notes Phys. 2002; 594: 201–230. doi: 10.1007/3-540-45646-5_11

31. Scionti G, Moral M, Toledano M, Osorio R, Duran JDG, Alaminos M, et al. Effect of the hydration on the biomechanical properties in fibrin-agarose tissue-like model. J Biomed Mater Res Part A. 2014; 102: 2573–2582. doi: 10.1002/jbm.a.34929

32. Alaminos M, Sanchez-Quevedo MC, Munoz-Avila JI, Serrano D, Medialdea S, Carreras I, et al. Construction of a complete rabbit cornea substitute using a fibrin-agarose scaffold. Invest Ophthalmol Vis Sci. 2006; 47: 3311–3317. pmid:16877396 doi: 10.1167/iovs.05-1647

33. Rodriguez IA, Lopez-Lopez MT, Oliveira AC, Sanchez-Quevedo MC, Campos A, Alaminos M, et al. Rheological characterization of human fibrin and fibrin-agarose oral mucosa substitutes generated by tissue engineering. J Tissue Eng Regen Med. 2012; 6: 636–644. doi: 10.1002/term.466. pmid:21916018

34. Viñuela-Prieto JM, Sánchez-Quevedo MC, Alfonso-Rodríguez CA, Oliveira AC, Scionti G, Martín-Piedra MA, et al. Sequential keratinocytic differentiation and maturation in a three-dimensional model of human artificial oral mucosa. J Periodontal Res. 2014; doi: 10.1111/jre.12247.

35. Thanikaivelan P, Narayanan NT, Pradhan BK, Ajayan PM. Collagen based magnetic nanocomposites for oil removal applications. Sci Rep. 2012; 2: 230. doi: 10.1038/srep00230. pmid:22355744

36. Jiles DC. Introduction to Magnetism and Magnetic Materials. 2nd ed. Boca Raton: Chapman & Hall/CRC, Taylor & Francis Group; 1998.

37. Rosensweig RE. Ferrohydrodynamics. Cambridge: Cambridge University Press; 1985.

38. Christensen RM. Mechanics of Composite Materials. Malabar: Krieger Publishing Company; 1991.

39. Jolly MR, Carlson JD, Muñoz BC, Bullions RA. The Magnetoviscoelastic Response of Elastomer Composites Consisting of Ferrous Particles Embedded in a Polymer Matrix. J Intell Mater Syst Struct. 1996; 7: 613–622. doi: 10.1177/1045389x9600700601

40. Ge L, Gong X, Fan Y, Xuan S. Preparation and mechanical properties of the magnetorheological elastomer based on natural rubber/rosin glycerin hybrid matrix. Smart Mater Struct. 2013; 22: 115029. doi: 10.1088/0964-1726/22/11/115029

41. Rodriguez MA, Lopez-Lopez MT, Duran JDG, Alaminos M, Campos A, Rodriguez IA. Cryopreservation of an artificial human oral mucosa stroma. A viability and rheological study. Cryobiology. 2013; 67: 355–362. doi: 10.1016/j.cryobiol.2013.10.003. pmid:24177233

Chapter 6

DIP TIPS AS A FACILE AND VERSATILE METHOD FOR FABRICATION OF POLYMER FOAMS WITH CONTROLLED SHAPE, SIZE AND PORE ARCHITECTURE FOR BIOENGINEERING APPLICATIONS

Naresh Kasoju[1], Dana Kubies[1], Marta M. Kumorek[1], Jan Kříž[2], Eva Fábryová[2], Luďka Machová[1], Jana Kovářová[3], and František Rypáček[1]

[1]Department of Biomaterials and Bioanalogous Polymer Systems, Institute of Macromolecular Chemistry, Academy of Sciences of the Czech Republic, v.v.i., Prague, Czech Republic

[2]Laboratory of Islets of Langerhans, Institute for Clinical and Experimental Medicine, Prague, Czech Republic

[3]Department of Polymer Processing, Institute of Macromolecular Chemistry, Academy of Sciences of the Czech Republic, v.v.i., Prague, Czech Republic

ABSTRACT

The porous polymer foams act as a template for neotissuegenesis in tissue engineering, and, as a reservoir for cell transplants such as pancreatic islets while simultaneously providing a functional interface with the host body. The fabrication of foams with the controlled shape, size and pore structure is of prime importance in various bioengineering applications. To this end, here we demonstrate a thermally induced phase separation (TIPS) based facile process for the fabrication of polymer foams with a controlled architecture. The setup comprises of a metallic template bar (T), a metallic conducting block (C) and a non-metallic reservoir tube (R), connected in sequence T-C-R. The process hereinafter termed as Dip TIPS, involves the dipping of the T-bar into a polymer solution, followed by filling of the R-tube with a freezing mixture to induce the phase separation of a polymer solution in the immediate vicinity of T-bar; Subsequent free-drying or freeze-extraction steps produced the polymer foams. An easy exchange of the T-bar of a spherical or rectangular shape allowed the fabrication of tubular, open- capsular and flat-sheet shaped foams. A mere change in the quenching time produced the foams with a thickness ranging from hundreds of microns to several millimeters.

And, the pore size was conveniently controlled by varying either the polymer concentration or the quenching temperature. Subsequent *in vivo* studies in brown Norway rats for 4-weeks demonstrated the guided cell infiltration and homogenous cell distribution through the polymer matrix, without any fibrous capsule and necrotic core. In conclusion, the results show the "Dip TIPS" as a facile and adaptable process for the fabrication of anisotropic channeled porous polymer foams of various shapes and sizes for potential applications in tissue engineering, cell transplantation and other related fields.

INTRODUCTION

Porous polymer foams are extensively used in various fields of science and technological applications including, but not limited to mechanical, thermal, acoustic and electrical insulations, chemical catalysis, filtration processes and medical devices [1]. In particular, a significant academic and commercial interest has been rising in recent years over the use of polymer foams as scaffolds, along with cells and biological factors, to develop biological substitutes that restore, replace or regenerate defective tissues [2]. For consideration in such bioengineering applications, the scaffolds should (a) be biocompatible, (b) be bioresorbable to provide void volume for neotissuegenesis and remodeling, (c) have an appropriate pore structure for efficient nutrient and metabolite exchange, and (e) provide adequate mechanical or structural stability [2], [3]. Polymers such as degradable polyesters (e.g. polylactide, polyglycolide), silk fibroin, either alone or as composites, and either with or without a functionalization, has been described as biocompatible and bioresorbable materials [4], [5], [6]. However, different tissues/organs in the body have a distinctive architecture in their native states, and thus a scaffold design suitable for all types of tissue engineering is impractical. Therefore, the fabrication of a scaffold with controlled shape, size and pore properties remain a thrust area of research in bioengineering [2].

The physical dimensions such as shape and size of the scaffold play a key role in engineering the desired tissue. For example, the reconstruction of vascular, neural or other tubular tissues requires a hollow tubular scaffold for acting as a physical template and guide neotissuegenesis [7], [8]. In such cases, the tubule thickness and inner lumen diameter should be designed to meet the requirements of the host tissue. The skin or other similar tissue reconstruction strategies demand flat sheet scaffolds [9], [10]. Here also, the thickness should be carefully controlled to avoid the development of any necrotic cores. In addition to regular tubular and flat sheet foams, capsular shaped polymer meshes have been recently reported for use as the matrices for pancreatic islet transplantation applications [11]. Besides, an important criterion that influences the efficiency of tissue reconstruction process is the pore architecture of the scaffold [3]. For instance, the scaffolds with regular isotropic pores often lead to the formation of a necrotic core owing to restriction on the cell penetration and nutrient exchange to the scaffold center caused by a rapid tissue formation on the outer edge of the scaffold [12]. While, the scaffolds with anisotropic pores inherently improve the cell infiltration and nutrient flow, both *in vitro* and *in vivo*, and thus do not lead to any necrotic core formation [12]–[13]. Recent studies also demonstrated that in contrast to the spherical porous scaffolds, the channeled porous scaffolds promote the guided cell infiltration and tissue ingrowth and thus yield enriched, homogenously distributed cell population with enhanced functionality [14]–[15].

Various technologies have been widely explored for the fabrication of foams with controlled architectures [3], [16]–[20]. Examples include, (a) solid free-form tools such as three-dimensional (3D) printing, stereo-lithography, laser sintering, (b) porogen involving processes such as gas foaming, phase separation, particulate leaching, and (c) fiber-based techniques such as electrospinning or fiber bonding [3], [16]–[20]. Amongst all, the phase separation process, particularly the thermally induced phase separation (TIPS), was efficient in the preparation of interconnected porous foams [21]. Additionally, by applying a unidirectional thermal gradient, it was possible to obtain the anisotropic channeled porous scaffold [21], [22]. The standard TIPS setups were used to prepare regular 3D foams with channeled pores, but without the limitation on the final shape and size [22]. The scaffolds in the form of hollow fibers or tubes (e.g. for reconstruction of vascular vessels or other tubular tissues) have also been fabricated [23], [24]. However, the developed methods were based on complex setups involving (i) several thermal conducting and insulating components, (ii) multiple systems to obtain differently shaped foams, and (iii) multiple adjustments to vary the foam thickness. The pores were usually axially oriented to the tube lumen and the outer surface of the foams often exhibited less-/non- porous skin that restricted the cell infiltration [22]–[26].

Here we demonstrate a TIPS-based efficient, facile and adaptable methodology, hereby termed as Dip TIPS, to obtain the polymer foams with a controlled shape, size and pore design. We tested the versatility of the method to yield the foams with (a) variable shapes such as tubes, open-end capsules and flat 3D sheets, (b) variable inner lumen diameters in the case of tubes and capsules, (c) variable thickness, ranging from hundreds of microns to several millimeters and with (d) controlled anisotropic interconnected channeled pores. The systematic investigations were performed to determine first the influence of polymer properties (such as polymer type, molecular weight, concentration), then process parameters (such as quenching temperature and time, coarsening duration) and finally mold properties (such as template diameter) on the final foam architecture. The feasibility of the scaffolds for use in bioengineering applications, such as guided tissue engineering, was tested by the *in vivo* implantation in the male brown Norway rats followed by the histochemical and immuno-histochemical analysis of the excised implants.

MATERIALS AND METHODS

Materials

We purchased L-lactide, ε-caprolactone, Tin(II) 2-ethylhexanoate, phosphate buffer saline (PBS) tablets from Sigma-Aldrich, Czech Republic, paraffin (histowax 56–58°C) from Bamed s.r.o., Czech Republic, hematoxylin and eosin from Roche s.r.o., Czech Republic, anti-CD31(cluster of differentiation 31, or also known as platelet endothelial cell adhesion molecule-1) antibody from Acris Antibody GmbH, Germany. All other reagents and chemicals were obtained from P-Lab a.s., Lach-Ner s.r.o. and Sigma-Aldrich Czech Republic, and were used as received.

Synthesis of Polymers

High molecular weight poly(L-lactide) (PLA), poly(ε-caprolactone) (PCL) and poly(L-lactide-*co*-ε-caprolactone) (PLCL) were synthesized by ring-opening polymerization or co-polymerization of the corresponding monomers (L-lactide, ε-caprolactone) in the presence of Tin(II) 2-ethylhexanoate as a catalyst in bulk as described previously [27], [28]. The molecular weight of the polymers was determined using a gel permeation chromatography (Waters Corporation) and the details are as follows: PLA: M_w=220 000 g/mol and M_n=98 000 g/mol; PCL: M_w=120 000 g/mol and M_n=80 000 g/mol; PLCL300: M_w=316 000 \g/mol and M_n=120 000 g/mol; PLCL150: M_w=162 000 g/mol and M_n=57 000 g/mol. The content of ε-caprolactone in both PLCL copolymers was found to be 7% mol as analyzed by the ^{1}H nuclear magnetic resonance analysis (DPX 300, Bruker).

Dip TIPS Setup

Figure 1 shows the experimental setup for the fabrication of polymer foams by dipping the template bar of a particular size and shape into a polymer solution followed by controlled cooling. The setup consists of (a) a thermally conductive metal template bar with variable macro-shapes and dimensions (hereby referred to as "*template*", dimensions: a cylindrical bar for tubular or capsular foams: 2, 3 or 4 × 40 mm diameter and height respectively; a planar bar for flat 3D foams: $3 \times 10 \times 40$ mm thickness, width and height respectively), (b) a thermally conductive metallic solid cylindrical block with pre-defined dimensions (hereby referred to as "*conductor*", 30×30 mm diameter and height respectively), along with (c) a thermally low/non-conductive non-metallic hollow tube used as a reservoir for the cooling mixture (hereby referred to as "*reservoir*", 30×120 mm diameter and height respectively). The *template* was attached at one end to the *conductor* block that was in turn bolted into the *reservoir* tube (*template* → *conductor* → *reservoir*). The whole setup was arranged properly onto a laboratory stand with the help of appropriate holders.

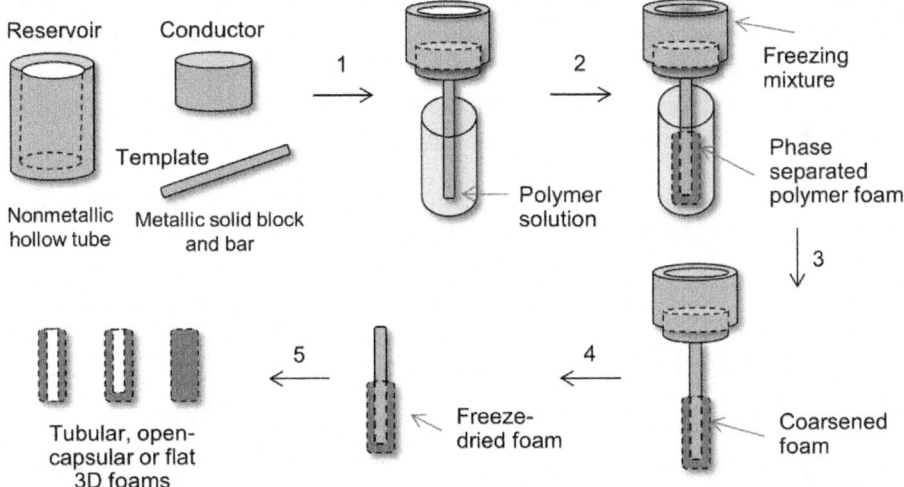

Figure 1. Dip TIPS scheme. An illustration of the essential components of the setup (*reservoir, conductor* and *template*) and the sequential steps involved in the Dip TIPS process (1: assembling, 2: quenching, 3: coarsening, 4: freeze-drying and 5: collection of the foam).

Dip TIPS Process

The fabrication process is schematically presented in Figure 1. The *template* and the *conductor* maintained in a water bath at 40°C were taken out and wiped with tissue paper and were then immediately assembled together along with the *reservoir*. First, the *template* was dipped into the polymer solution at ambient temperature. Then, the *reservoir* tube was filled with an appropriate cooling mixture to quench the polymer solution in the immediate vicinity of the *template*. After a preset quenching time, the *template* with the frozen polymer foam was removed from the polymer solution and was allowed to coarsen for a defined period. The coarsened foams were then freeze-dried under vacuum in the dry ice/ethanol bath for initial 1-2 days and then in ambient temperature for at least another 1 day. Alternatively, the coarsened foams were subjected to the freeze-extraction process by immersing into pre-cooled ethanol for 2–3 days with intermittent solvent exchange. The scaffolds were then collected from the *template* and kept in a desiccator until further use.

Ethanol with a controlled addition of dry ice, dry ice/ethanol and liquid nitrogen baths were used as the cooling mixtures to achieve the temperatures of −25, −80 and −196°C, respectively. The experimental conditions were tested in the order as they are listed in Table 1. After each experiment, the tested parameter leading to appropriate scaffold parameters was fixed for further test. First, the effect of the polymer type was tested and the polymer giving the optimal results was selected for the following experiment. Then, the effect of molecular weight was tested and the polymer with appropriate results was selected for the test of the polymer concentration. Having selected polymer parameters, we likewise performed the systematic experiments to optimize various Dip TIPS process conditions.

Table 1. Parameters under Dip TIPS study with the information about tested variables and other constant conditions followed* (n=6).

Variable parameter	Details	Constant experimental conditions
Polymer type	PLA, PCL, **PLCL**	Polymer concentration: 5% (w/v)
		Quenching temperature: −80°C
		Quenching time: 30 s
		Coarsening time: None
Polymer molecular weight	162000 g/mol (PLCL150)	Polymer concentration: 5% (w/v)
	316000 g/mol (**PLCL300**)	Quenching temperature: −80°C
		Quenching time: 30 s
		Coarsening time: None
Polymer concentration	3, **5**, 7, 10% (w/v)	Polymer type: PLCL300
		Quenching temperature: −80°C
		Quenching time: 30 s
		Coarsening time: None
Quenching temperature	−25, **−80**, −196°C	Polymer type: PLCL300
		Polymer concentration: 5% (w/v)
		Quenching time: 30 s
		Coarsening time: None
Quenching time	15, **30**, 45, 60 s	Polymer type: PLCL300
		Polymer concentration: 5% (w/v)
		Quenching temp: −80°C
		Coarsening time: None
Coarsening duration	**0**, 30, 60, 120 min	Polymer type: PLCL300
		Polymer concentration: 3% (w/v)
		Quenching temperature: −25°C
		Quenching time: 30 s
Mold diameter (for tubular and open-end capsular foams)	2, **3**, 4 mm	Polymer type: PLCL300
		Polymer concentration: 5% (w/v)
		Quenching temperature: −80°C
		Quenching time: 30 s
		Coarsening time: None

* First, the effect of the polymer type was tested and the polymer giving the optimal results was selected for the subsequent experiment. Next, the effect of molecular weight was tested and the polymer with best results was selected for the test of the polymer concentration. Having selected polymer parameters, we then progressively optimized the process conditions. The parameter fixed after each step is marked in bold font.
doi:10.1371/journal.pone.0108792.t001

Scaffold Characterization

Morphological properties.

The morphological features of the pores and the pore patterns were examined by a scanning electron microscope (SEM, Vega, Tescan; n=6). Typically, a foam was cut carefully with a fine razor to expose the outer and inner surfaces, and the cross and longitudinal sections. Prior to the analysis, all samples were coated with Platinum in a sputter coater (SCD050, Leica Microsystems) for 120 s at 40 mA current and pressure below 10^{-1} mBar. The diameter of the pores was determined from SEM images using *Image J*freeware. At least 25 random pores were measured from each image to calculate the average diameter.

Porosity and surface area analysis.

The PLCL300 foams prepared from a 5% w/v solution by quenching at -25, -80 and $-196°C$ for 30 seconds were analyzed to explore the typical pore properties and their relationship with the processing conditions (n=3). First, to determine the open-porous character, the foams were subjected to mercury intrusion porosimetry analysis (Pascal 140 and 440, Thermo Finigan, Rodano, Italy). A mercury tension of 480 mN/m and a contact angle of 141.3° were imposed for all measurements. The applied pressure of mercury was in the range of 0.01–400 MPa allowing the determination of meso- and macro- pores from 4 nm to 116 μm. The pore volume and the most frequent pore diameter were calculated from the cumulative pore volume curves by the Pascal program with the use of Washburn equation under the assumption of the cylindrical pore model [29]. The porosity was calculated according to the equation (1), where V is the cumulative pore volume (ml/g) and ρ is density of the used polymer.

$$Porosity(\%) = \frac{V \times 100}{V + \left(1/\rho\right)} \times 100 \tag{1}$$

The specific surface area of the foams was measured by a gas adsorption technique using nitrogen as the adsorbate and liquid nitrogen (77 K) as a cooling medium (Gemini VII 2390, Micromeritics Instruments Corp.). The surface area was calculated from the Brunauer-Emmett-Teller (BET) plot of the adsorption/desorption isotherm using the software supplied with the instrument. Prior to the porosimetry and surface area analysis, the samples were dried under vacuum at 40°C overnight. For all calculations, the polymer density (ρ) of 1.3 g/cm^3 was used.

Thermal properties characterization.

The PLC300 foams prepared from a 5% w/v solution by quenching at -25, -80 and $-196°C$ for 30 seconds were subjected to differential scanning calorimetry (DSC, Pyris 1, Perkin-Elmer) analysis (n=3). The degree of crystallinity was calculated following the equation (2), where, X_c (%) refers to the percentage of crystallinity, ΔH_f refers to the heat of fusion of the sample, while, ΔH_f° refers to the theoretical heat of fusion of 100% crystalline sample [30]. Due to the lack of ΔH_f° value of the copolymer under study, the literature proposed to consider as ΔH_f° the ΔH_f° value of the major portion of the copolymer [30], [31]. Accordingly, in the current study, since the PLCL300 has 93% (w/w) of lactide content, the heat of fusion of pure PLA (i.e., 93 J/g) was considered as the ΔH_f° value.

$$X_c(\%) = \frac{\Delta H_f}{\Delta H_f^\circ} \times 100$$

(2)

In Vivo Studies

Ethics Statement.

This study was carried out in strict accordance with the recommendations for the care and use of laboratory animals of the Institute for Clinical and Experimental Medicine (ICEM), Prague, Czech Republic. The Animal Care Committee of the ICEM and the Ministry of Health, Czech Republic approved all the protocols related to this study. Animals were kept according to the European Convention on Animal Care in a controlled temperature, humidity and 12/12 light/dark regimen, with a free access to the sterile food pellets and water. All surgical procedures were done under the total anesthesia induced by a mixture of medetomidine and ketamine injected intramuscularly. At the end of the study, the test samples were excised from animals under the general anesthesia induced by a mixture of medetomidine and ketamine injected intramuscularly and subsequently, the animals were euthanized using exsanguination. During the entire study, all efforts were made to minimize suffering for the animals.

In Vivo Implantation

The PLCL300 foams prepared with a convenient pore size and physical strength prepared at the optimized conditions (5% w/v in dioxane, quenched at −80°C for 30 s) were used in the in vivo study. The control samples were products of ELLA-CS, Ltd. Czech Republic and were made from monofilament polydioxanone fibers by knitting, with a fiber thickness of ~200 μm and a mesh size between 500 to 700 μm. Prior to the implantation, all scaffolds were sterilized by 70% ethanol treatment for 1 h and were then thoroughly washed with sterile distilled water. The foams were implanted into the greater omentum of model brown Norway rats (male, aged between 2–3 months, 250–270 g, n=6). After placement of implants, the incisions were sutured in two levels with 4-0 vicryl absorbable sutures.

Histochemical and Immuno-Histochemical Staining

After four weeks of implantation, the rats were euthanized and the implants were harvested. For histological analysis, the implants were washed in PBS, fixed with 4% formaldehyde in PBS overnight, dehydrated through a graded series of ethanol, embedded in paraffin and sectioned at a thickness of 5 μm. The sections were then de-paraffinized, rehydrated with a graded series of ethanol and stained with the following stains as per the standard protocols: hematoxylin and eosin (H&E, to display the cytoplasmic and nuclear features of the tissue), masson›s trichrome (TRI, to display extracellular matrix components, particularly collagen) and anti-CD31 antibody (CD31, to display the presence of vascular endothelial cells).

Sample Size and Statistical Analysis

The sample size in SEM analysis and *in vivo* studies was 6, and in porosimetry, BET and DSC analysis was 3. The data presented was a representative of respective 'n'. The quantitative values were averaged and expressed as mean ± standard deviation (SD). The statistical differences were determined by the Student›s t-test and the differences were considered as statistically significant at P<0.01. The quantitative data was also subjected to Pearson›s correlation analysis to deduce the relationship between two properties. The coefficients (R) of −1 and +1 were considered to represent the inverse and direct correlation respectively, while the 0 represents no correlation. The closer the coefficient is to either −1 or +1, the stronger the correlation between the variables.

RESULTS AND DISCUSSION

Typical Features of Pore Architecture

The gross appearance and SEM images of the foams are presented in Figure 2. As may be seen, the current methodology readily enabled the fabrication of foams in shapes such as open-end capsules, tubules and flat 3D sheets, and with variable foam thickness and inner lumen diameters (Figure 2a). The cross section image (Figure 2c) shows the lengthwise cut pores made by the solvent crystals formed perpendicularly to the lumen. The pores are long and nearly continuous from one end to the other with intermittent branches also indicating the channeled structure. The anisotropic nature of the pores with a gradual increase in the pore size from inside to outside is evident as well. A high thickness of the analyzed sample did not show the open-cells in this section. However, the longitudinal section of the tubular scaffold clearly depicted its open-porous and interconnected nature (Figure 2d). The images of the scaffold surface showed bigger pores on the outer surface of the foam (Figure 2e) and relatively smaller pores on the inner surface that was in direct-contact with the *template* (Figure 2g), and thus confirmed an anisotropic pore structure. Further, the inner pores were found to be randomly organized, whereas, the outer pores exhibited a well-organized honeycomb shaped channeled network. A vertical cut in the middle of the foam revealed the well-organized honeycomb shaped pore structure under the outer surface also (Figure 2f). Remarkably, the overall observations revealed that the channels were without any transverse cross walls, as in contrast to previous reports describing the foams with a significant amount of transverse ladder-like cross walls that would plausibly obstruct the guided cell infiltration and nutrient flow [24], [32].

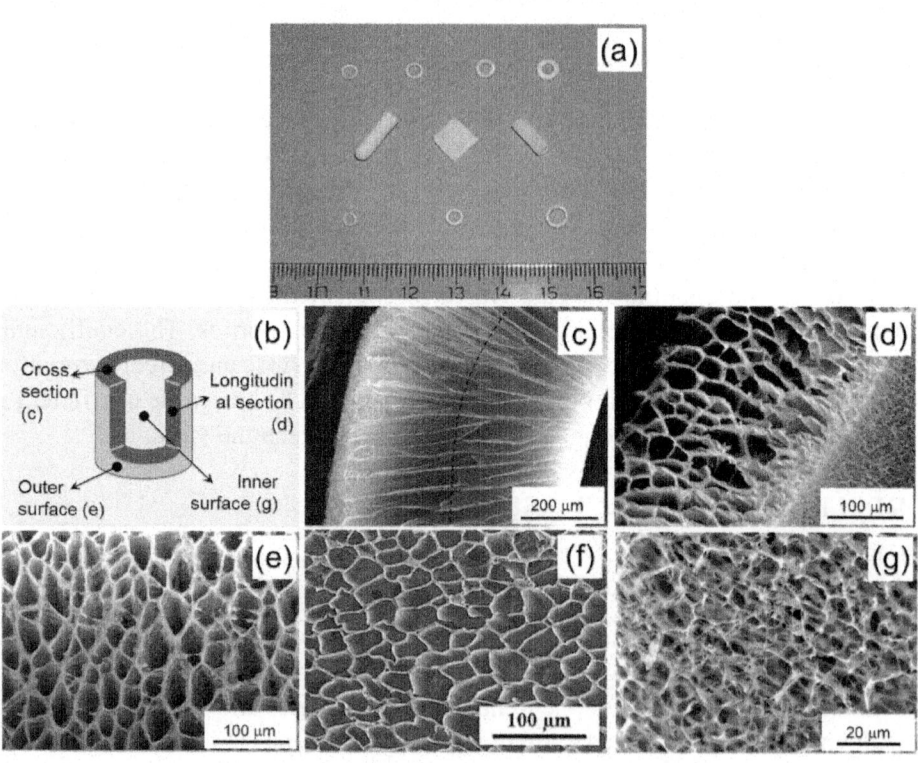

Figure 2. Macro- and micro- morphological features of the foams. (a) gross appearance of the open-end capsular, tubular, flat 3D porous PLCL300 scaffolds (5% w/v,

quenched at −80°C) with variable foam thickness and inner lumen diameters; (b) schematic of different sections of the scaffold analyzed under SEM; typical SEM images of (c) cross section of the scaffold showing the lengthwise cut elongated pores in direction of the applied thermal gradient (pore walls and overall channeled character of pores are clearly visible), (d) longitudinal section of the scaffold showing interconnected open-cells between particular channels, and (e) outer surface and (g) inner surface of the scaffold revealing the anisotropic nature of the pores. Panel (f) is the middle section of the foam's cross section (black dotted line in the panel c) showing an internal honey-comb like pore architecture.

Influence of Polymer Properties on Pore Architecture

Polymer Type

To understand the influence of the polymer type on pore architecture, we prepared PLA, PCL and PLCL foams under same experimental conditions (Table 1). The SEM images showing the pore morphology of foams are presented in Figure 3. It was observed that the PCL foam resulted in a poorly-ordered pore structure and was too soft and elastic to handle. This could be attributed majorly to low glass transition temperature (T_g, −60°C) of the polymer and its consequent impact on the overall phase separation phenomenon at the applied quenching temperature of −80°C [33]. On the other hand, PLA with T_g of 60°C successfully yielded the well-oriented foam at the same quenching temperature. However, a detailed examination of the inner surface of the foam that was in direct-contact with the *template* revealed micro-cracks and a significantly reduced porosity. The development of such micro-cracks (or often referred to as crazes) could be attributed to the inherent chain stiffness of PLA [25], [34]. In contrast, the PLCL foam with a PLA:PCL ratio of 93:7 mol/mol exhibited a well-ordered pore morphology without any crazes and with tough yet flexible mechanical properties compared to relatively brittle PLA scaffolds. Such improved features could be attributed to the polymer properties (molecular weight, chain stiffness and T_g value of 30°C), and the final quench depth (the temperature difference between the melting point of the solvent or T_g of the polymer or the cloud point of the polymer solution and the applied quenching temperature). Thus, it was evident that in principle the current methodology could be applicable to any polymer type, but, inherent properties of the polymer would influence the pore architecture and mechanical strength of the resulting foam. Since PLCL was found to yield favorable features of the foams, further studies were carried out using this polymer.

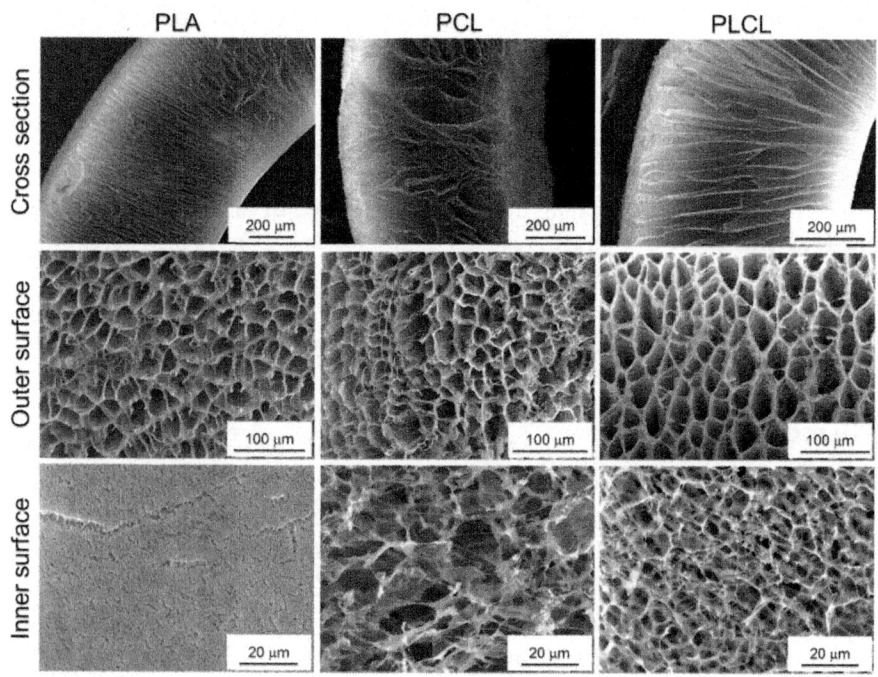

Figure 3. Influence of the polymer type. SEM images of the cross section, the outer and inner surfaces of the foams prepared from PLA, PCL and PLCL300 (5% w/v, quenched at −80°C for 30 s) revealed the relatively superior pore morphology without any micro-cracks of the PLCL foam as compared to that of pure PLA and PCL foams.

Polymer Molecular Weight

To investigate the effects of the polymer molecular weight on the pore morphology, we prepared the foams from PLCL of two different molecular weights, i.e. M_w=316 000 g/mol (PLCL300) and M_w=162 000 g/mol (PLCL150) under same experimental conditions (Table 1). SEM images of the cross section and outer surface of the scaffolds are presented inFigure 4. In contrast to the PLCL150 foams, the PLCL300 foams had well-organized pore structure with significantly thicker pore walls and enhanced toughness. Also, the PLCL300 foams exhibited higher overall foam thickness (612±22 μm) as compared to that of PLCL150 (469±25 μm). Thus, despite the same concentration and phase separation conditions, the order of the pores, the pore wall thickness, the overall foam thickness and toughness (by physical examination) were directly proportional to the increased polymer molecular weight, while, the pore size was inversely related. The observations comply with those of previous studies of PLA-based TIPS foams, where the increasing polymer molecular weight was suggested to reduce the polymer-solvent interactions and thereby to increase the cloud point or the freezing temperature [35], [36]. Additionally, the increasing viscosity along with increasing polymer-rich phase were to be accounted, at least partially, for the enhanced order in the pore structure of foams prepared from higher molecular weights [35], [36]. Due to the favorable features of the foams, PLCL300 was used for following investigations.

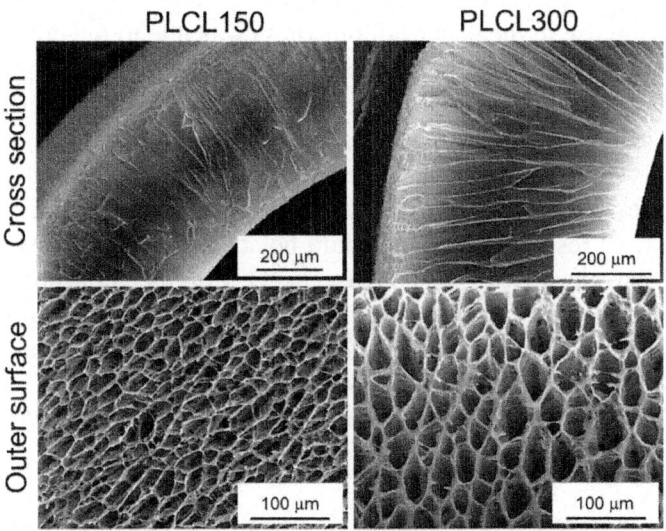

Figure 4. Influence of the polymer molecular weight. SEM images of the cross section and the outer surface of the foams prepared from PLCL solution (5% w/v, quenched at $-80°C$ for 30 s) of variable molecular weights showed the well-organized pore morphology and increased overall foam thickness in PLCL300 (M_w=316,000 g/mol and M_n=120,000 g/mol) as compared to that of PLCL150 (M_w=162,000 g/mol and M_n=57,000 g/mol).

Polymer Concentration

The effect of the polymer concentration on the foam morphology was investigated using the PLCL300 polymer. Four concentrations were tested: 3, 5, 7 and 10% (w/v), respectively.Figure 5 presents SEM images of cross sections and the outer surface of PLC300 foams along with a plot displaying the trend in the foam thickness and the outer pore size. As evident, the foams prepared from 3% (w/v) PLCL solution exhibited irregular and undefined pore architecture mainly due to deficiency of a polymer-rich phase. In contrast, the foams with higher polymer content demonstrated the well-organized channeled pores. There was a gradual decrease in the outer pore size from 53 ± 6 to 35 ± 5 to 19 ± 3 μm with an increasing polymer concentration from 5, 7 to 10%, respectively. SEM observations of the outer pore morphology also revealed a gradual thickening of the pore wall in direct relation to the polymer concentration. And, the pores on the inner side which was in a direct contact with the *template* were randomly organized with the size ranging between 5-10 μm (Figure 2g), and were following a decreasing trend with respect to the increasing polymer concentration (data not presented). As reported previously, such decrease in the pore size was attributed to reduction in the solvent crystallite phase that was more often interrupted by the polymer phase. While, an increase in the pore wall thickness was due to the possible spinodal phase separation including the exclusion of the solvent from the polymer phase to stabilize the overall system in terms of thermodynamic interfacial energy [35], [32], [37], [38]. In the current study, SEM images of cross sections also showed a clear increase in the overall foam thickness of 405±9, 612±22, 708±8 and finally 756±9 μm with increasing polymer concentration from 3, 5, 7 to 10% (w/v) respectively. This could be attributed to the gradual decrease in the solvent phase with an increase in the polymer concentration and its subsequent influence on the overall phase separation process under the same applied quenching temperature. Besides, as obvious, the physical examination of the foams suggested an increased toughness with an increase in the polymer content. To optimize Dip TIPS process conditions, the 5% (w/v) solution of PLCL300 was selected for the following experiments.

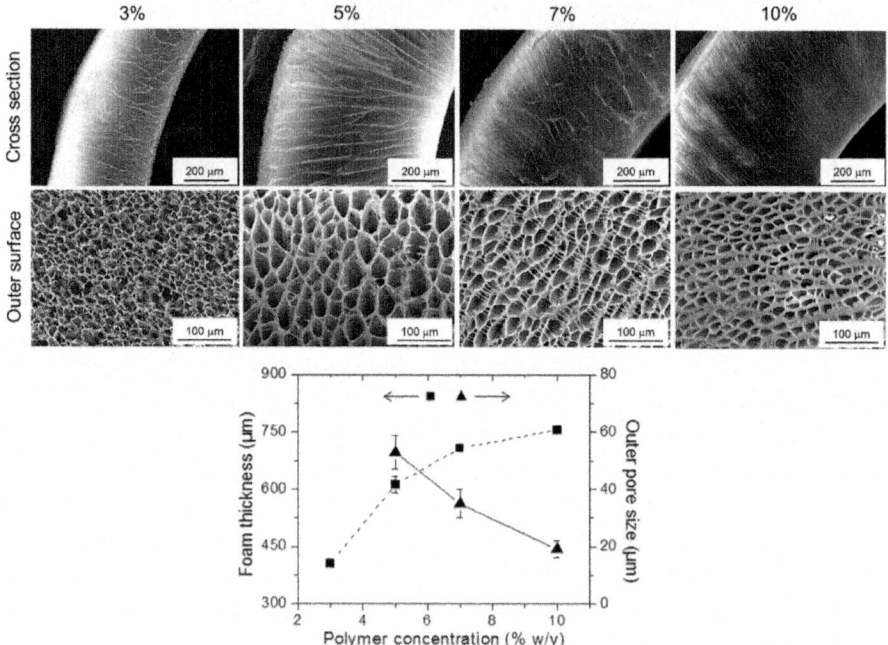

Figure 5. Influence of the polymer concentration. SEM images of the cross section and the outer surface of the PLCL300 scaffolds prepared from variable concentration

(3, 5, 7 and 10% w/v, quenched at −80°C for 30 s) demonstrated that the pore size was inversely proportional, and the pore wall thickness and the overall foam thickness was directly proportional to increase in the polymer concentration. Measurements were performed by *Image J* (n=25). The differences in the foam thickness or the pore size between any two groups were found to be statistically significant. The correlation coefficients between the polymer concentration and the outer pore size and the foam thickness were calculated to be −0.99 and +0.92, respectively.

Influence of Processing Conditions on Pore Architecture

Quenching Temperature.

The ability to control the solvent crystallization is crucial because the crystallite geometry serve as a template for macro and micro structure of the pores. We investigated and compared the influence of three different quenching temperatures (all lower than the melting point of 1,4-Dioxane) on the pore architecture of PLCL300 foams with a constant polymer concentration (5% w/v). SEM images of the outer surface revealed that the average pore sizes of the foams quenched at −25, −80 and −196°C were 64±9, 53±6 and 20±5 µm, respectively (Figure 6). There was a clear indication of gradual reduction in the outer pore size with decreasing quenching temperature or, in other words, with increasing quenching depth. The overall foam thickness increased from 494±28 to 612±22 µm when the quenching temperature decreased from −25 to −80°C. However, further decrease in the quenching temperature causes only a slight change in the thickness (565±23 µm, at −196°C). The PLCL300 solution subjected to a higher temperature (−25°C) exhibited slow crystallization and an active phase coalescence by decreasing interfacial energy, and resulted in bigger pores. While, the solution subjected to lower temperature (−196°C) underwent fast crystallization and arrest of phase nucleation, and hence resulted in relatively smaller pores. These observations correspond with the data reported in the scientific literature [33], [35], [32], [39]. The foams prepared at −80°C showed a well-developed honey-comb shaped pore structure; therefore the cooling temperature of −80°C was the fixed process parameter for the following tests.

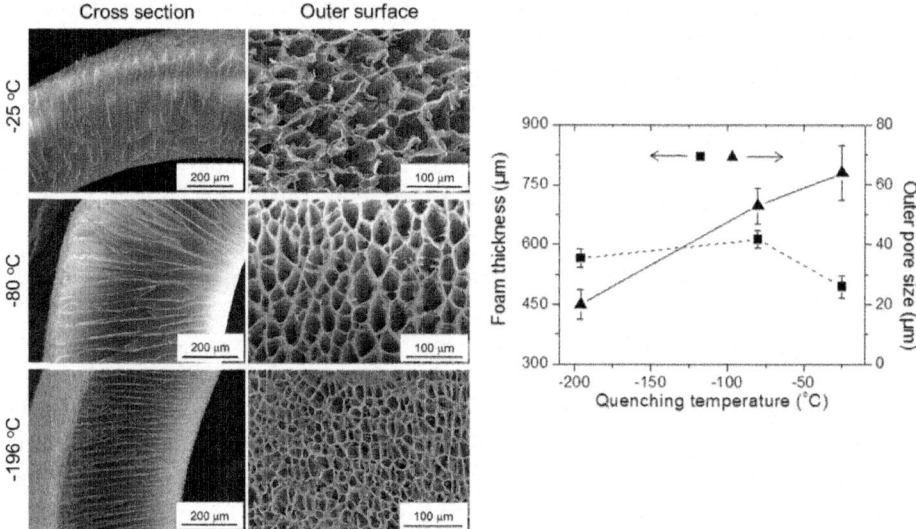

Figure 6. Influence of the quenching temperature. SEM images of the cross section and the outer surface of PLCL300 foams (5% w/v) prepared at various quenching temperatures (−25, −80 and −196°C) for 30 s revealed that the increase in the quenching depth promoted the organization of pores with a significant decrease in the average pore size, but with a slight alteration in the overall foam thickness. Measurements were done by *Image J* ($n=25$). The differences in the foam thickness or the pore size between any two groups were found to be statistically significant. The correlation coefficients between the quenching temperature and the outer pore size and the foam thickness were calculated to be −0.99 and +0.42, respectively.

Quenching Time

The influence of four different quenching times (15, 30, 45 and 60 s) on the pore morphology of PLCL300 foams (5% w/v, in 1,4-Dioxane, quenched at −80°C) was assessed. The SEM micrographs of cross section and outer surface morphologies of the foams quenched for various time intervals are presented in Figure 7. The average thickness of the phase separated foams fabricated with the quenching times of 15, 30, 45 and 60 s were found to be 395±25, 612±22, 852±20 and 1208±26 μm, respectively. Such gradual increase in the polymer foam thickness could be attributed to the gradual increase in the amount of the phase separated polymer over the mold with the increasing quenching time. However, since there was no change in either the polymer concentration or the applied quench depth, there was a negligible effect on the mean outer pore sizes of the foams prepared at the selected quenching times. The increasing trend in the outer pore size at higher quenching times may be attributed to the decreasing gradient of quench strength from the source point (*template*) to the end point (the outer surface of the foam) [24], . Besides, as a matter of fact, the physical examination of the foams suggested the improved mechanical toughness due to the increased foam thickness. Overall, it was evident that merely by changing the quenching times, the current Dip TIPS method enabled the fabrication of foams with a variable thickness while maintaining the outer pore size, thus avoiding any adjustments in the setup (e.g. the size of the mold).

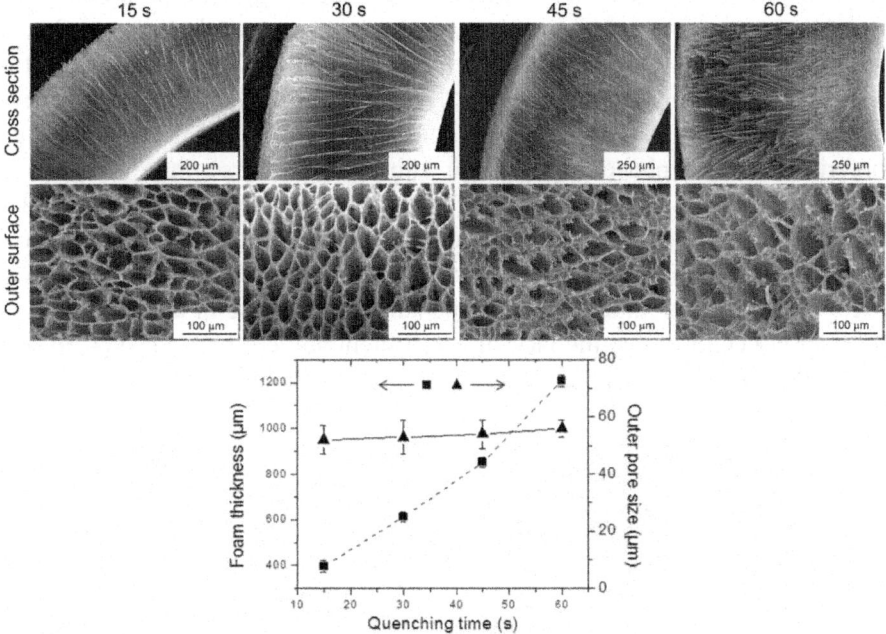

Figure 7. Influence of the quenching time. SEM images of the cross section and the outer surface of PLCL300 (5% w/v) foams prepared at −80°C for different quenching times (15, 30, 45 and 60 s) demonstrated the facile fabrication of foams of variable thickness without any significant change in the average pore size but with a slight thickening of the pore wall. Measurements were performed by *Image J* (*n*=25). The differences in the outer pore sizes were statistically not significant, but the differences in the thickness between any two groups were statistically significant. The correlation coefficients between the quenching time and outer pore size and foam thickness were calculated to be +0.98 and +0.99, respectively.

Coarsening Time

The morphology evolution of the PLCL-dioxane binary phase systems in relation to increasing coarsening time was also investigated. The SEM micrographs showing the pore morphology of the PLCL300 scaffold (3% w/v, quenched at −25°C for 30 s) coarsened for 0, 30, 60 and 120 min) are presented in Figure 8. The observations clearly demonstrated that the foams with longer coarsening times yielded the well-ordered pore architecture in comparison with the foams coarsened for a shorter time. However, when foams were prepared from higher polymer concentrations (i.e., 5, 7 or 10% w/v) or at lower quenching temperatures (−80 or −196°C), no significant changes in the pore morphology were observed in relation to the coarsening time (data not presented). Our observations agree with the spinodal phase separation theories of polymer solutions, wherein it was suggested that under lower quench depth and lower polymer concentration, even though the initial spatial configurations of the phases were nearly random shortly after quenching, an anisotropic system develops strong spatial correlations along the elastically soft crystallographic directions of the phases during the subsequent coarsening. Thus, as the coarsening continues the system undergoes infinitesimal alignment to minimize the total free energy and yield evolved micro-structure of the phases [41]–[43]. On the other hand, the system undergoes instant crystallization and arrest of the phases under a higher quench depth. While in the case of higher polymer concentrations, the lack of a sufficient solvent phase leaves no scope for further fine tuning of the phases.

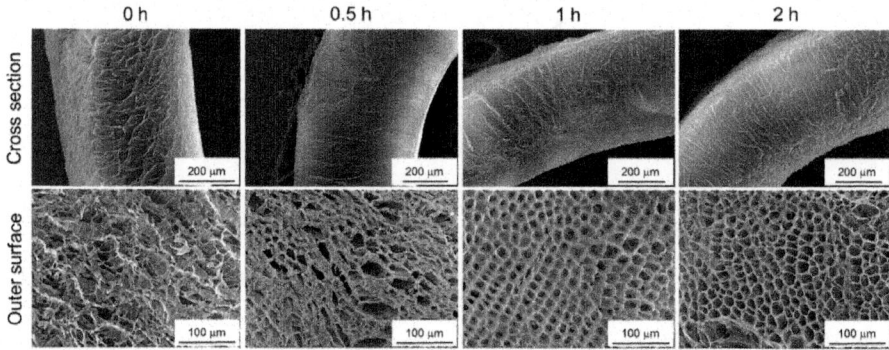

Figure 8. Influence of the coarsening time. SEM images of the cross section and the outer surface of the PLCL300 (3% w/v) foams prepared by quenching at −25°C for 30 s and coarsening for various times (0, 0.5, 1 and 2 h) suggested that an increase in the coarsening time resulted in better organization of the solvent rich phase what after solvent removal led to well-ordered pores.

Influence of the Mold Diameter on Pore Architecture

There were two metallic components in the Dip TIPS setup (Figure 1), i.e. the *conductor* with defined dimensions and the *template* of variable shapes and sizes. Hypothetically, any significant change in the *conductor* block would cause alterations in the final quench strength and thereby influence the resultant foam structure. However, since the *conductor* dimensions were predefined and kept unchanged for all the investigations, we have not explored this parameter in the current study. Instead, we investigated the effect of diameter of the *template* (2, 3, and 4 mm) on the final pore architecture. The morphological observations are presented in Figure 9. The formation of anisotropic oriented interconnected channeled pores was successful in all cases. As evident from the images, the increase in the mold diameter from 2, 3 to 4 mm lead to a slight decrease in the overall foam thickness from 653±39, 612±22 to 588±21 μm respectively. On the other hand, there was a small increase in the average pore size and the pore wall thickness. This can be attributed to the fact that, in the case of a lower diameter mold, the quench strength was plausibly higher and hence led to the increased phase separation of the polymer over the *template* accounting for the increased foam thickness. Also, perhaps the quench rate was quicker in the case of a lower diameter *template* and thus resulted in relatively smaller pores. However, the increase in the pore wall thickness with an increasing *template* diameter may be attributed to the possible spinodal phase separation of the solvent from the polymer phase associated with lower quench strength and slower quench rate.

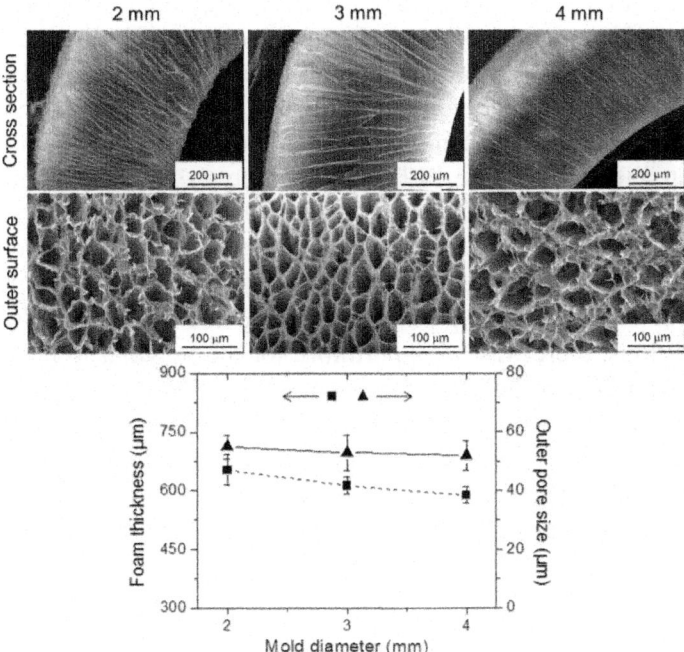

Figure 9. Influence of the mold diameter. SEM images of the cross section and the outer surface of the PLCL300 (5% w/v) foams prepared with molds of 2, 3 and 4

mm diameter at −80°C for 30 s demonstrated the ability to fabricate foams with variable inner lumen diameters without any significant change in the average pore size but with a slight thickening of the pore wall and decrease in the overall foam thickness. Measurements were performed by *Image J* (*n*=25). The differences between any two groups were statistically not significant. The correlation coefficients between the mold diameter and outer pore size and foam thickness were calculated to be −0.92 and −0.98, respectively.

Thermal Characteristics of PLCL300 Foams

The aim of the DSC analysis was to characterize thermal properties of the PCLC300 foams (5% w/v) and to follow possible changes in the polymer crystallinity during the foam processing potentially induced by change in the quenching temperature. It was hypothesized that higher quench strength would yield lower crystallinity due to a rapid arrest of polymer and solvent phases, and vice versa. The results obtained for dried polymer foams are presented in Table 2; In general, there were no significant changes in the studied thermal characteristics for quenching temperatures −25, −80 and −196°C, and all tested samples showed a crystallinity of ~30%. However, the melting temperature (T_m) of the PLLA part from the PLCL300 copolymer and overall crystallinity of the processed foams exhibited a decreasing trend with respect to the increasing quench depth. Such trend was not observed in the second run due to the erase of thermal history. A similar behavior was observed by *Goh* and *Ooi* during the phase separation of a pure poly(l-lactide) (PLLA) by quenching the polymer solution in dioxane from room temperature to −25 or −80°C. No significant difference in the PLLA crystallinity before and after processing was observed (~18%), although a slight crystallinity decrease with respect to increasing quench depth was detected [32]. The PLCL300-dioxane system undergoes the solid-liquid phase separation when quenching temperatures are much lower than the melting point of dioxane and T_g of the polymer. Under such conditions, there was no opportunity for the polymer to undergo further crystallization during the foam processing [33], [32]. On the other hand, the decreasing trend in the crystallinity with respect to the decreasing quenching temperature could be attributed to the fact that the nucleation and growth of the PLCL crystallites at lower quench depth (e.g. −25°C) was reduced to a lower extent than in the case of systems prepared at higher quench depth (−80°C, −196°C) [32], [44].

Table 2. DSC analysis of PLCL300 before processing (control) and PLCL300 foams (5% wt, 30 s) prepared under various quenching temperatures (n=3).

Quenching temperature	1st run#			2nd run					
	T_m	ΔH_f	X_c	T_g	T_c	ΔH_c	T_m	$\Delta H_f X_c$	
	(°C)	(J/g)	(%)	(°C)	(°C)	(J/g)	(°C)	(J/g)	(w)
Control*	164.1	31.1	34	30.2	84.9	−19.1	163.4	31.4	34
25°C	162.3	31.4	34	33.5	89.0	−18.0	163.3	30.8	33
−80°C	163.0	29.1	32	34.9	90.6	−18.3	163.4	30.9	33
−196°C	162.5	28.6	31	31.3	92.8	−19.1	163.4	31.5	34

the cold crystallization peak (T_c and corresponding ΔH_c) was not observed in the first run; also, the T_g was not calculated in the first run.
* After polymer isolation.
doi:10.1371/journal.pone.0108792.t002

Porosity and Surface Area Properties of PLCL300 Foams

The aim of porosity studies was to characterize the porosity and surface area properties of the PCLC300 foams used for *in vivo* study and to follow possible changes in the porosity due to the change in the quenching temperature. The obtained data for the PLCL300 (5% w/v) foams prepared by quenching for 30 seconds at −25, −80 and −196°C are presented in Table 3. All the PLC300 foams were found to have a high porosity of about 90% which was comparable with the porosity of pure PLLA and PCL foams prepared by the standard TIPS but analyzed mostly by gravimetric methods [26], [32], [33], [35]. The mean pore diameter observed was ~25 µm and the specific surface area varied between 4.4–4.9 m²/g. The foam porosity and the mean pore diameter had decreasing trend whereas the specific surface area increased with increasing quench depth. However, the changes observed were minimal and were considered as insignificant. In contrast, Guarino *et al.* [33] observed almost a doubled increase in the mean pore size for the PCL foams (5% wt, dioxane) from 25 to 50 µm when quenching temperature increased from −18 to 4°C. In the case of PLA foams prepared by TIPS, the pore size was characterized mainly by the microscopic methods (as also performed in the present study) and not giving the information about the mean pore size [24], [26], [32], [40]. As expected, the determined pore volume was relatively high (7–8.5 ml/g, Table 3) and reflected the pore diameter values together with high porosities. The effect of the quenching temperature was prominent over the pore volume; the pore volume distinctively decreases with decreasing quenching temperature in accordance with decreasing trends in the porosity and the mean pore size.

Table 3. Mercury intrusion porosimetry and BET surface area analysis of PLCL300 foams (5% wt, 30 s) prepared at various quenching temperatures (n=3).

Quenching temperature	Mean pore diameter (μm)*	Pore volume (ml/g)	Porosity (%)	BET surface area (m²/g)
−25°C	26	8.5	90	4.4
−80°C	25	7.1	88	4.8
−196°C	23	7.0	87	4.9

* Pore range considered: 0.2 and 116 μm.
doi:10.1371/journal.pone.0108792.t003

Figure 10 shows a typical cumulative pore volume curve and a derivative pore size distribution observed for the analyzed PLCL300 foams. Generally, the pores are characterized by a broad distribution that can be attributed to strongly anisotropic character of the channeled pores observed by SEM (Figure 2); the determined pore size distribution (expressed in a logarithm scale as the $dV/d\log(d)$ ratio) ranged from 0.2 to 116 μm and the pores with the size from 10 to 70 μm were found to be the most frequent.

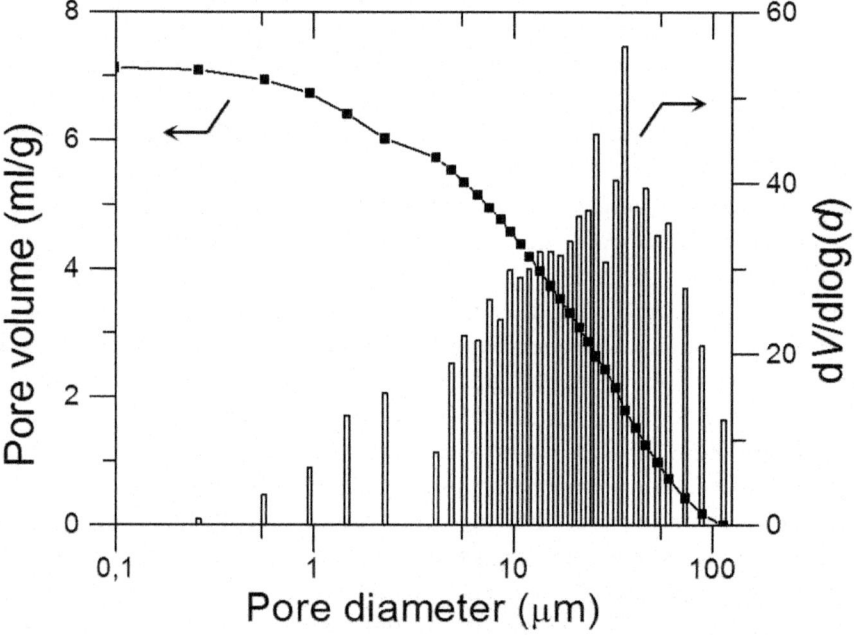

Figure 10. Mercury porosity analysis. The cumulative pore volume (line with markers) and derivative pore size distribution (vertical columns) of PLCL300 foam prepared at −80°C for 30 s (pore range: 0.2 to 116 μm).

The mean pore size calculated by the porosimetry is not comparable with the outer and inner pore size obtained by the SEM analysis; the porosimetry analysis considered for calculations all the pores ranging from 0.2 to 116 μm throughout the foam, whereas SEM calculations were performed by considering the pores visible on the outer surface only. As a matter of fact, the gas/fluid intrusion based methods solely allow the evaluation of the open-porous and interconnected network and do not yield any results in case of the closed-porous foams [33], [45]. Thus, the determined 90% porosity for PLCL300 foams straightway depicts a highly interconnected open porous nature of the foams fabricated by Dip TIPS. This feature of the foam morphology is an essential parameter for the successful colonization of foams by the cells and formation of the tissue in the *in vivo* conditions [3]. However, the data obtained from porosimetry analysis did not enable to deduce a correlation between Dip TIPS process parameters and pore parameters. The data obtained was not significant enough in this regard. Thus, we followed the SEM-based pore size analysis to deduce the possible correlation (in earlier sections).

In vivo Behavior of PLCL300 Foams

Since polylactide products are biocompatible and biodegradable polymers that have long been approved by the United States Food and Drug Administration for use in medical applications [46], we did not consider re-establishing its biocompatibility in general. However, based on our previous experiences, the implanted scaffolds can induce a temporary fluid accumulation and mechanical irritation of surrounding tissue [11]. To this end, the commonly performed *in vitro* studies do not allow a proper cell ingrowth into the scaffold, especially under static conditions [15]. Therefore, in the current study, we have studied the influence of the scaffold architecture on the cell infiltration, extracellular matrix synthesis and vascularization *in vivo* using a rat animal model. Accordingly, the PLCL300 foams (5% w/v in dioxane, quenched at −80°C for 30 s) and the control macroporous scaffolds (made from monofilament polydioxanone fibers, by knitting) were implanted into the greater omentum of healthy brown Norway rats. The scaffolds were engrafted by a gentle fibrous membrane (including vessels) in one week and did not cause any side effect such as inflammation or an excessive fibrotic reaction (data not presented). After 4 weeks, all the rats with the PLCL300 survived the procedure and were no different from the controls. The implants were excised and analyzed for the basic morphology (H&E staining), production of fibrous tissue (TRI staining) and the presence of endothelial cells (CD31 staining) representing mature as well as newly formed blood capillaries. The results are presented in Figure 11. Based on the macroscopic observations, both the tested PLCL300 and the control macroporous scaffolds maintained their geometrical shape and structural integrity during the implantation, engraftment and excision (Figure 11a, 11f).

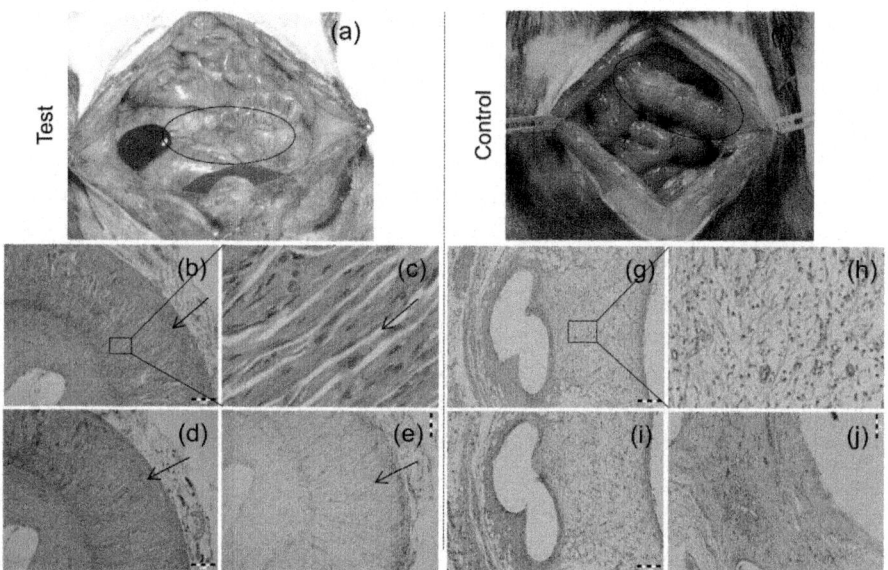

Figure 11. *In vivo* behavior of the test (a–e) and control (f–j) scaffolds. (a, f) 4-week old anastomosed scaffolds as seen in the omentum of the model animal; (b, g) low magnification and (c, h) high magnification H&E stained sections showing the host cell infiltration and cell distribution (deep blue-purple nuclei, pink cytoplasmic and extracellular proteins); (d, i) TRI stained sections showing the synthesis of extracellular collagen (blue or green) by the invading cells; and (e, j) anti-CD31 stained sections showing the infiltration of microvascular endothelial cells (brown). The black arrow in the panels (b–e) represents the direction of host cell/tissue infiltration. Scale: 200 μm.

The H&E staining provides information about the general morphology of samples under examination. The cross section images of the H&E stained samples of the PLCL300 foams depicted the guided infiltration of the cells coming from the surface to the center and the homogenous distribution of the cells throughout the foam (Figure 11b). A high magnification image clearly revealed a guided infiltration of the host cells through the oriented channeled pores of the microporous PLCL300 scaffolds (Figure 11c). On the other hand, the fibrous tissue was randomly spread across the control macro-porous scaffold (Figure 11g, 11h). The TRI staining usually produces blue or green collagen, light red or pink cytoplasm and dark brown or black cell nuclei. The TRI stained cross section analysis showed the active synthesis of extracellular matrix components, particularly collagen, by the invading host cells (preferentially the cells of the connective tissue) in the PLCL300 foam (Figure 11d); in contrast, the macroporous scaffold analysis revealed a poor matrix synthesis by cells (Figure 11i). Apart from the cell infiltration and extracellular matrix synthesis, another important factor required for the successful tissue regeneration is the scaffold›s ability to support angiogenesis. The CD31 staining is a widely used immuno-histochemistry method to demonstrate the presence of vascular endothelial cells that have an abundant CD31 surface marker. In the current study, the CD31 stained cross section images showed that not only the fibroblast-like cells but also the vascular endothelial cells and microvascular network (Figure 11e, brown colored) were present on the surface of the implant; however, they did not migrate towards the internal surface of the scaffold. On the other hand, the control scaffold showed the scattered presence of endothelial cells (Figure 11j).

Overall, the preliminary *in vivo* investigations showed that the anisotropic radially oriented channeled pores of adjusted pore-size parameters successfully offered the guidance for the host cell infiltration and provided convenient conditions (for exchange of nutrients, gases, secretions, etc.) for supporting higher cell density and uniform cell distribution. Importantly, there was no sign of any fibrous capsule formation around the implant, thus suggesting the compatibility of the implant material with the surrounding tissue. Our results correlate with the findings in several earlier investigations using, for example, the PLA scaffold with aligned channeled pores prepared by super critical fluid processing [47], or PLA scaffolds with the anisotropic channeled pores [24], as well as the chitosan scaffold with uniaxial tubular pores prepared by TIPS [48].

Features of Dip TIPS

The polymer foams with anisotropic interconnected channeled pores are increasingly gaining importance in the guided tissue engineering and other related applications. However, till now the preparation of anisotropic channeled porous foams by TIPS was done by using complex setups [24]–[26], [33], [40], [48], [49]. For example, to prepare PLA tubular foams with lumen diameters up to 3 mm and the foam thickness from 1 to several millimeters, the molds were assembled by inserting a thermally conductive cylindrical*template* into a thermally non-/less- conductive capillary tube [24], [49]. To obtain a uniform foam thickness, the *template* was held tightly within the capillary tube by tapes or sleeves at both ends [49]. The fabrication of PLA tubular foams for nerve regeneration with a variable inner lumen diameter (>3 mm) or wall thickness (>0.5 mm) involved complex adjustments including additional metal molds in the setup [49]. For the construction of flat 3D foams, the molding setup included a tailored thermally non-/less- conductive container with single (at bottom) or double (at top and bottom) plate(s) of high thermal conductivity [33]. Hence, in general, the successful fabrication of anisotropic foams by the conventional TIPS setups described above requires a number of accessories, different setups for preparation of differently shaped foams and skillful hands for careful and precise maneuver.

In the current study, we demonstrate a process termed as Dip TIPS that fundamentally relies on the principle of unidirectional TIPS (Figure 12). When the *template* that was dipped in the polymer solution was subjected to quenching using a cooling mixture, the polymer solution in the immediate vicinity of the *template* has underwent unidirectional phase separation along the direction of thermal quenching [21], [35]. In Dip TIPS, similar to the conventional TIPS, the phase separation proceeds through either the solid-liquid or the liquid-liquid phase separation phenomenon depending on the applied quenching depth and composition of the system [33], [35], [32]. However, in contrast to the previous methods, the Dip TIPS methodology allowed the fabrication of tubular, open-end capsular and flat 3D foams with a variable pore size, foam thickness and inner lumen diameters, without complex adjustments. A summary of the results obtained is presented in Table 4. A comparison of Dip TIPS with the state of the art methods for the fabrication of anisotropic porous foams of various shapes and sizes with controlled pore architecture is presented inTable 5.

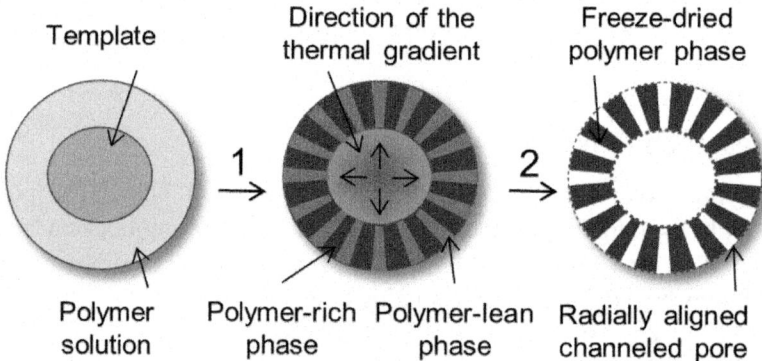

Figure 12. Dip TIPS working principle. A schematic illustration of the mechanism of the formation of anisotropic oriented interconnected channeled pores (1: quenching, 2: freeze-drying).

doi:10.1371/journal.pone.0108792.g012

Table 4. Summary of the effects of various process parameters on the foam properties (n=6).

Parameter studied	Observations
Polymer type (PLA, PCL, PLCL)	Pore size: PLA<PLCL<PCL; Foam thickness: PLA>PLCL>PCL; PLA foams were rigid and brittle with prominent micro-cracks. PCL foams were soft and elastic with collapsed pore architecture upon manipulations. PLCL foams were tough and without micro-cracks.
Polymer molecular weight (PLCL150, PLCL300)	Pore size: PLCL150>PLCL300; Foam thickness: PLCL150<PLCL300; The PLCL300 foams had consistently well-organized pore structure with significantly thicker pore walls and enhanced toughness in contrast to the PLCL150 foams
Polymer concentration (3, 5, 7 and 10% w/v)	Pore size: 3>5>7>10; Foam thickness: 3<5<7<10; In contrast to the foams prepared from concentrated PLCL solution (5% or higher), the foams from 3% exhibited irregular and undefined pore architecture. A gradual thickening of pore walls in a direct correlation with the polymer concentration was also observed.
Quenching temperature (−25, −80, −196°C)	Pore size: −25>−80>−196; Foam thickness: −25<−80<−196; The physical examination revealed that the mechanical strength of the capsules increased with an increasing quench depth.
Quenching time (15, 30, 45, 60 s)	Pore size: no significant changes; Foam thickness: 15<30<45<60; An increase in the quenching time led to the thickening of the foam that in turn led to enhanced mechanical strength (as per the physical examination).
Coarsening duration (0, 30, 60, 120 min)	The effects observed only for 3% (w/v) PLCL300 solution quenched at −25°C.
Mold diameter (2, 3, 4 mm)	Pore size: no significant changes; Foam thickness: no significant changes; A gradual thickening of pore walls in a direct correlation with the mold diameter was noted.

doi:10.1371/journal.pone.0108792.t004

Table 5. Summary of the practical advantages of Dip TIPS in comparison with the state of the art method for the fabrication of anisotropic porous foams of various shapes for various applications.

Foam type	Potential applications	State of the art methodology	Dip TIPS methodology
Porous open-end capsular foams	Cell transplantation	No method reported till now	The setup involves a set of easy-to-assemble *template*, *conductor* and *reservoir*, and enables the fabrication of open-capsules with variable inner lumen diameter, wall thickness and with controlled pore architecture.
Porous tubular foams	Vascular, nerve or other tubular tissue engineering	Typical setup [24,49]. Molds contain one inner metallic bar and one outer non-metallic cylinder with helical locks at both ends, or with metallic bottom; requires another setup with appropriate dimensions for controlling both lumen diameter and foam thickness. the outer surface is often prone to the skin-effect with low/no porosity.	Post-fabrication cutting of the closed end of the open-capsule leads to a tubular foam; fabrication of tubular foams with a variable inner lumen diameter is achieved by a simple exchange of the *template* of a desired size; fabrication of tubular foams with a variable thickness is possible by a mere change in the quenching time.
Porous flat foams	Guided tissue engineering	Typical setup [14,33]. Molds contain a dish with metallic bottom but with non-metallic walls; obtaining homogenous foam thickness, especially in the case of low thickness foams, is difficult due to concave meniscus of the polymer solution in the mold; the outer or top surface is often prone to the skin-effect with low/no porosity.	The same mold as for open-capsular/tubular foams, except the use of a flat *template* instead of a cylindrical one; the thickness of flat foams is nearly homogenous; preparation of flat foams with a variable thickness is possible by a mere change in the quenching time; there is skin-effect, but it is not a process related error, rather it is a manual error (such as the exposure of the just phase separated frozen sample to environment, due to a delay during the transfer from the conductor to a freezer or freeze drying).

doi:10.1371/journal.pone.0108792.t005

The conventional setups follow the thermal conductivity directly from the primary source, while Dip TIPS follows the thermal conductivity from the extended surface of the primary source (known as the "fin"). Hence, the heat transfer principles governing the conventional and Dip TIPS are different. A detailed description of these mechanisms has been described elsewhere [50], [51]. In brief, the fins on the base surface are made either by extrusion, welding or simple mechanical fixing to enhance or extend the heat transfer from a given surface. The thermal conductivity properties and dimensions of the fin as well as the resistance in the joint between the primary source and the fin determine the thermal profile[50], [51].

In the context of Dip TIPS, the shape, size and material composition of the fin used affects the formation of the foams and the properties there-of. In the current study, cylindrical and rectangular Dural fins with a thickness of 3 mm and a length of 40 mm were used; nearly uniform thermal profile (indicated by a nearly-uniform foam thickness for a foam length of 15 mm) was observed. Further, the solution properties, in particular the solvent properties profoundly affect the initial nucleation process and homogeneity of the phase separation along the length of the fin. In our experience in this regard, we observed that the organic solvents such as dioxane was readily able to undergo nucleation, but it was difficult to achieve in the water system; This could be attributed to differences in the enthalpy of crystallization of various solvents or solvent systems. Thus, although the presented Dip TIPS setup can be in principle applied for the controlled preparation of any polymer foams, we anticipate that the fin, polymer and solvent properties could potentially influence the foam formation and its properties.

CONCLUSIONS

We demonstrated a facile methodology termed as "Dip TIPS" for the fabrication of polymer foams with anisotropic interconnected channeled pores with an ascending gradient pore size perpendicular to the mold. The method works on the principle of unidirectional TIPS of a polymer solution that involves the separation of the polymer and solvent phases along the direction of the thermal gradient. In comparison to other complex methods, the process readily enabled the fabrication of PLA based foams in shapes such as tubules, open-end capsule and flat 3D sheets. The foams with thickness between 395 and 1208 µm were obtained merely by changing the quenching times (15, 30, 45 and 60 s). The foams with inner lumen diameters of 2, 3 and 4 mm were obtained easily by changing the mold diameter. On the other hand, the pore size (between 20 to 65 µm) was controlled by changing either the quenching temperature (−25, −80 and −196°C) or the polymer concentration (3, 5, 7 or 10% w/v). The current study confirmed the previously published data that suggested an inverse relation between the pore size, and the concentration and molecular weight of the polymer, and a direct relation between the pore size and the applied quenching temperature. The preliminary *in vivo* investigations in brown Norway rats showed that the selected PLCL300 scaffolds were biocompatible as there was no inflammation or an excessive fibrotic reaction observed and that the character of the pore structure supported the guided cell infiltration and homogenous cell distribution within the scaffolds in comparison to the control macroporous scaffold. Further studies focused on the enhancement of the surface morphology of the scaffold, the encapsulation of bioactive factors and the subsequent evaluation of its *in vivo* potential are in progress.

ACKNOWLEDGMENTS

We thank *Dr. Silvia Grama* and *Ms. Jana Koubkova* (IMC, Prague) for porosimetry measurements, *Dr. Eduard Brynda, Dr. Daniel Horak, Dr. Miroslav Šlouf* (IMC, Prague) and*Dr. Daniel Jirak* and *Dr. David Habart* (ICEM, Prague) for helpful discussions.

AUTHOR CONTRIBUTIONS

Conceived and designed the experiments: NK DK. Performed the experiments: NK MMK J. Kříž EF J. Kovářová. Analyzed the data: NK DK J. Kříž FR. Contributed reagents/materials/analysis tools: NK LM. Wrote the paper: NK DK J. Kříž.

REFERENCES

1.   Shastri VP, Martin I, Langer R (2000) Macroporous polymer foams by hydrocarbon templating. Proc Natl Acad Sci USA 97: 1970–1975. doi: 10.1073/pnas.97.5.1970

2.   Berthiaume F, Maguire TJ, Yarmush ML (2011) Tissue Engineering and Regenerative Medicine: History, Progress, and Challenges. Annu Rev Chem Biomol Eng 2: 403–430. doi: 10.1146/annurev-chembioeng-061010-114257

3.   Liu C, Xia Z, Czernuszka JT (2007) Design and development of three-dimensional scaffolds for tissue engineering. Chem Eng Res Des 85: 1051–1064. doi: 10.1205/cherd06196

4.   Xiao L, Wang B, Yang G, Gauthier M (2012) Poly(Lactic Acid)-Based Biomaterials: Synthesis, Modification and Applications. Biomedical Science, Engineering and Technology, Prof. Dhanjoo N. Ghista (Ed.), ISBN: 978-953-307-471-9, InTech, DOI: 10.5772/23927.

5.   Kasoju N, Bora U (2012) Silk Fibroin in Tissue Engineering. Adv Healthcare Mater 1: 393–412. doi: 10.1002/adhm.201200097

6.   Sakiyama-Elbert SE, Hubbell JA (2001) Functional biomaterials: design of novel biomaterials. Ann Rev Mater Res 31: 183–201. doi: 10.1146/annurev.matsci.31.1.183

7.   Matsumura G, Nitta N, Matsuda S, Sakamoto Y, Isayama N, et al. (2012) Long-term results of cell-free biodegradable scaffolds for in situ tissue-engineering vasculature: in a canine inferior vena cava model. PLoS One 7: e35760. doi: 10.1371/journal.pone.0035760

8.   Masaeli E, Morshed M, Nasr-Esfahani MH, Sadri S, Hilderink J, et al. (2013) Fabrication, characterization and cellular compatibility of

poly(hydroxy alkanoate) composite nanofibrous scaffolds for nerve tissue engineering. PLoS One 8: e57157. doi: 10.1371/journal.pone.0057157

9. Gugerell A, Kober J, Laube Y, Walter T, Nürnberger S, et al. (2014) Electrospun Poly(ester-Urethane)- and Poly(ester-Urethane-Urea) Fleeces as Promising Tissue Engineering Scaffolds for Adipose-Derived Stem Cells. PLoS One 9: e90676. doi: 10.1371/journal.pone.0090676

10. Wang H-M, Chou Y-T, Wen Z-H, Wang Z-R, Chen C-H, et al. (2013) Novel Biodegradable Porous Scaffold Applied to Skin Regeneration. PLoS One 8: e56330. doi: 10.1371/journal.pone.0056330

11. Kriz J, Vilk G, Mazzuca DM, Toleikis PM, Foster PJ, et al. (2012) A novel technique for the transplantation of pancreatic islets within a vascularized device into the greater omentum to achieve insulin independence. Am J Surg 203: 793–797. doi: 10.1016/j.amjsurg.2011.02.009

12. Mitchell GR, Tojeira A (2013) Role of Anisotropy in Tissue Engineering. Procedia Eng 59: 117–125. doi: 10.1016/j.proeng.2013.05.100

13. Vrana NE, Dupret A, Coraux C, Vautier D, Debry C, et al. (2011) Hybrid Titanium/Biodegradable Polymer Implants with an Hierarchical Pore Structure as a Means to Control Selective Cell Movement. PLoS ONE 6: e20480. doi: 10.1371/journal.pone.0020480

14. Ma PX, Zhang R (2001) Microtubular architecture of biodegradable polymer scaffolds. J Biomed Mater Res 56: 469–477. doi: 10.1002/1097-4636(20010915)56:4<469::aid-jbm1118>3.0.co;2-h

15. Kennedy JP, McCandless SP, Rauf A, Williams LM, Hillam J, et al. (2011) Engineered channels enhance cellular density in perfused scaffolds. Acta Biomater 7: 3896–3904. doi: 10.1016/j.actbio.2011.06.037

16. Patel H, Bonde M, Srinivasan G (2011) Biodegradable polymer scaffold for tissue engineering. Trends Biomater Artif Organs 25: 20–29.

17. Chan BP, Leong KW (2008) Scaffolding in tissue engineering: general approaches and tissue-specific considerations. Eur Spine J 17 Suppl 4: 467–479. doi: 10.1007/s00586-008-0745-3

18. Kasoju N, Bora U (2010) Antheraea assama Silk Fibroin-Based Functional Scaffold with Enhanced Blood Compatibility for Tissue Engineering Applications. Adv Eng Mater 12: B139–B147. doi: 10.1002/adem.200980055

19. Chen G, Ushida T, Tateishi T (2002) Scaffold Design for Tissue Engineering. Macromol Biosci 2: 67–77. doi: 10.1002/1616-5195(20020201)2:2<67::aid-mabi67>3.0.co;2-f

20. Kasoju N, Bora U (2012) Silk fibroin based biomimetic artificial

extracellular matrix for hepatic tissue engineering applications. Biomed Mater 7: 045004. doi: 10.1088/1748-6041/7/4/045004

21. Martínez-Pérez CA, Olivas-Armendariz I, Castro-Carmona JS, García-Casillas PE (2011) Scaffolds for Tissue Engineering Via Thermally Induced Phase Separation. In: Wislet-Gendebien S, editor. Advances in Regenerative Medicine: InTech. pp.275–294.

22. Kim JW, Taki K, Nagamine S, Ohshima M (2009) Preparation of porous poly(L-lactic acid) honeycomb monolith structure by phase separation and unidirectional freezing. Langmuir 25: 5304–5312. doi: 10.1021/la804057e

23. Moriya A, Maruyama T, Ohmukai Y, Sotani T, Matsuyama H (2009) Preparation of poly(lactic acid) hollow fiber membranes via phase separation methods. J Membr Sci 342: 307–312. doi: 10.1016/j.memsci.2009.07.005

24. Ma H, Hu J, Ma PX (2010) Polymer Scaffolds for Small-Diameter Vascular Tissue Engineering. Adv Funct Mater 20: 2833–2841. doi: 10.1002/adfm.201000922

25. Yang F, Qu X, Cui W, Bei J, Yu F, et al. (2006) Manufacturing and morphology structure of polylactide-type microtubules orientation-structured scaffolds. Biomaterials 27: 4923–4933. doi: 10.1016/j.biomaterials.2006.05.028

26. Hu X, Shen H, Yang F, Bei J, Wang S (2008) Preparation and cell affinity of microtubular orientation-structured PLGA(70/30) blood vessel scaffold. Biomaterials 29: 3128–3136. doi: 10.1016/j.biomaterials.2008.04.010

27. Kubies D, Rypacek F, Kovarova J, Lednicky F (2000) Microdomain structure in polylactide-block-poly(ethylene oxide) copolymer films. Biomaterials 21: 529–536. doi: 10.1016/s0142-9612(99)00219-7

28. Kotek J, Kubies D, Baldrian J, Kovarova J (2011) Biodegradable polyester nanocomposites: The effect of structure on mechanical and degradation behavior. Eur Polym J 47: 2197–2207. doi: 10.1016/j.eurpolymj.2011.09.005

29. Rigby SP, Barwick D, Fletcher RS, Riley SN (2003) Interpreting mercury porosimetry data for catalyst supports using semi-empirical alternatives to the Washburn equation. Appl Catal A 238: 303–318. doi: 10.1016/s0926-860x(02)00348-4

30. Zhai W, Ko Y, Zhu W, Wong A, Park CB (2009) A study of the crystallization, melting, and foaming behaviors of polylactic acid in compressed CO_2. Int J Mol Sci 10: 5381–5397. doi: 10.3390/ijms10125381

31. Fernandez J, Etxeberria A, Sarasua JR (2012) Synthesis, structure and properties of poly(L-lactide-co-epsilon-caprolactone) statistical copolymers. J Mech Behav Biomed Mater 9: 100–112. doi: 10.1016/j.jmbbm.2012.01.003

32. Goh YQ, Ooi CP (2008) Fabrication and characterization of porous poly(L-lactide) scaffolds using solid-liquid phase separation. J Mater Sci Mater Med 19: 2445–2452. doi: 10.1007/s10856-008-3366-9

33. Guarino V, Guaccio A, Guarnieri D, Netti PA, Ambrosio L (2012) Binary system thermodynamics to control pore architecture of PCL scaffold via temperature-driven phase separation process. J Biomater Appl 27: 241–254. doi: 10.1177/0885328211401056

34. Bhardwaj R, Mohanty AK (2007) Modification of brittle polylactide by novel hyperbranched polymer-based nanostructures. Biomacromolecules 8: 2476–2484. doi: 10.1021/bm070367x

35. Chen JS, Tu SL, Tsay RY (2010) A morphological study of porous polylactide scaffolds prepared by thermally induced phase separation. J Taiwan Inst Chem Eng 41: 229–238. doi: 10.1016/j.jtice.2009.08.008

36. Hua FJ, Park TG, Lee DS (2003) A facile preparation of highly interconnected macroporous poly(D,L-lactic acid-co-glycolic acid) (PLGA) scaffolds by liquid-liquid phase separation of a PLGA-dioxane-water ternary system. Polymer 44: 1911–1920. doi: 10.1016/s0032-3861(03)00025-9

37. Beysens D, Jayalakshmi Y (1995) Kinetics of phase separation under a concentration gradient. Physica A 213: 71–89. doi: 10.1016/0378-4371(94)00149-n

38. Lacasta AM, Sancho JM, Yeung C (1994) Phase Separation Dynamics in a Concentration Gradient. Eur Phy Lett 27: 291. doi: 10.1209/0295-5075/27/4/007

39. Yang MC, Perng JS (1998) Effect of quenching temperature on the morphology and separation properties of polypropylene microporous tubular membranes via thermally induced phase separation. J Polym Res 5: 213–219. doi: 10.1007/s10965-006-0059-2

40. Kim J-W, Taki K, Nagamine S, Ohshima M (2008) Preparation of poly(L-lactic acid) honeycomb monolith structure by unidirectional freezing and freeze-drying. Chem Eng Sci 63: 3858–3863. doi: 10.1016/j.ces.2008.04.036

41. Zhu J, Chen L, Shen J (2001) Morphological evolution during phase separation and coarsening with strong inhomogeneous elasticity Model Simul Mater Sci Eng. 9: 499. doi: 10.1088/0965-0393/9/6/303

42. Pang YY, Dong X, Zhao Y, Han CC, Wang DJ (2011) Phase Separation Induced Morphology Evolution and Corresponding Impact Fracture Behavior of iPP/PEOc Blends. J Appl Polym Sci 121: 445–453. doi: 10.1002/app.33686

43. Wang H, Composto RJ (2000) Understanding morphology evolution and roughening in phase-separating thin-film polymer blends. Europhys Lett 50: 622–627. doi: 10.1209/epl/i2000-00315-2

44. Ravari F, Mashak A, Nekoomanesh M, Mobedi H (2013) Non-isothermal cold crystallization behavior and kinetics of poly(l-lactide): effect of l-lactide dimer. Polym Bull 70: 2569–2586. doi: 10.1007/s00289-013-0972-6

45. Nam YS, Park TG (1999) Biodegradable polymeric microcellular foams by modified thermally induced phase separation method. Biomaterials 20: 1783–1790. doi: 10.1016/s0142-9612(99)00073-3

46. Xiao L, Wang B, Yang G, Gauthier M (2012) Poly(Lactic Acid)-Based Biomaterials: Synthesis, Modification and Applications, Biomedical Science, Engineering and Technology, Dhanjoo N. Ghista (Ed.),. ISBN: 978-953-307-471-9, InTech, DOI: 10.5772/23927.

47. Silva MMCG, Cyster LA, Barry JJA, Yang XB, Oreffo ROC, et al. (2006) The effect of anisotropic architecture on cell and tissue infiltration into tissue engineering scaffolds. Biomaterials 27: 5909–5917. doi: 10.1016/j.biomaterials.2006.08.010

48. Jana S, Cooper A, Zhang M (2013) Chitosan scaffolds with unidirectional microtubular pores for large skeletal myotube generation. Adv Healthcare Mater 2: 557–561. doi: 10.1002/adhm.201200177

49. Sun C, Jin X, Holzwarth JM, Liu X, Hu J, et al. (2012) Development of channeled nanofibrous scaffolds for oriented tissue engineering. Macromol Biosci 12: 761–769. doi: 10.1002/mabi.201200004

50. Thirumaleshwar M (2009) Heat Transfer from Extended Surfaces FINS. In: Fundamentals of Heat and Mass Transfer. Pearson Education India. pp. 221–265.

51. Nagarani N, Mayilsamy K, Murugesan A, Kumar GS (2014) Review of utilization of extended surfaces in heat transfer problems. Renew Sust Energ Rev 29: 604–613. doi: 10.1016/j.rser.2013.08.068

Chapter 7

NEW BIOSORBENT MATERIALS: SELECTIVITY AND BIOENGINEERING INSIGHTS

George Z. Kyzas[1,2], Jie Fu[3], and Kostas A. Matis[1]

[1]Laboratory of General & Inorganic Chemical Technology, Department of Chemistry, Aristotle University of Thessaloniki, Thessaloniki GR 541 24, Greece

[2]Department of Petroleum and Natural Gas Technology, Technological Educational Institute of Kavala, Kavala GR 654 04, Greece

[3]Environmental Engineering Program, Department of Civil Engineering, Auburn University, Auburn, AL 36849, USA

ABSTRACT

Many researchers have studied the biosorption of different pollutants. However, a quite limited number of works focus on selectivity, which may be characterized as specific property for each biosorbent. Two main criteria need to be adopted for the selection and synthesis of modern biosorbents, such as their rebinding capacity and selectivity for only one target, molecule, ion, *etc.* Selective biosorption could be achieved using in synthesis an innovative technique termed molecular imprinting; the idea applied through specific polymers (Molecular Imprinted Polymers (MIPs)) was used in many fields, mainly analytical. In the present work, also isotherm and kinetic models were reviewed highlighting some crucial parameters, which possibly affect selectivity. A critical analysis of the biosorption insights for biosorbents, mostly selective, describes their characteristics, advantages and limitations, and discusses various bioengineering mechanisms involved.

INTRODUCTION

Worldwide environmental problems are becoming more and more acute. It is known, for example, that many specific industrial wastewater streams with large flows contain toxic metals in concentrations up to 500 mg/L, which have to be removed prior to water recycling, indirect discharge into the sewage system or direct discharge into surface waters [1]. When discharged directly into rivers, polluted wastewater poses a great risk to the aquatic ecosystem, whilst discharge into the sewage system negatively affects bio-sludge activity and leads to contamination of the excess sludge to be disposed of. As a result of the standards specified in the Water Resources Act, industry takes precautions against these risks by treating dangerous components in a partial stream, *i.e.*, before being mixed with other types of wastewater. For centuries, water has been a manufacturing tool that industry has taken for granted, because it is inexpensive and plentiful. However, population growth, globalization, and climate change are shepherding in a new water-constrained era. Good, clean water just cannot be replaced and it is becoming harder to come by [2].

Therefore, research was focused, among other things, on the development of highly selective bonding agents, including the biosorbents, with fast reaction kinetics for the removal of toxic substances. The latter may led to a better use of the capacity of the bonding agents, resulting in smaller units and low residual concentration of pollutants in the treated water streams, to comply with individual standards for water re-use or discharge. The ability of microorganisms to remove metal ions is a well-known phenomenon; biosorption was called the process that makes use of dead biomass (in comparison to bioaccumulation), a separation technique usually applied to fermentation wastes or byproducts. This process has been recently reviewed in depth [3]. Several biomass types were investigated, such as bacteria (*Streptomyces clavuligerus* or *Actinomycetes AK61/JL322*), yeast (*Saccharomyces cerevisiae* or *carlsbergensis*) fungi (*Penicillium Chrysogenum*), as well as biomass from a biological wastewater treatment plant after anaerobic digestion and grape stalks (a by-product of the winery industry).

As an example, the use of *Aeromonas caviae* biomass is given in the following (*i.e.*, in the kinetics study) for the removal of cadmium and/or chromate ions; this microorganism is a Gram-negative bacterium, isolated from raw water wells near Thessaloniki [4,5]. An advantage of the proposed operation is that its basic unit processes are rather conventional and widely applied in the field [6]. Biosorbents can be regenerated for multiple reuse, offering in addition and meanwhile the metal recovery possibility from concentrated wash solutions, *i.e.*, by electrochemical methods. Non-living biomass showed generally greater metal binding capacities than the respective living bacterium. From a comparison between biosorption and other metal separation methods, as filtration, centrifugation, *etc.*, it was found that in terms of the removal efficiency and applicability at lower (acidic) pH values, the former was favored [2,7]. In the latter, biosorption was studied for a mixture of copper, zinc and nickel.

A common feature in biotechnology is of course the presence of suspended particles, living or disrupted microorganisms (generally, having low density), which are difficult or time-consuming to remove by filtration and on the other hand, centrifugation is apparently more expensive. The possibility of applying downstream biomass flotation has been extensively reviewed in this volume; observed recoveries were reaching almost 100% [8]. The efficiency of combined "biosorptive flotation" process has been proved for the treatment of toxic metals' mixture, even when applying a multi-cycle biosorption-flotation operation [2]. A flowsheet of the proposed (two-stage countercurrent) biosorptive flotation process was presented [9].

The microbial biosorption of metals has attracted the interest of scientists as a treatment method, especially during the last two decades. Although the biological treatments are a removal process for some organic compounds, their products of biodegradation may also be hazardous [10].

SELECTIVITY

Generally, metal recovery or removal from solution may involve the following pathways: (i) The binding of metal cations to cell surfaces, or within the cell wall, where microprecipitation may enhance uptake; (ii) Translocation of the metal into the cell, possibly by active (metabolic energy dependent) transport; the active uptake or concentration of metal by living microbial cells; (iii) The formation of metal-containing precipitates, by reaction with extracellular polymers or microbially produced anions such as sulfide or phosphate ("bioprecipitation"); (iv) The volatilization of the metal by biotransformation— see Hughes and Poole [11]. The metal binding properties of Gram-positive bacteria, including the actinomycetes, according to Hancock [12] are largely due to specific anionic polymers in the cell wall structure.

Equilibrium and kinetic analyses classically lead to the appropriate rate expressions, characteristic of the possible reaction mechanism(s). The results of titration experiments suggested the presence of carboxylic and phosphate groups on the bacterial cell wall. These types of acidic sites can remove metallic ions, usually cations (cadmium), from aqueous solutions through the application of different mechanisms, such as cell surface sorption (complexation, surface precipitation *etc.*), as well as by extracellular and intracellular accumulation [13].

As for the removal of hexavalent chromium oxyanions (by *Aeromonas caviae*) at low pH values may be attributed to their attraction/affinity toward positively charged surface groups of biomass or reduction of Cr(VI) to Cr(III), followed by its bonding to the negatively charged biosorbent. The characterization of our biomass, *Aeromonas caviae*, including zeta-potential measurements, supports clearly this argument [5]. Thousand tons of residual biomass are produced each year from fermentation industries and also from biological wastewater treatment plants; hence, it could be considered as suitable biosorbents, perhaps with certain modification or treatment [14].

A selectivity factor "f" was defined [15], when considering two metals, A and B, as:

$$f = \frac{\left(C_A / C_B\right)_{biosorbed}}{\left(C_A / C_B\right)_{remaining}}$$

(1)

in order to describe the effectiveness of biosorption as a separation process, similar to the one used in ion exchange or solvent extraction processes. For the system Zn/Cd, where some selective separation was apparent, the value off reached around 40 in the pH range 8 to 9. Selectivity is of interest specifically if recovery of metals is sought from a mixture of metal ions, which most of the practical cases of wastes are. Selectivity was said to be a problem generally with biosorption systems, but this may be minimized depending on the relative concentrations of the various metals present [16].

As also discussed by Zouboulis *et al.* [7], the biosorption results for copper did worth mentioning, showing a selectivity of the process for copper; it is further noted that this selective separation was obtained in only one stage operation. A good explanation for that can be found in the literature [17].

A two cycles operation was attempted with alternative addition of dodecylamine surfactant; both the metals (copper, nickel, zinc) removal due to biosorption on (zetag-modified) *Streptomyces rimosus* industrial biomass, and also flotation behavior of the system, was investigated as a function of solution pH. Again a pronounced indication for possible selective recovery of copper (at a pH value of around 6.5) was observed [18].

The selective removal of Cu(II), Cr(III) and Ni(II) by strains of exopolysaccharide-producing cyanobacteria was assessed and the interaction of sorption in solutions with multiple-metals was investigated [19]. Experimental results elsewhere indicated that the uptake capacity and biosorption yield of one metal ion were reduced by the presence of the other metal ion; the selectivity order of $Pb^{2+} > Cu^{2+} > Zn^{2+}$ was found [20]. Although biosorption for reclaiming single precious metal was frequently reported, the actual subsistent adsorptive competition among different metal ions sometimes shows diverging reinforcement or prohibition for different species. Another study tried to screen bacteria that are able to absorb certain precious metals with high selectivity under competitive conditions. For binary metal system, the adsorption parameters of extended-Langmuir model were modified by introducing a selectivity factor of the solute [21].

A mass action law was able to predict the ion exchange equilibrium with Na-loaded algae, considering a ternary system $Na^+/H^+/Cd^{2+}$ or $Na^+/H^+/Pb^{2+}$ [22]. The selectivity coefficients of the Na-loaded algae increases in the following order: $Na^+ < H^+ < Cd^{2+} < Pb^{2+}$, which indicates that carboxylic and sulfonic groups have a higher preference (affinity) to Pb^{2+}, followed by Cd^{2+}, H^+ and Na^+. The higher affinity of lead ion to sulfonic groups was attributed to the hard and soft acid and base theory. A mass transfer model, considering that the ion exchange limiting step is the intraparticle ion diffusion, was then able to fit the concentration profile of all ionic species at the liquid and solid phases.

Adsorption behaviors of non-conventional and cost-effective adsorbent prepared from orange waste has been investigated for various metal ions [23]. Separation factors for Fe(III) and Zr(IV) over Zn(II) at around pH 2, derived from individual adsorption isotherm by fitting a linear curve, suggested that there was an excellent selectivity for transition metals over alkaline/alkaline earths. The selectivity of a bio-based dithiocarbamate modified chitosan, using Pb(II) as imprinted ions and the non-imprinted beads for lead ions over other metal ions were evaluated from the selectivity coefficient, defined as the ratio of the distribution ratios of the Pb(II) ions and other coexistent metal ions [24]. Cross-linked imprinted chitosan polymer has been recently prepared from chitosan, using citric acid-cadmium complex as template and glutaraldehyde as the cross-linker [25]. Therefore, this may explain the following attempt and proposal.

MIPs as Alternative Biosorbent Candidates

One of the hot topics of recent research is the reuse of some compounds existed as pollutants in environment. These compounds (molecules, ions, complexes, *etc.*) are of high-added value and it will be ideal to selectively bind them with any environmental application and reuse them in their initial or modified form. The latter could be achieved using selective biosorbents with a special technique, which is called molecular recognition. Molecular recognition is realized with molecular imprinting which is an emerging technique to create high affinity polymeric matrices (MIPs) for target molecules. Many papers in literature refer monomers (or their derivatives) used in molecular imprinting. Detailed studies (as that of Mayes and Whitcombe) presents especially those used in non-covalent technique [26]. Some of the widely used monomers are: (i) methacrylic acid or acrylic acid; (ii) 4-vynilpyridine; (iii) diethylaminoethyl methacrylate; (iv) acrylamides; (v) 2-hydroxyethyl methacrylate; (vi) acrylamide, *etc.* The other crucial reagent in MIP preparation is the cross-linker which samely presents variety. There are the acrylated-based cross-linkers (ethyleneglycol dimethacrylate, trimethylolpropane trimethacrylate, *etc.*), those which are structurally based on styrene and its derivatives (*i.e.*, divinylbenzene), and those which are soluble in water (ethylenebisacrylamide).

Molecular recognition is a process occurred everywhere. We can call that molecular recognition exists when two molecules has the spatially same geometry but each molecule can selectively interact with only one functional site [27]. Therefore, a specific technology has been bloomed and re-designed in the last 40 years, called molecular imprinting (MI). The whole process is based on adsorption technology, which is already one of the most successful techniques for pollutants removal [28,29,30,31,32,33,34].

MI is not a recent science. The first track of imprinting was recorded in 1930 from Polyakov [35]. His target was to prepare silica gels (not only one but a series of those). Finally, he understood that the silica prepared showed selective capacity (binding) for a particular solvent in which the synthesis has been done. In 1955, a senior student of Linus Pauling, Frank Dickey, observed that after the removal of "patterning" dye the silica would re-bind the same dye in preference to the others [36]. However, in 1972, a step change in molecular imprinting occurred when the group of Wulff reported that they had successfully prepared a molecularly imprinting organic polymer (MIP) [37], using what is now termed a "covalent approach", to prepare an organic molecularly imprinted polymer capable of discriminating between the enantiomers of glyceric acid. The technique, which is widely used for MIP preparation, is based on reactions of condensation that can be characterized as reversible. Characteristic examples are the use of (i) boronate ester [38]; (ii) ketal/acetal [39]; (iii) formation of Schiff's base [40], in order to synthesize different combinations between templates and monomers. In more recent decades (1970s and 1980s), the research group of Wulff used this technique/approach with different templates and prepared numerous specialized MIPs.

The second major breakthrough in organic polymer imprinting occurred in 1981 when Arshady and Mosbach reported that they had prepared an organic MIP using non-covalent interactions only [41]. This approach was termed the "non-covalent approach", as opposed to the covalent approach favored by Wulff, and it was this, with its simple, seemingly trivial methodology that triggered the explosion in molecular imprinting, occurring during the 1990s. Contrarily, the non-covalent technique is based on some attractive bonds among the molecules (hydrogen bonding, ion-pairs, forces of dipole-dipole, van der Waals bonds). All the aforementioned forces produce and stabilize the template molecule and the monomer (after selection) in the solution (solvent). The basic difference between covalent and non-covalent technique is that in latter the additives are not stable during the imprinting process. To this day, the non-covalent *versus* covalent debate continues with both sides being championed. However, it is generally accepted that there are pros and cons to both approaches. Therefore, in 1995, Whitcombe reported an intermediate approach that combine the advantages of both [42]. Importantly, in order to improve subsequent non-covalent binding geometry, Whitcombe's approach incorporated a sacrificial spacer group that was designed to be lost during template removal. The non-covalent approach however is still by far the most widely used approach in MIP synthesis. Several of its drawbacks can be overcome by the use of stoichiometrically associating monomer-template systems [43]. This has resulted in a range of receptors exhibiting high capacity and effective recognition properties in aqueous media.

It is interesting to prepare/design materials, which only selectively remove carcinogenic pollutants from wastewaters, as ions, phenols and drugs/pharmaceuticals. Nowadays, MIPs are designed in such way in order to be stable in extreme conditions (pH *etc.*). Therefore, a high cross-linking is required. Another interesting point is the turn of researchers on the more environmental-based application. To achieve this, a high selectivity is required to bind only the templates, employed in separation processes of environmental pollutants (chromatography, solid-phase extraction, membrane separations, adsorption), artificial antibodies and sensors recognition elements [40]. Many examples of template molecules have been reported; mention can be given in environmental targets as dyes (see Figure 1), ions, metals, drugs, phenols, *etc.*

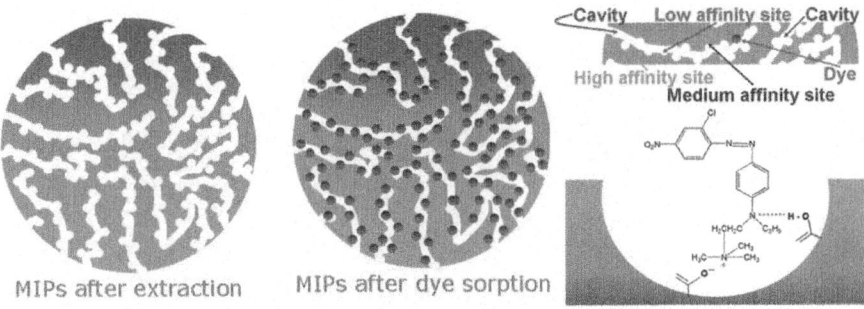

MIPs after extraction   MIPs after dye sorption

Figure 1. Example for the synthesis of Molecular Imprinted Polymers (MIPs) for capturing/binding dye molecules.

The simplicity of use, the relatively low cost and the broad range of possible guest molecules (small organic molecules, ions but also biological macro-molecules) have since led to the important development of this technique, as illustrated by the increasing numbers of publications over recent years. This review aims to gather and report the bioengineering insights regarding the rebinding (adsorption) using MIPs along with discussion for the importance of the models for fitting.

Limitations

The engineering part is based on the selection of the suitable model for fitting of rebinding experiments either of equilibrium (isotherms) or kinetics. However, similarly as in the case of all biosorbents, each system of MIP (adsorbent) and target molecule (adsorbate) is unique. Modifying the conditions in polymer "cookery" (synthesis/polymerization, cross-linking, template extraction), the product will be completely different. The latter can be confirmed with scanning electron micrographs (SEM) of the prepared MIPs. For example, a recent study investigated the synthesis for selectively binding dyes, but having obvious surface changes due to the different solvent used (organic or aqueous) (Figure 2).

An important parameter regarding the possible porosity of MIPs is the solvent [45]. The type of solvent (or else "porogen") demonstrates some morphological properties of porosity and surface area. There are two possible cases: (i) the use of solvents with low solubility phase, which can be rapidly separated and give adequate large pores, but MIPs with lower surface areas; (ii) the use of solvents with high solubility phase, which can be separated later and give smaller pore size distributions, but MIPs with higher surface area. It does not appear, however, that binding and selectivity in MIPs is dependent on a particular porosity.

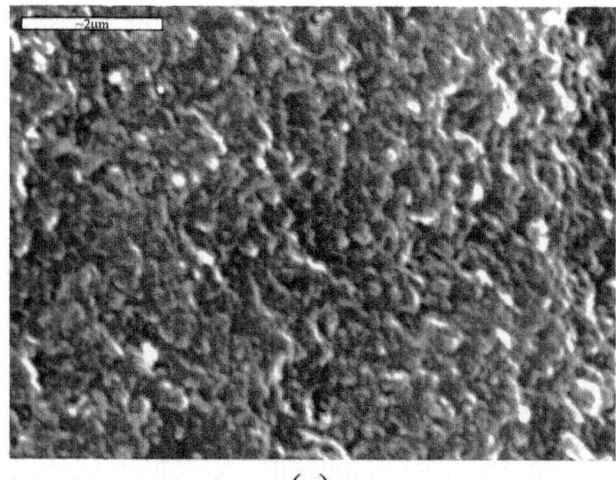

(a)

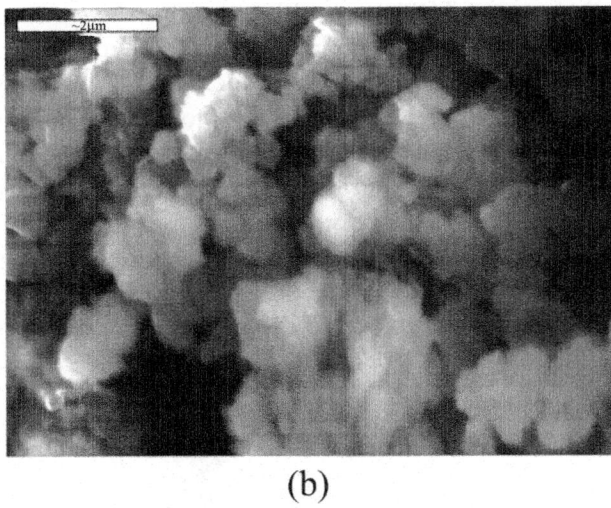

(b)

Figure 2. SEM micrographs of dye-MIPs using (**a**) aqueous and (**b**) organic solvent. Reproduced with permission from George Z. Kyzas [44], published by Elsevier, 2009.

In fact, optimum results are often obtained when chloroform is used. In this case, the polymers prepared did not present adequate porosity or surface area (BET measurements), they were highly solvated and MIPs made without any porogen did not exhibit any selectivity, because substrate could not access the polymer. Thus, diffusion of substrates through the MIP appears to be fast enough through the chloroform solvated polymers without requiring porosity. Therefore, there is no big chance to repeat the data of literature. Researchers have understood the latter and studied uniquely each system of MIPs and for this reason, they have tested many isotherm models to predict the affinity or theoretical capacity of MIPs.

Apart from the synthesis limitations, as described above, another crucial factor which influences the engineering behavior of MIPs is the limitations during extraction of template molecules from the polymeric matrix, after synthesis. A 100% removal of the template was not achievable despite sequential attempts, using mainly Soxhlet apparatus. The latter is presented because some regions of MIP are highly cross-linked and therefore, the insertion/accessibility to them is limited. Another possible scenario is that in many cases, the template molecule does not present enough solubility in the porogen and therefore, cannot participate in interactions with the cavity of MIP [46,47]. The results from the above are not simple: (i) the most possible is a reduction of the total number of cavities suitable for rebinding (Figure 3); (ii) the template can be "escaped" during the last step of elution mainly in MIPs used in columns for solid phase extraction [48] or during analysis [49].

Even in the case of MIPs prepared with non-covalent or self-assembly technique, the binding of the template to the components of the imprinted cavity can be so strong that extraction under drastic conditions is required [51]. Extreme pH or temperature applied for a long time can lead to distortion and even rupture of the cavity during removal, resulting in MIPs of poor selectivity and recovery [46]. Furthermore, changes in the degree of swelling of the MIP network during extraction and subsequent desiccation can result in the collapse of the cavity, sterically hindering the entrance of target molecule, or in a distortion of the binding points or the strength of interactions [52,53].

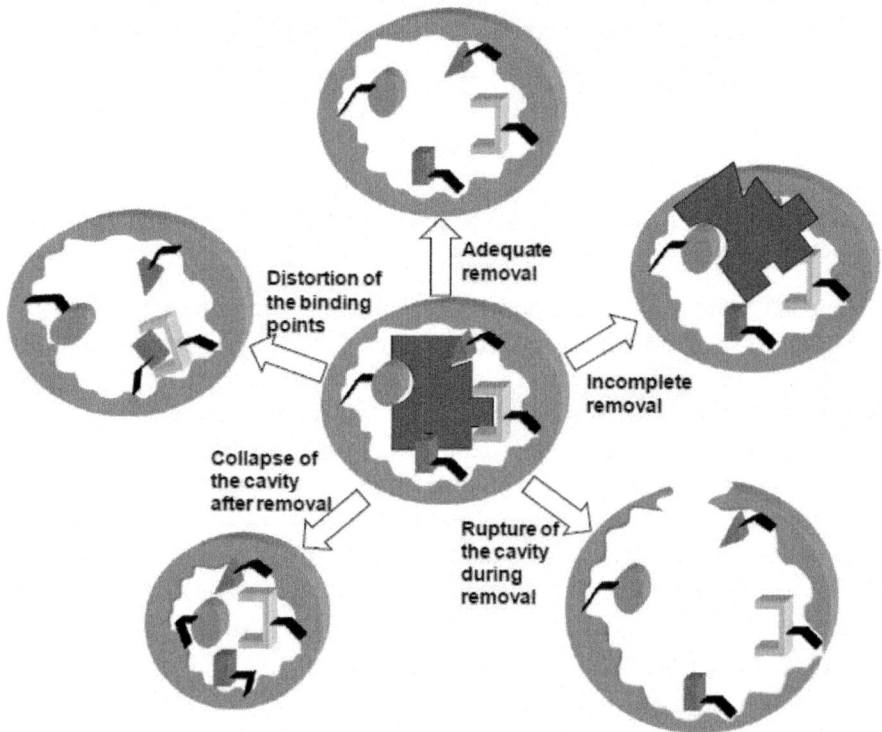

Figure 3. Example for the synthesis of MIP for capturing/binding dye molecules. Reproduced with permission from Rosa A. Lorenzo [50], published by MDPI AG, 2011.

One of the key assumptions in the analysis of binding data is that these are gathered after equilibrium between the template and the imprinted polymer is reached. Usually, this is accomplished by serial incubation of a known amount of imprinted polymer with different concentrations of the template during a specified period of time, necessary to reach equilibrium. The incubation time for most assays is the time required for 90% of the template to bind.

ISOTHERM MODELS

Studies of biosorbents contain mainly factors such as: (i) the isotherm models and (ii) the affinity distribution analysis (selectivity). An adsorption isotherm is a measure of the relationship between the equilibrium concentrations of bound and free guest over a certain concentration range and is readily generated from equilibrium batch rebinding studies or chromatographic frontal-zone analysis. Binding properties can be calculated from the binding isotherm by fitting the adsorption. It is a fact that the main theories are the same compared to the commonly-used biosorbents. However, some changes in the symbols and the physical meanings differentiate the models and give other potential to the whole engineering part. Models are used everywhere for simulating any possible process [54,55,56,57,58,59,60,61,62,63,64,65,66]. The main models, which will be discussed in following, are the Freundlich, Langmuir, and Langmuir-Freundlich (L-F) equations. In general, the model chosen to explain the particular performance of a biosorbent is the simplest and most statistically significant. For example, if the data fit a model with three different binding sites better than a model with one or two kind of binding sites, the three-binding site model is often chosen, unless other independent data suggest using a different model (tetra-modal, exponential, *etc.*). Before accepting a given n-site fit it is advisable to test whether the improvement is statistically significant.

The Freundlich isotherm is an empirical power function for non-ideal sorption on heterogeneous surfaces as well as for multilayer sorption and is expressed by the equation:

$$B = aC^m \tag{2}$$

where B is the amount of adsorbed pollutant at equilibrium; a is the Freundlich adsorption coefficient (related with the adsorption capacity (N_t) and the average affinity(K_0)); m is the Freundlich constant which represents the heterogeneity index and varies from zero to one (values approaching to zero indicate increasingly heterogeneity and one being homogeneous); C is the equilibrium concentration of template. The term B in Equation (2) was calculated from the simple mass balance equation as follows:

$$B = \frac{(C_0 - C)V}{M} \tag{3}$$

where C_0 is the initial pollutant concentration, C is the pollutant concentration at equilibrium, V is the volume of and M is the mass of biosorbent. The linearized form of Equation (2) was obtained by taking log on both sides:

$$\log(B) = \log(a) + m \cdot \log(C)$$

(4)

therefore, the plot of log(B) *versus* log(C) was employed to generate the intercept value of a and the slope of m. The Freundlich equation has been derived by assuming an exponentially decaying adsorption site energy distribution.

The data given by this model can be explained, in most cases, taking into account that the Freundlich model is a generalization of the Langmuir model applied to a heterogeneous surface with an energy distribution corresponding to an exponential decrease. Although the Freundlich model predicts that there is an indefinite increase of the adsorbed solute increasing its concentration in solution, this empirical equation is suitable for highly heterogeneous surfaces [67,68,69,70] and often represents typical adsorption data over a restricted range of concentration. In spite that the Freundlich isotherm is suitable to describe the dependence between the coverage degree (θ) and the adsorption energy, it does not follow the fundamental thermodynamic basis since it does not reduce to Henry's law at lower concentrations nor predicts the monolayer saturation at higher concentrations. Even so, several methods have been developed in order to estimate the exponential distribution of the isotherm.

On the other hand, the Langmuir sorption isotherm assumes that adsorption takes place at specific homogeneous sites within the material. The isotherm equation is derived from simple mass action kinetics, assuming chemisorption. Also, it assumes that once a template occupies a site, no further adsorption can take place at that site, all sites are energetically equivalent and there is no interaction between molecules adsorbed on neighboring sites. A saturation value should be reached beyond which no further sorption can take place.

While the Langmuir model assumes that there is only a single class of binding sites, the bi-Langmuir model assumes that there are two classes of sites within the imprinted material. It is straightforward to implement the Langmuir and bi-Langmuir models using Scatchard plots to determine the binding parameters, the binding affinity (K) and the number of binding sites (N_t), using the general expression:

$$\frac{B}{C} = KN_t - KB$$

(5)

where B is the amount of adsorbed pollutant at equilibrium; N_t is the total number of accessible adsorption sites; C is the equilibrium concentration of template; K is the Langmuir isotherm equilibrium constant.

In homogeneous systems with only one type of binding sites, by plotting B/C against B, it is possible to obtain the value of N from the x-intercept and the value of K from the slope. In heterogeneous systems, Scatchard plots are not linear and the simplest model in this case is a material with two different kinds of adsorption sites. Langmuir equation is then extended to an equation with two Langmuir terms (bi-Langmuir equation):

$$B = \frac{N_1 K_1 C_1}{1 + K_1 C_1} + \frac{N_2 K_2 C_2}{1 + K_2 C_2} \tag{6}$$

Thus, the plot B/C *versus* B is composed of two straight lines, from which two sets of binding parameters (K_1, N_1 and K_2, N_2) for the two classes of binding sites within the imprinted polymer can be obtained. The steeper line corresponds to the high-affinity sites while the flatter line measured the low-affinity ones.

Furthermore, another isotherm model can be used which is the combination of Langmuir and Freundlich equations namely Langmuir-Freundlich (L-F) isotherm. This model, first described by Sips [71,72] was introduced for the biosorbents by the groups of Shimizu *et al.* [69,70,73] and Guiochon *et al.* [74,75,76]. The model describes an equilibrium relationship between the concentration of a bound template (B) and the equilibrium template concentration in solution (C) such that (where N_t is the total number of binding sites and K_0 is the median binding affinity):

$$B = \frac{N_t K_0^m C^m}{1 + K_0^m C^m} \tag{7}$$

The variable a is related to K_0 via $K_0 = a^{1/m}$. The fitting parameter "m" is identical to the heterogeneity index of site energies from the Freundlich isotherm. The difference between the L-F model and the Freundlich one is evident at high adsorbate concentrations, for which the L-F model is able to represent the saturation behavior. At low adsorbate concentrations, the L-F equation reduces to the classical Freundlich equation. On the other hand, as m approaches unity, indicative of a completely homogeneous adsorbent surface (*i.e.*, energetic equivalence of all binding sites) the L-F equation reduces to the classical Langmuir equation. Thus, the hybridised L-F isotherm is able to model adsorption of solutes at high and low concentrations onto homogeneous and heterogeneous biosorbents. Although a linear analysis is not possible for a three-parameter isotherm, the L-F isotherm can be fitted to the experimental data following the method of Shimizu *et al.*[4,5] in which a solver function may be used to maximize the coefficient of determination (R^2) by iteratively varying the three fitting parameters N_t, a and m. R^2 is calculated from the sum of residuals (*i.e.*, the difference between the experimental model and model-predicted bound concentrations).

Linear regression is frequently used to determine the most fitted isotherm for two-parameter isotherms. The idea is to transform the data to create a linear graph and use the method of least squares to find the parameters of the isotherm. Examples include Scatchard plots of binding data [70,77,78] and linearized forms of Freundlich and Langmuir equations [69,75,79,80]. It is very common to express the isotherm models in linear form. A drawback resulting from linearization ($y = a + bx$) is that some assumptions of linear regression are violated. In particular, the analysis of linear regression shows that the experimental data/points located around the fitting line has a Gaussian trend regarding their distribution. Furthermore, for each value of x, the analysis with standard deviation is the same. Also, in some transformations, the relationship between x and y are altered. For example, when a Scatchard plot is created, the measured value of bound template winds up on both the x-axis (which plots bound) and the y-axis (which plots bound/free). In spite of these drawbacks, linearizing methods are a good starting point for generating initial values for non-linear regression.

Examples

Some characteristic examples of literature will be given below. It is interesting that in many cases the adsorption results were fitted in two or more models comparing the fitting parameters. Tsai and Syu [81] studied the preparation of MIP-poly(4-vinylpyridine-co-divinylbenzene) (poly(4-VP-co-DVB)) as the specific receptor of creatinine by heated polymerization. The monomer used in that case was 4-Vinylpyridine. The other reagents for synthesis were creatinine (template) and divinylbenzene (cross-linker). The equilibrium rebinding data were fitted using Langmuir equation and gave 11.95 mg/g maximum theoretical capacity.

Milojkovic *et al.* [82] developed a novel synthesis procedure for MIPs. The polymerization was initiated by γ-radiation, but using as template molecule (±)-menthol. The evaluation of the adsorption results were done comparing the isotherms camphor (model molecule for testing) and menthol from *n*-hexane. The results isotherms seemed to be as those of Langmuir.

Hsu *et al.* [83] prepared a molecularly imprinted polymer of morphine was prepared through thermal radical copolymerization of methacrylic acid and ethylene glycol dimethacrylate. A MIP assay was also synthesized (using mainly colorimetric reporter) was in order to observe and record the adsorption isotherm of morphine imprinted polymer binding. The adsorption isotherms fitted to Langmuir equation.

Baggiani and co-workers [84] investigated the adsorption isotherms of polymers prepared by imprinting them with 2,4,5-trichlorophenoxyacetic acid (2,4,5-T). The polymers were prepared by thermoinduced polymerization of template mixtures, 4-vinylpyridine and ethylene dimethacrylate. The experimental adsorption isotherms were fitted by using several isotherm models, and the L-F model was found to give the best fitting.

Sajonz *et al.* [75] studied the adsorption isotherms of d- and l-phenylalanine anilide (PA) on an l-phenylalanine anilide imprinted stationary phase have been determined using staircase frontal analysis. It was found that the adsorption data fit well to both the Freundlich and the Bi-Langmuir isotherm models. Examination of the best values of the numerical coefficients of the Bi-Langmuir model shows that the site class representing the binding sites with the highest binding energy exhibits a very low saturation capacity for the non-imprinted enantiomer, indicating a high selectivity for the imprinted l-enantiomer.

Hwang and Lee [85] synthesized cholesterol-imprinted polymers in bulk polymerization by the methods of covalent and non-covalent imprinting. For the covalent imprinting, the combination of template/monomer was cholesteryl (4-vinyl)phenyl carbonate, while for the non-covalent imprinting the respective combination was methacrylic acid or 4-vinylpyridine. The equilibrium data were successfully fitted to L-F model.

Lehmann *et al.* [86] investigated the binding of l-Boc-phenylalanine anilide (BFA) and l-Boc-phenylalanine (phe) to molecularly imprinted and non-imprinted polymer nanoparticles consisting of poly[(ethylene glycol) dimethacrylate)-co-(methacrylic acid)] by adsorption experiments and mathematical modeling. The isotherms have been fitted using the Freundlich, L-F, bi-Langmuir, Langmuir and extended Langmuir model.

AFFINITY DISTRIBUTION ANALYSIS

A property of sorbents that has limited their wider applicability is their heterogeneity. The drawback, for instance, of the MIP technique is its low fidelity, which increases the distribution of association constants [87]. Therefore, a first target the improvement of heterogeneity and change the so-called distribution in higher affinity sites. The majority of papers face the MIPs with homogeneity. Their surfaces are homogeneous where all functional sites can be estimated as one (Langmuir model) or two (bi-Langmuir model) general classes [88,89]. Therefore, we cannot base on these models in order to compare the possible changes of distributions. A possible solution for the latter is the analysis of limiting slopes according to scatchard plots, which can be characterized as type of bi-Langmuir equation [90]. Hence, the comparison of binding properties of different or even of the same MIP by homogeneous models is difficult [78].

Umpleby and co-workers [69] beginning from the Freundlich equation (Equation (2)), express the affinity distribution, calculating the total number of binding sites (N) (Equation (8)):

$$N = \int_{\ln K_{min}}^{\ln K_{max}} N(K_i)d(\ln K) = \frac{K_{fr}\sin(\pi n)}{\pi}(K_{min}^{-n} - K_{max}^{-n})$$

(8)

To find the number average binding constant (for a specified range of $K_{min} - K_{max}$), the sum of all sites N_i multiplied by the corresponding affinity constant, K_i, is divided by the sum of N_i, which is the total number of sites N Equation (9):

$$\sum N_i K_i / \sum N_i = \sum N_i K_i / N$$

(9)

The term $\sum N_i K_i$ of the Equation (8) can be shifted using the integration of the number of binding sites with its corresponding association constant each time. When this is divided by the number of binding sites N from Equation (10), the number average association constant (K_{av}) is obtained.

$$K_{av} = \frac{\int_{\ln K_{min}}^{\ln K_{max}} N(K_i)K_i d(\ln K)}{\int_{\ln K_{min}}^{\ln K_{max}} N(K_i)d(\ln K)}$$

(10)

After substitution and followed by integration, we get the following solution for the number average association constant (Equation (11)):

$$K_{av} = \left(\frac{n}{1-n}\right)\frac{\left(K_{max}^{1-n} - K_{min}^{1-n}\right)}{\left(K_{min}^{-n} - K_{max}^n\right)}$$

(11)

From Equation (11), the number average association constant can be calculated using a binding isotherm that is modeled by the Freundlich equation (Equation (2)).

KINETICS

The process is describing, by definition, the attachment of charged species (like the toxic metal ions) from a solution to a coexisting biosolid surface. Kinetics may be controlled by several independent processes that can act in series or in parallel. These sorption (a general term) processes fall in one of the following general categories: (i) bulk diffusion; (ii) external mass transfer (film diffusion); (iii) chemical reaction (chemisorption) and (iv) intraparticle diffusion. Kinetic analyses not only allow estimation of sorption rates but also lead to suitable rate expressions characteristic of possible reaction mechanisms [91].

Many studies engaged so far to examine sorption phenomena involved analysis of batch experiments where data were sampled at even time intervals over the entire course of the process. As a result, fast changing kinetic data characteristic of the phenomena just after the onset of sorption could not be accurately depicted in an adequately short time scale. The model selection criteria proposed by Ho et al. concerning sorption of pollutants in aqueous systems were used herein, as a guideline [92].

For equilibrium and kinetic modeling, usually an overall mass balance of the sorbate across the biosorbent surface is initially written. The used example below deals with an investigation of the removal and depletion of cadmium and chromates from aqueous solutions by biosorption on *Aeromonas cavia*; this microorganism is often present in groundwater and general in aquatic environments. From the data, evidence was provided that the examined system was a complex process. More than one sorption models were often reported to describe correctly a case study [93].

From the chemical reaction category (chemisorption), the best fit for the data sets of this study is achieved by 2nd order-type chemical reactions [94]. The solution of the standard 2nd order reaction based on a constant stoichiometry of one metal ion per binding site is:

$$C_t = \frac{C_0}{1 - \left(\dfrac{C_0}{C_e}\right)\exp\left(-k_1 C_e t\right)}$$

(12)

where k_1 is the reaction rate constant [L × (mg^{-1} of metal) × min^{-1}]; C is the metal bulk concentration (mg·L^{-1}). Subscripts 0 and t denote conditions at the beginning and any other instant (time, t) of the process, respectively; and the subscript e denotes equilibrium conditions.

This adsorption model has been very effective in describing the kinetics of adsorption of gases on solids. Nevertheless, when the data were plotted as a figure, it was shown that Equation (12) clearly fails to capture the steep concentration gradient of the early removal stage. This was a direct indication that adsorption on solids from a liquid phase is a different process than adsorption from a gas phase where traditionally the remaining bulk concentration dictates the kinetics.

If the rate of sorption depends not on bulk concentration but on uptake by the sorbent this can be described by the so-called Ritchie 2nd order equation according to which one metal ion occupies two binding sites [95]:

$$q_t = q_e \left(1 - \left(\frac{1}{1 + k_2 t} \right) \right)$$

(13)

where q is the specific metal uptake (mg of metal per g of sorbent) and k_2 is the reaction rate constant (min^{-1}). When in the above treatment it is not necessarily q_e to dictate the sorbate uptake then a pseudo 2nd order rate expression is more appropriate:

$$\frac{t}{q_t} = \frac{1}{k_m q_m^{\,2}} + \left(\frac{1}{q_m} \right) t$$

(14)

where k_m is the reaction rate constant [g of sorbent $\times$ (mg^{-1} of metal) $\times$ min^{-1}] and q_m is a numerically determined parameter which under ideal 2nd order rate control corresponds to q_e. It is noted that in the literature [92] various other kinetic equations have been attempted: zero, first (forward or reversible) order, Langmuir-Hinshelwood, Elovich-type, etc.

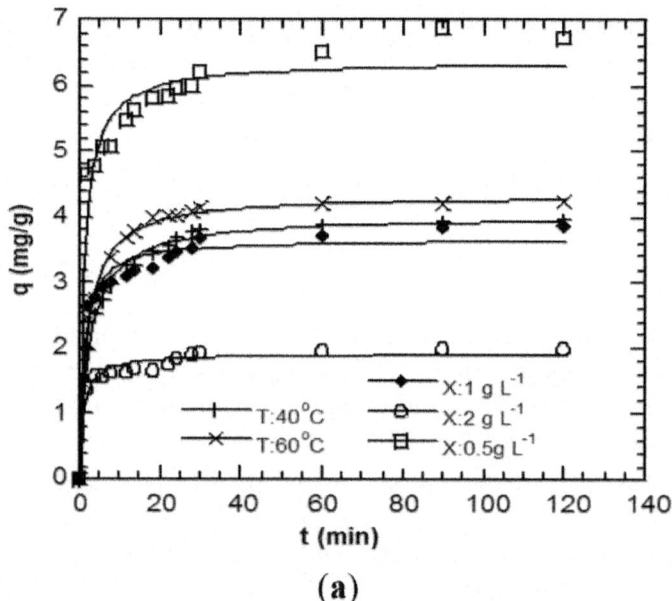

(a)

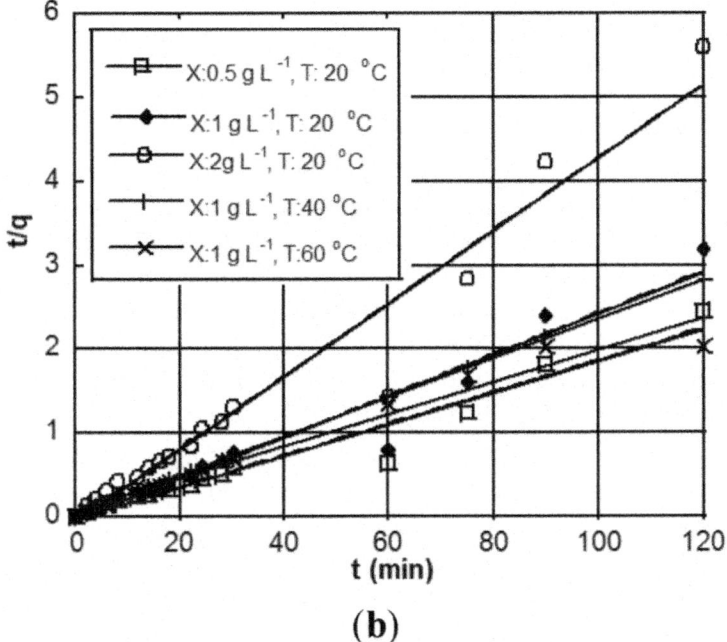

(b)

Figure 4. Comparison of experimental removal curves against theoretical predictions based: **(a)** on the Ritchie 2nd order equation (at initial cadmium concentration of 5 mg·L⁻¹) and **(b)** on the pseudo 2nd order equation (at initial cadmium concentration of 50 mg·L⁻¹). Reprinted with permission from reference [94]; copyright (2005) Taylor & Francis.

Equations (13) and (14) provided a quite suitable description of data for advancing time (see Figure 4). It is noteworthy that both models adequately capture the rapid rate of adsorption during the first minutes of the experiments. This already implies that the metal uptake by the sorbent is a satisfactory rate-controlling parameter under a 2nd order reaction mechanism.

For intraparticle diffusion, Crank [96] proposed a model, which takes into account the continuously decreasing bulk concentration due to sorbate removal. This gives rise to a time dependent boundary condition for the concentration at the surface of the sorbent particle. The solution of the diffusion equation for such a boundary condition and a concentration independent diffusivity is:

$$\alpha = 1 - 6 \sum_{n=1}^{\infty} \frac{exp\left(-\xi p_n^2 t\right)}{9\Lambda/\left(1-\Lambda\right) + \left(1-\Lambda\right) p_n^2} \tag{15}$$

where p_n is given by the non-zero roots of

$$\tan(p_n) = \frac{3p_n}{3 + p_n^2/(1-\Lambda)}$$

(16)

and $\Lambda \equiv (C_0 - C_\infty)/C_0$ is the fraction of metal ultimately adsorbed by the sorbent.

Equation (15) can be solved numerically to determine ξ, the effective diffusional time constant, which for the case of particle (also called micropore) diffusion control equals to D_c/R_c^2, D_c and R_c being the intraparticle diffusion coefficient (m²·s⁻¹) and mean particle radius (m), respectively. The same expression is the solution of the diffusion equation for a (macro) pore diffusion control but only in cases where the equilibrium isotherm is linear for the concentration range under investigation.

External mass transfer has been customary analyzed in literature by adopting a pseudo first-order reaction model [97]. This approach tacitly assumes that the sorbate concentration at the sorbent surface is zero at all times. However, this is not true particularly in cases where a significant quantity of sorbate is adsorbed rapidly at the beginning of the process. A more realistic model should consider instead a rapid equilibrium being established between the sorbate at the interface and that present on the sorbent surface [98] and this concept has been adopted.

If one combines the mass balance across the sorbent surface, the Langmuir adsorption isotherm and the rate equation of change in the bulk concentration one ends up after some algebra with:

$$\frac{dC_t}{dt} = -K_m S \left(C_t - C_t^s \right)$$

(17)

$$\frac{dC_t^s}{dt} = \left(\frac{K_m S}{X q_{max} b} \right) \left[\left(C_t - C_t^s \right) \left(1 + b C_t^s \right)^2 \right]$$

(18)

where K_m is the external mass transfer coefficient (m·s⁻¹), S is the specific surface area of the sorbent particles per unit volume of the reactor (m²·m⁻³) and X is the sorbent feeding per unit volume of solution (g·L⁻¹); dimensionless variables could be also used. The conversion a system of two first-order ordinary differential equations that must be solved simultaneously [99]. The values of Λ, ξ and the computed values of D_c (being the intraparticle diffusion coefficient, $m^2 \cdot s^{-1}$) were displayed in the form of a table.

Equations (15)–(16) and (17)–(18) were solved numerically to determine ξ and $K_m S$, respectively. The non-linear numerical regression to fit experimental data to those equations is performed by the Levenberg-Marquardt method, which gradually shifts the search for the minimum of the sum of the errors squared, from steepest descent to quadratic minimization—i.e., Gauss-Newton [100]. Figure 5a presents the results of fitting Equation (15) to biosorption data obtained with different initial concentrations, solids loads and temperatures. It is apparent that despite some scatter in measurements the finite volume diffusion model can describe fairly well the entire range of data, including also the steep concentration gradient at short times. Such behavior has been customary met as a consequence of the decreasing slope of a non-linear equilibrium curve, e.g., Langmuir isotherm, which causes the diffusivity to increase rapidly with increasing concentration [93].

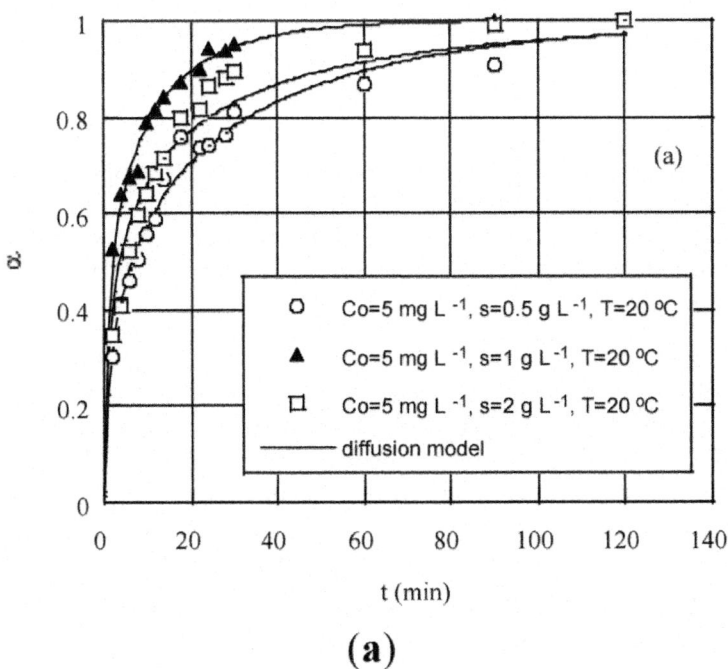

(a)

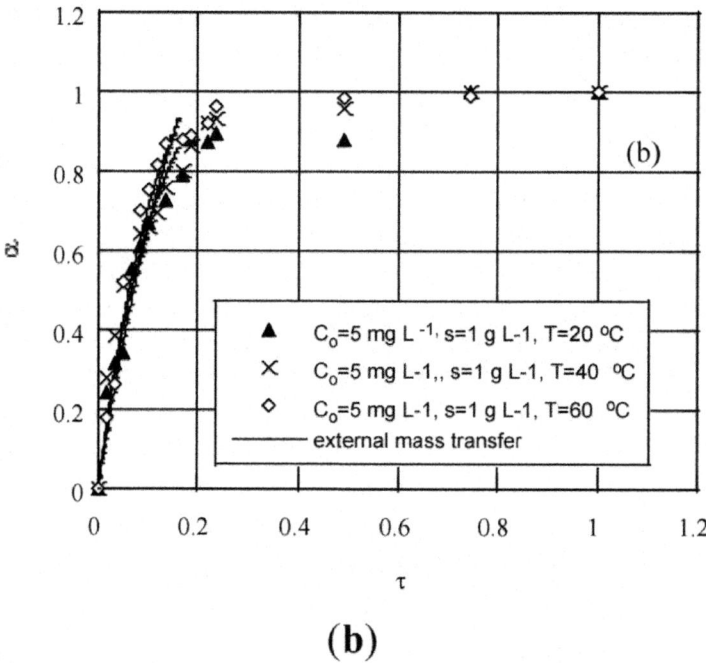

(b)

Figure 5. Experimental degree of conversion, α, against predictions based on the solution of the: **(a)** diffusion equation, for various adsorbent loads and **(b)** mass transfer equation, for various temperatures (both at initial chromium concentration of 5 mg·L^{-1}). Reprinted with permission from Ref. [99]; copyright (2004) American Chemical Society.

A way to check further on the possibility of a pore diffusion-controlled mechanism is to perform desorption kinetic tests with adsorbent previously used for sorption. For the case of a non-porous sorbent particle, transport of solute inside the particle may be neglected and it can be assumed that biosorption occurs mainly at the particle surface. This idea can be effectively extended to cases of relatively large macropores, where the metal ions may have a ready access to react with internal surface sites.

It was argued that at the beginning of the process that chromium is sorbed according to a quite fast and highly favorable chemical mechanism, such as ion-exchange, but soon external film diffusion comes into play. By this account, if one ignores the very first minute of sorption, the remaining curves were fitted pretty well by the model Equations (17) and (18). Figure 5b displays these results. Near the end of sorption a much slower process, e.g., intraparticle diffusion, becomes gradually the rate-controlling step. Yet, this is a regime of no practical significance [91,101]. Rather contradictory indications on the subject were pointed out [3].

CONCLUSIONS

The engineering of selective biosorbents is characterized as rather chaotic by many researchers given the number of assumptions and scenarios which are necessary. Nevertheless, in recent years, more and more combinations of reagents exist and the selective sorbents produced are numerous. In this review article some examples were given, *i.e.*, presenting some limitations in the synthesis of MIPs (porogens, cross-linkers, extraction, *etc.*) and also in the models, both isotherm and kinetic, used for the description of binding capacity. The major models from the literature have been discussed.

REFERENCES

1. Erwe, T.; Mavrov, V.; Peleka, E.N.; Matis, K.A. *Bonding of Toxic Metal Ions*; Wiley & Sons: Hoboken, NJ, USA, 2005.

2. Peleka, E.N.; Matis, K.A. Water separation processes and sustainability. *Ind. Eng. Chem. Res.* 2011, *50*, 421–430.

3. Loukidou, M.X.; Peleka, E.N.; Karapantsios, T.D.; Matis, K.A. Biosorption of metal ions. *Trends Chem. Eng.* 2011, *13*, 53–64.

4. Loukidou, M.X.; Karapantsios, T.D.; Zouboulis, A.I.; Matis, K.A. Diffusion kinetic study of cadmium(II) biosorption by *Aeromonas caviae*. *J. Chem. Technol. Biotechnol.* 2004, *79*, 711–719.

5. Loukidou, M.X.; Zouboulis, A.I.; Karapantsios, T.D.; Matis, K.A. Equilibrium and kinetic modeling of chromium(VI) biosorption by *Aeromonas caviae*. *Colloid. Surface A* 2004, *242*, 93–104.

6. Butter, T.J.; Evison, L.M.; Hancock, I.C.; Holland, F.S.; Matis, K.A.; Philipson, A.; Sheikh, A.I.; Zouboulis, A.I. The removal and recovery of cadmium from dilute aqueous solutions by biosorption and electrolysis at laboratory scale.*Water Res.* 1998, *32*, 400–406.

7. Zouboulis, A.I.; Rousou, E.G.; Matis, K.A.; Hancock, I.C. Removal of toxic metals from aqueous mixtures. Part 1: Biosorption. *J. Chem. Technol. Biotechnol.* 1999, *74*, 429–436.

8. Kyzas, G.Z.; Matis, K.A. Flotation of biological materials. *Processes* 2014, *2*, 293–310.

9. Zamboulis, D.; Peleka, E.N.; Lazaridis, N.K.; Matis, K.A. Metal ion separation and recovery from environmental sources using various flotation and sorption techniques. *J. Chem. Technol. Biotechnol.* 2011, *86*, 335–344.

10. Aksu, Z. Application of biosorption for the removal of organic pollutants: A review. *Process Biochem.* 2005, *40*, 997–1026.

11. Hughes, M.N.; Poole, R.K. *Metals and Microorganisms*; Chapman and Hall: London, UK, 1989.

12. Hancock, I.C. The use of Gram-positive bacteria for the removal of metals from aqueous solution. In *Trace Metal Removal from Aqueous Solution*; Thompson, R., Ed.; Royal Society of Chemistry: London, UK, 1986; pp. 25–43.

13. Esposito, A.; Pagnanelli, F.; Lodi, A.; Solisio, C.; Veglio, F. Biosorption of heavy metals by Sphaerotilus natans: An equilibrium study at different pH and biomass concentration. *Hydrometallurgy* 2001, *60*, 129–141.

14. Zouboulis, A.I.; Matis, K.A.; Hancock, I.C. Biosorption of metals from dilute aqueous solutions. *Sep. Purif. Methods* 1997, *26*, 255–295.

15. Solari, P.; Zouboulis, A.I.; Matis, K.A.; Stalidis, G.A. Removal of toxic metals by biosorption onto nonliving sewage sludge. *Sep. Sci. Technol.* 1996, *31*, 1075–1092.

16. Gadd, G.M. Biosorption: Critical review of scientific rationale, environmental importance and significance for pollution treatment. *J. Chem. Technol. Biotechnol.* 2009, *84*, 13–28.

17. Zouboulis, A.I.; Kydros, K.A.; Matis, K.A. Adsorbing flotation of copper hydroxo precipitates by pyrite fines. *Sep. Sci. Technol.* 1992, *27*, 2143–2155.

18. Zouboulis, A.I.; Matis, K.A.; Rousou, E.G.; Kyriakidis, D.A. Biosorptive flotation for metal ions recovery. *Water Sci. Technol.* 2001, *43*, 123–129.

19. Micheletti, E.; Colica, G.; Viti, C.; Tamagnini, P.; De Philippis, R. Selectivity in the heavy metal removal by exopolysaccharide-producing cyanobacteria. *J. Appl. Microbiol.* 2008, *105*, 88–94.

20. Şengil, A.; Özacar, M. Competitive biosorption of Pb^{2+}, Cu^{2+} and Zn^{2+} ions from aqueous solutions onto valonia tannin resin. *J. Hazard. Mater.* 2009, *166*, 1488–1494.

21. Soetaredjo, F.E.; Kurniawan, A.; Ki, O.L.; Ismadji, S. Incorporation of selectivity factor in modeling binary component adsorption isotherms for heavy metals-biomass system. *Chem. Eng. J.* 2013, *219*, 137–148.

22. Hackbarth, F.V.; Girardi, F.; de Souza, S.M.A.G.U.; de Souza, A.A.U.; Boaventura, R.A.R.; Vilar, V.J.P. Marine macroalgae *Pelvetia canaliculata* (Phaeophyceae) as a natural cation exchanger for cadmium and lead ions separation in aqueous solutions. *Chem. Eng. J.* 2013, *242*, 294–305.

23. Ghimire, K.N.; Inoue, J.I.; Inoue, K.; Kawakita, H.; Ohto, K. Adsorptive separation of metal ions onto phosphorylated orange waste. *Sep. Sci. Technol.* 2008, *43*, 362–375.

24. Liu, B.; Lv, X.; Meng, X.; Yu, G.; Wang, D. Removal of Pb(II) from aqueous solution using dithiocarbamate modified chitosan beads with Pb(II) as imprinted ions. *Chem. Eng. J.* 2013, *220*, 412–419.

25. Liang, P.; Wang, D.; Qi, H.; Liu, X.; Xu, Y. Biosorption of citric acid-cadmium complex by imprinted chitosan polymer.*Desalin. Water Treat.* 2013, *51*, 3754–3761.

26. Mayes, A.G.; Whitcombe, M.J. Synthetic strategies for the generation of molecularly imprinted organic polymers. *Adv. Drug Del. Rev.* 2005, *57*, 1742–1778.

27. Chen, B.; Piletsky, S.; Turner, A.P.F. Molecular recognition: Design of "keys". *Comb. Chem. HighThroughput Screen.*2002, *5*, 409–427.

28. Srinivasan, R. Advances in application of natural clay and its composites in removal of biological, organic, and inorganic contaminants from drinking water. *Adv. Mater. Sci. Eng.* 2011, *2011*, 872531.

29. Sasaki, H.; Kobashi, Y.; Nagai, T.; Maeda, M. Application of electron beam melting to the removal of phosphorus from silicon: Toward production of solar-grade silicon by metallurgical processes. *Adv. Mater. Sci. Eng.* 2013, *2013*, 857196.

30. Radenović, A.; Malina, J.; Sofilić, T. Characterization of ladle furnace slag from carbon steel production as a potential adsorbent. *Adv. Mater. Sci. Eng.* 2013, *2013*, 198240.

31. Alahmadi, S.M.; Mohamad, S.; Jamil Maah, M. Preparation of organic-inorganic hybrid materials based on MCM-41 and its applications. *Adv. Mater. Sci. Eng.* 2013, *2013*, 634863.

32. Balogh, A.G.; Baba, K.; Cohen, D.D.; Elliman, R.G.; Ensinger, W.; Gyulai, J. Modification, synthesis, and analysis of advanced materials using ion beam techniques. *Adv. Mater. Sci. Eng.* 2012, *2012*, 431297.

33. Jiang, G.; Chen, T.; Yang, Q. Photocatalytic materials. *Adv. Mater. Sci. Eng.* 2012, *2012*, 186948.

34. Mobarak, Y.; Bassyouni, M.; Almutawa, M. Materials selection, synthesis, and dielectrical properties of PVC nanocomposites. *Adv. Mater. Sci. Eng.* 2013, *2013*, 149672.

35. Polyakov, M.V. Adsorption properties and structure of silica gel. *J. Phys. Chem.* 1931, *2*, 799–805.

36. Dickey, F.H. Specific adsorption. *J. Phys. Chem.* 1955, *59*, 695–707.

37. Wulff, G.; Sarhan, A. Use of polymers with enzyme-analogous structures for the resolution of racemates. *Angew. Chem. Int. Ed. Engl.* 1972, *11*, 341–344.

38. Sellergren, B.; Andersson, L.I. Molecular recognition in macroporous polymers prepared by a substrate-analog imprinting strategy. *J. Org. Chem.* 1990, *55*, 3381–3383.

39. Shea, K.J.; Sasaki, D.Y. An analysis of small-molecule binding to functionalized synthetic polymers by 13C CP/MAS NMR and FT-IR spectroscopy. *J. Am. Chem. Soc.* 1991, *113*, 4109–4120.

40. Wulff, G. Enzyme-like catalysis by molecularly imprinted polymers. *Chem. Rev.* 2002, *102*, 1–27.

41. Arshady, R.; Mosbach, K. Synthesis of substrate-selective polymers by host-guest polymerization. *Makromol. Chem.*1981, *182*, 687–692.

42. Whitcombe, M.J.; Rodriguez, M.E.; Villar, P.; Vulfson, E.N. A new method for the introduction of recognition site functionality into polymers prepared by molecular imprinting-synthesis and characterization of polymeric receptors for cholesterol. *J. Am. Chem. Sci.* 1995, *117*, 7105–7111.

43. Sellergren, B. Imprinted dispersion polymers: A new class of easily accessible affinity stationary phases. *J. Chromatogr. A* 1994, *673*, 133–141.

44. Kyzas, G.Z.; Bikiaris, D.N.; Lazaridis, N.K. Selective separation of basic and reactive dyes by molecularly imprinted polymers (mips). *Chem. Eng. J.* 2009, *149*, 263–272.

45. Lloyd, L.L. Rigid macroporous copolymers as stationary phases in high-performance liquid chromatography. *J. Chromatogr. A* 1991, *544*, 201–217.

46. Ellwanger, A.; Berggren, C.; Bayoudh, S.; Crecenzi, C.; Karlsson, L.; Owens, P.K.; Ensing, K.; Cormack, P.; Sherrington, D.; Sellergren, B. Evaluation of methods aimed at complete removal of template from molecularly imprinted polymers. *Analyst* 2001, *126*, 784–792.

47. Shea, K.J.; Sasaki, D.Y.; Stoddard, G.J. Fluorescence probes for evaluating chain solvation in network polymers. An analysis of the solvatochromic shift of the dansyl probe in macroporous styrene-divinylbenzene and styrene-diisopropenylbenzene copolymers. *Macromolecules* 1989, *22*, 1722–1730.

48. Lanza, F.; Sellergen, B. The application of molecular imprinting technology to solid phase extraction. *Chromatographia*2001, *53*, 599–611.

49. Szumski, M.; Buszewski, B. Molecularly imprinted polymers: A new tool for separation of steroid isomers. *J. Sep. Sci.*2004, *27*, 837–842.

50. Lorenzo, R.A.; Carro, A.M.; Alvarez-Lorenzo, C.; Concheiro, A. To remove or not to remove? The challenge of extracting the template to make the cavities available in molecularly imprinted polymers (mips). *Int. J. Mol. Sci.* 2011,*12*, 4327–4347.

51. Martin, P.D.; Jones, G.R.; Stringer, F.; Wilson, I.D. Comparison of normal and reversed-phase solid phase extraction methods for extraction of β-blockers from plasma using molecularly imprinted polymers. *Analyst* 2003, *128*, 345–350.

52. Fu, G.Q.; Yu, H.; Zhu, J. Imprinting effect of protein-imprinted polymers composed of chitosan and polyacrylamide: A re-examination. *Biomaterials* 2008, *29*, 2138–2142.

53. Yungerman, I.; Srebnik, S. Factors contributing to binding-site imperfections in imprinted polymers. *Chem. Mater.*2006, *18*, 657–663.

54. Bunin, G.; François, G.; Bonvin, D. A real-time optimization framework for the iterative controller tuning problem.*Processes* 2013, *1*, 203–237.

55. Chiavazzo, E.; Gear, C.; Dsilva, C.; Rabin, N.; Kevrekidis, I. Reduced models in chemical kinetics via nonlinear data-mining. *Processes* 2014, *2*, 112–140.

56. Donato, D.; Napoli, I.; Catapano, G. Model-based optimization of scaffold geometry and operating conditions of radial flow packed-bed bioreactors for therapeutic applications. *Processes* 2014, *2*, 34–57.

57. Ji, G.; Wang, G.; Hooman, K.; Bhatia, S.; da Costa, J. Scale-up design analysis and modeling of cobalt oxide silica membrane module for hydrogen processing. *Processes* 2013, *1*, 49–66.

58. Kapoor, K.; Powell, K.; Cole, W.; Kim, J.; Edgar, T. Improved large-scale process cooling operation through energy optimization. *Processes* 2013, *1*, 312–329.

59. Klemuk, S.; Vigmostad, S.; Endapally, K.; Wagner, A.; Titze, I. A multiwell disc appliance used to deliver quantifiable accelerations and shear stresses at sonic frequencies. *Processes* 2014, *2*, 71–88.

60. Lakerveld, R.; Benyahia, B.; Heider, P.; Zhang, H.; Braatz, R.; Barton, P. Averaging level control to reduce off-spec material in a continuous pharmaceutical pilot plant. *Processes* 2013, *1*, 330–348.

61. Rogers, A.; Hashemi, A.; Ierapetritou, M. Modeling of particulate processes for the continuous manufacture of solid-based pharmaceutical dosage forms. *Processes* 2013, *1*, 67–127.

62. Schaschke, C.; Fletcher, I.; Glen, N. Density and viscosity measurement of diesel fuels at combined high pressure and elevated temperature. *Processes* 2013, *1*, 30–48.

63. Sen, M.; Barrasso, D.; Singh, R.; Ramachandran, R. A multi-scale hybrid CFD-DEM-PBM description of a fluid-bed granulation process. *Processes* 2014, *2*, 89–111.

64. Shahmoon, A.; Zalevsky, Z. Electrical model for analyzing chemical kinetics, lasing and bio-chemical processes.*Processes* 2013, *1*, 12–29.

65. Song, H.-S.; Ramkrishna, D. Complex nonlinear behavior in metabolic processes: Global bifurcation analysis of*Escherichia coli* growth on multiple substrates. *Processes* 2013, *1*, 263–278.

66. Travis, C.; Adomaitis, R. Dynamic modeling for the design and cyclic operation of an Atomic Layer Deposition (ALD) Reactor. *Processes* 2013, *1*, 128–152.

67. Rampey, A.M.; Umpleby Ii, R.J.; Rushton, G.T.; Iseman, J.C.; Shah, R.N.; Shimizu, K.D. Characterization of the imprint effect and the influence of imprinting conditions on affinity, capacity, and heterogeneity in molecularly imprinted polymers using the freundlich isotherm-affinity distribution analysis. *Anal. Chem.* 2004, *76*, 1123–1133.

68. Rushton, G.T.; Karns, C.L.; Shimizu, K.D. A critical examination of the use of the Freundlich isotherm in characterizing molecularly imprinted polymers (MIPs). *Anal. Chim. Acta* 2005, *528*, 107–113.

69. Umpleby Ii, R.J.; Baxter, S.C.; Bode, M.; Berch, J.K., Jr.; Shah, R.N.; Shimizu, K.D. Application of the Freundlich adsorption isotherm in the characterization of molecularly imprinted polymers. *Anal. Chim. Acta* 2001, *435*, 35–42.

70. Umpleby Ii, R.J.; Baxter, S.C.; Rampey, A.M.; Rushton, G.T.; Chen, Y.; Shimizu, K.D. Characterization of the heterogeneous binding site affinity distributions in molecularly imprinted polymers. *J. Chromatogr. B* 2004, *804*, 141–149.

71. Sips, R. On the structure of a catalyst surface. *J. Chem. Phys.* 1948, *16*, 490–495.

72. Sips, R. On the structure of a catalyst surface. II. *J. Chem. Phys.* 1950, *18*, 1024–1026.

73. Umpleby Ii, R.J.; Baxter, S.C.; Chen, Y.; Shah, R.N.; Shimizu, K.D. Characterization of molecularly imprinted polymers with the Langmuir-Freundlich isotherm. *Anal. Chem.* 2001, *73*, 4584–4591.

74. Miyabe, K.; Guiochon, G. Kinetic study of the concentration dependence of the mass transfer rate coefficient in enantiomeric separation on a polymeric imprinted stationary phase. *Anal. Sci.* 2000, *16*, 719–730.

75. Sajonz, P.; Kele, M.; Zhong, G.; Sellergren, B.; Guiochon, G. Study of the thermodynamics and mass transfer kinetics of two enantiomers on a polymeric imprinted stationary phase. *J. Chromatogr. A* 1998, *810*, 1–17.

76. Szabelski, P.; Kaczmarski, K.; Cavazzini, A.; Chen, Y.B.; Sellergren, B.; Guiochon, G. Energetic heterogeneity of the surface of a molecularly imprinted polymer studied by high-performance liquid chromatography. *J. Chromatogr. A* 2002, *964*, 99–111.

77. Quiñones, I.; Cavazzini, A.; Guiochon, G. Adsorption equilibria and overloaded band profiles of basic drugs in a reversed-phase system. *J. Chromatogr. A* 2000, *877*, 1–11.

78. Umpleby Ii, R.J.; Bode, M.; Shimizu, K.D. Measurement of the continuous distribution of binding sites in molecularly imprinted polymers. *Analyst* 2000, *125*, 1261–1265.

79. Andersson, L.I.; Müller, R.; Vlatakis, G.; Mosbach, K. Mimics of the binding sites of opioid receptors obtained by molecular imprinting of enkephalin and morphine. *Proc. Natl. Acad. Sci. USA* 1995, *92*, 4788–4792.

80. Vlatakis, G.; Andersson, L.I.; Muller, R.; Mosbach, K. Drug assay using antibody mimics made by molecular imprinting. *Nature* 1993, *361*, 645–647.

81. Tsai, H.A.; Syu, M.J. Synthesis and characterization of creatinine imprinted poly(4-vinylpyridine-co-divinylbenzene) as a specific recognition receptor. *Anal. Chim. Acta* 2005, *539*, 107–116.

82. Milojković, S.S.; Kostoski, D.; Čomor, J.J.; Nedeljković, J.M. Radiation induced synthesis of molecularly imprinted polymers. *Polymer* 1997, *38*, 2853–2855.

83. Hsu, H.C.; Chen, L.C.; Ho, K.C. Colorimetric detection of morphine in a molecularly imprinted polymer using an aqueous mixture of Fe^{3+} and $[Fe(CN)_6]^{3-}$. *Anal. Chim. Acta* 2004, *504*, 141–147.

84. Baggiani, C.; Giraudi, G.; Giovannoli, C.; Tozzi, C.; Anfossi, L. Adsorption isotherms of a molecular imprinted polymer prepared in the presence of a polymerisable template: Indirect evidence of the formation of template clusters in the binding site. *Anal. Chim. Acta* 2004, *504*, 43–52.

85. Hwang, C.C.; Lee, W.C. Chromatographic characteristics of cholesterol-imprinted polymers prepared by covalent and non-covalent imprinting methods. *J. Chromatogr. A* 2002, *962*, 69–78.

86. Lehmann, M.; Dettling, M.; Brunner, H.; Tovar, G.E.M. Affinity parameters of amino acid derivative binding to molecularly imprinted nanospheres consisting of poly[(ethylene glycol dimethacrylate)-co-(methacrylic acid)]. *J. Chromatogr. B* 2004, *808*, 43–50.

87. Katz, A.; Davis, M.E. Investigations into the mechanisms of molecular recognition with imprinted polymers.*Macromolecules* 1999, *32*, 4113–4121.

88. Scatchard, G. The attraction of proteins for small molecules and ions. *Ann. N. Y. Acad. Sci.* 1949, *51*, 660–672.

89. Kermode, J.C. The curvilinear scatchard plot. Experimental artifact or receptor heterogeneity? *Biochem. Pharmacol.*1989, *38*, 2053–2060.

90. Spivak, D.; Gilmore, M.A.; Shea, K.J. Evaluation of binding and origins of specificity of 9-ethyladenine imprinted polymers. *J. Am. Chem. Soc.* 1997, *119*, 4388–4393.

91. Karapantsios, T.D.; Loukidou, M.X.; Matis, K.A. *Sorption Kinetics*; Wiley & Sons: New York, NY, USA, 2005.

92. Ho, Y.S.; Ng, J.C.Y.; McKay, G. Kinetics of pollutant sorption by biosorbents: Review. *Sep. Purif. Methods* 2000, *29*, 189–232.

93. Smith, E.H. Uptake of heavy metals in batch systems by a recycled iron-bearing material. *Water Res.* 1996, *30*, 2424–2434.

94. Loukidou, M.X.; Karapantsios, T.D.; Zouboulis, A.I.; Matis, K.A. Cadmium(II) biosorption by *Aeromonas caviae*: Kinetic modeling. *Sep. Sci. Technol.* 2005, *40*, 1293–1311.

95. Ritchie, A.G. Alternative to the Elovich equation for the kinetics of adsorption of gases on solids. *J. Chem. Soc. Farad. Trans.* 1977, *73*, 1650–1653.

96. Crank, J. *The Mathematics of Diffusion*; Oxford University Press: London, UK, 1975.

97. Dzul Erosa, M.S.; Saucedo Medina, T.I.; Navarro Mendoza, R.; Avila Rodriguez, M.; Guibal, E. Cadmium sorption on chitosan sorbents: Kinetic and equilibrium studies. *Hydrometallurgy* 2001, *61*, 157–167.

98. Puranik, P.R.; Modak, J.M.; Paknikar, K.M. A comparative study of the mass transfer kinetics of metal biosorption by microbial biomass. *Hydrometallurgy* 1999, *52*, 189–197.

99. Loukidou, M.X.; Karapantsios, T.D.; Zouboulis, A.I.; Matis, K.A. Diffusion Kinetic Study of Chromium(VI) Biosorption by Aeromonas caviae. *Ind. Eng. Chem. Res.* 2004, *43*, 1748–1755.

100. Bates, D.M.; Watts, D.G. *Nonlinear Regression Analysis and Its Applications*; Wiley & Sons: New York, NY, USA, 1988.

101. Zouboulis, A.I.; Lazaridis, N.K.; Karapantsios, T.D.; Matis, K.A. Heavy metals removal from industrial wastewaters by biosorption. *Int. J. Environ. Eng. Sci.* 2010, *1*, 57–78.

Chapter 8

BIOMATERIALS FOR CARDIAC TISSUE ENGINEERING

M. Arnal-Pastor[1], J. C. Chachques[2], M. Monleón Pradas[1, 3] and A. Vallés-Lluch[1]

[1]Center for Biomaterials and Tissue Engineering, Universitat Politècnica de València, Cno. de Vera s/n, Valencia, Spain

[2]Department of Cardiovascular Surgery, Laboratory of Biosurgical Research, Georges Pompidou European Hospital, Paris, France

[3]Networking Research Center on Bioengineering, Biomaterials and Nanomedicine (CIBER-BBN), Valencia, Spain

INTRODUCTION

Cardiovascular Diseases

Cardiovascular diseases (CVD) are a leading death cause in developed countries (1 of every 3 deaths in the United States in 2008) [1]. Changes in diet and habits are causing CVD to become major mortality pathologies in developing countries too [2] (they are already responsible for a 30% of the world deaths). This group of diseases constitutes a great burden for the national health systems, consuming great percentages of the health systems budgets. In the particular case of the coronary heart diseases (CHD), 3,8 million men and 3,4 million women die a year worldwide because of them [3]. In the United States 1 of every 6 deaths in 2008 was caused by CHD [1].

The heart is a complex organ that pumps 7000 liters of blood to all the tissues in the body per day [4]. This pumping function precisely determines its anatomy. Heart tissue basically is formed by cardiac myocytes (contractile elements) [5], smooth muscle cells, fibroblasts, blood vessels, nerves and the extracellular matrix components (cardiac interstitium and collagen) [6] organized in a very particular way. Myocytes form muscular fibers with changing orientation across the ventricular wall up to 180° [7]. At the same time, muscular fibers are organized into myocardial laminas 4-6 myocytes thick separated from neighboring laminas by extracellular collagen [8]. The particular arrangement of the ventricular myocytes influence the mechanical and electrical function of the heart and small changes in it can lead to severe changes in these functions [9].

The extracellular matrix (ECM) connects the cells into a 3D architecture allowing the coupling of the forces produced by the myocytes. The anatomical model proposed by Torrent-Guasp [8], which considers the heart one muscle band plied in a double helical loop, explains how the ventricles contract and get an efficient pumping in every heart beat, achieving an ejection fraction of the 60% when sarcomeres individually contract 15% only [10].

Myocytes are intimately connected, forming a functional syncytium [8]. Each myocardial cell is coupled in average to $9,1 \pm 2,2$ [11] myocytes, by 99 [12] gap junctions where the transfer of ionic currents takes place. Gap junctions are a specialized form of cell connection; they are formed by a cluster of ionic channels essential to the rapid propagation of the action potential. The action potential is the electrical impulse responsible for the contraction of the cells [13]. A proper electrical coupling of the cells is critical to avoid arrhythmias and reentries and essential for the contraction to spread as a wave front.

Acute myocardial infarction (AMI) occurs when a coronary artery is clogged, in 80% of the cases, by coronary atherosclerosis with superimposed luminal thrombus [14]. This occlusion leaves the downstream zone of the heart without blood supply, what means lack of oxygen, nutrients and metabolites wash for the affected zone. As a consequence, the aerobic metabolism changes to anaerobic glycolysis [14], leading to a decrease in the pH and reduction in the contractile function. Within 20 to 40 minutes without blood supply cells start to die and as times passes more myocardial tissue is compromised. There is also a zone of the heart affected by the infarction, where myocytes remain viable but lower their activity to reduce the metabolism and oxygen consumption to survive under hypoxic conditions; they can recover their contractibility after revascularization [15].

Clinical practices aim to limit the severity and extension of the AMI by rapidly restoring the blood flow (reperfusion), alleviating the oxygen demand [16] and reducing reperfusion injury. This can be done with different treatments or combinations of them. Pharmacological approaches involve the use of anticoagulant therapies and thrombolytic drugs to eliminate the clot. Vasodilatators like nitrates are also used to favor the dilation of the vessels, aspirin to avoid platelet aggregation, betabloqueants to reduce the heart pace, as well as morphine to reduce the pain are employed. Another group of therapies are the percutaneous coronary interventions; they physically reopen the vessel via catheterization. There are different techniques: the regular angioplasty uses a catheter with a balloon that is inflated in the place of the thrombus to reopen the lumen [17], or allows the permanent implantation of a stent in the vessel to keep it open. There is a wide variety of these devices depending on their composition, whether they release drugs or are biodegradable or not, etc [18, 19].

These therapies restore the blood flow to the infarcted zone; but reperfusion therapy is not exempt of risks: it is a complex process that can induce apoptosis by the microenvironmental changes that the recovery of the blood supply induces (formation of free radicals, calcium release, neutrophils, etc.) [20]. So it has to be done carefully and there is always a compromise between limiting the infarction extension due to the time without oxygen and the induced apoptosis due to the reperfusion. Reperfusion done soon after the onset of the ischemia is very advantageous, saving more tissue by restoring the blood flow than the tissue that will be lost because of the toxic substances released in the reperfusion. All the aforementioned treatments basically limit the damage of the acute episode but do not regenerate the damaged tissue and do not avoid the subsequent ventricular remodeling following an AMI.

In the infarcted area there is a great number of dead myocytes, and the host response to the injury consists in activating the inflammatory response and producing cytokines [21]. Thereupon neutrophils, monocytes and macrophages migrate into this area to remove the necrotic tissue [22]. Then, matrix metalloproteases (MMPs) are activated, which have a deleterious effect on the collagen matrix of the heart and in the surrounding coronary vasculature by degrading them [23]. The weakening of the collagen leads to wall thinning and ventricular dilation, as well as mural realignment of myocytes bundles [24]. After the inflammatory phase and the resorption of the necrotic tissue, there is an increase in the deposition of cross-linked collagen in the infarcted area that leads to scar tissue formation. During the remodelling process a change in the collagen composition occurs, the type I collagen fraction is reduced from 80% to 40% and the collagen III is increased [25].

Against what it was thought, this scar is a living tissue with a fibroblast-like cell population nourished by a neovasculature; these cells regulate the collagen turnover of the scar tissue [22]. The scar tissue has a reduced or absent contractility as compared with the original healthy myocardium [26], what leads to a reduction in the overall cardiac function [27].

The remodeling process initially is a compensatory mechanism to overcome the loss of contractile tissue. But with time this adaptative process of overload becomes maladaptative [15]. To compensate the additional effort, the remaining beating tissue hypertrophies trying to overcome the reduction in the cardiac function. This overload leads to myocyte slippage and fibrotic interstitial growth and to a degenerating process that may end in heart failure. The heart remodeling produces in the ventricles a set of anatomical and functional changes, including increased wall stress, slimming of the wall, chamber dilation, increase of the sphericity, and a significant loss of cardiac function.

The ventricular shape change from elliptical to spherical reduces its ejection fraction, because of a change in the apical loop fiber orientation [28]. Another problem caused by the shape change is that the papillary muscles are separated, what leads to regurgitation, contributing to the overload of the heart [24]. Besides, remodeled hearts are more prone to suffer arrhythmias as the membrane potential is altered and because of the interstitial fibrotic growth that may affect conductivity [15].

The end stage of the degeneration is the heart failure, when the heart is unable to pump enough blood to match the metabolic needs of the tissues. Current treatments aim to avoid reaching this point. Pharmacological treatments aspire to reduce the work load and to protect the cardiac tissues from the accumulated harmful substances [29]. Surgical therapy involves different techniques with different objectives: to restore a proper blood flow in areas that lack it (by-pass surgery), to restore the normal elliptical geometry (Dor and Batista procedures), to restore the wall stress to normal (Dynamic Cardiomyoplasty), to limit the pathologic dilation, etc [10].

Cell Therapy and Cardiac Tissue Engineering

For many years, the heart has been considered a fully differentiated organ, with no myocyte regeneration after birth [30]. Recently it has been proved that myocytes have a limited regenerative capacity, around 1% of the cells per year at the age of 20 and it is reduced to 0,3% at the age of 75 [31]. This regenerative capacity is achieved thanks to a small population of cardiac stem cells [32]. Nevertheless, their regenerative capacity is limited and in any case it is not enough to regenerate the heart if it suffers severe damage, like the one provoked by a myocardial infarction. New therapies under development like cell therapy or tissue engineering, aim to boost this limited regenerative potential of the native tissue by employing cells, drugs, factors or patches.

The aim of cardiac cell therapy is to heal the damaged infarcted tissue by the implantation of cells into or onto the pathologic myocardium by different techniques (figure 1 a). In tissue engineering strategies, different types of cells have been combined with materials and with bioactive molecules if necessary to again try to recover the injured tissue. The employed materials will support cells, provide them 3D organization, protect them, stimulate and guide its growth, maintain them in the site of interest, etc.; in sum, they will act as an artificial extracellular matrix during the regeneration process. But the use of materials either injectable, or *ex vivo* conformed (gels –patches- or scaffolds) (figure 1 b) has an additional and important effect: the implantation of a material in the scarred ventricular wall, increases its thickness and by Laplace's law, this increase leads to a reduction in the wall stress. This side-effect could be by itself very positive, even although regeneration did not arrive to happen, to limit ventricular remodeling and improve the quality of life of cardiac patients [29].

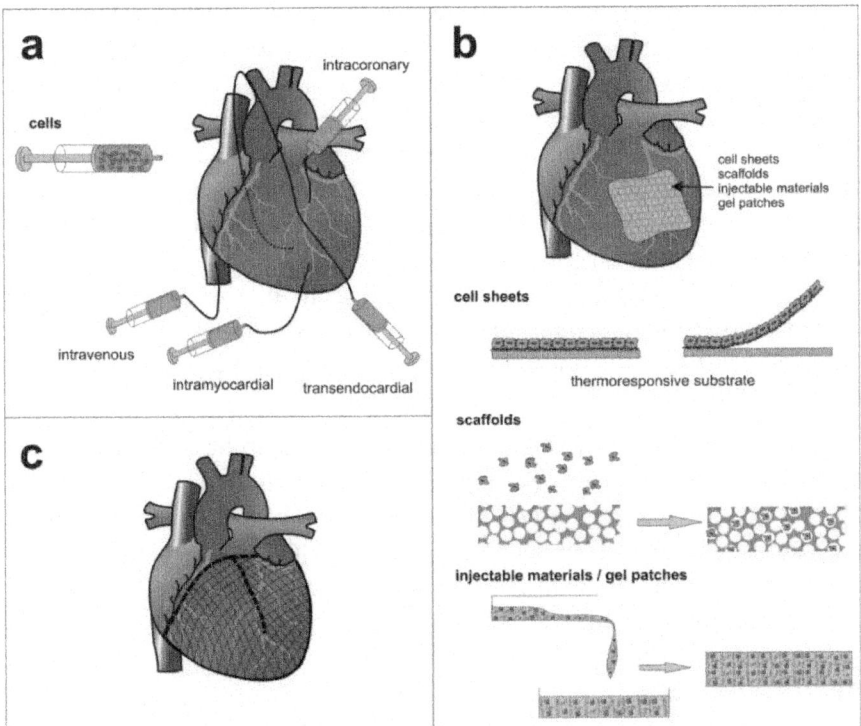

Figure 1. (a) Classical cell therapy in the heart (*freely inspired* in Strauer BE, Kornowski R, *Circulation* 2003; 107: 929-934). (b) Tissue engineering approaches with cell sheets, scaffolds or injectable materials (*freely inspired in* Masuda S *et al, Adv. Drug Del. Revs* 2008; 60(2): 277-85). (c) Ventricular restrain device.

CARDIOMYOPLASTY

Need for Cell Cardiomyoplasty

Cardiomyoplasty has evolved from "dynamic" to "cellular cardiomyoplasty".

The term dynamic cardiomyoplasty is referred to a surgical procedure developed in 1987 [33] to wrap the heart with the latissimus dorsi muscle, aiming to support the heart beating and limit the remodeling. Nevertheless, the obtained results were not as good as expected. With the advances in cell therapy, cellular cardiomyoplasty appeared as a promising therapeutical approach. This name encloses the therapies that use the injection of cells, from different origins, directly into the heart to try to obtain an improvement in the reduced heart function after an ischemic insult (figure 1 a).

The injected cells are envisaged to induce angiogenesis, inhibit apoptosis, help to recover hibernating myocardium, activate endogenous repair mechanisms, and create new contractile tissue that will replace the damaged one. Also they are expected to reverse the remodeling process that provoked ventricular dilation [34]. Many cells have been employed and the initial promising results obtained in animal models made this technique moved very fast to clinical trials, even if the mechanisms involved in the observed improvements were unknown. Unfortunately, the results obtained from the clinical trials were not as good as expected, and some were contradictory between them. One possible contributing cause to this discrepancy is that studies are carried out in young healthy animals, while patients susceptible to receive these treatments normally are aged people and in many cases with other co-morbidities [35].

Different ways to deliver cells into the damaged heart have been explored: intracoronary infusion (with the hope that cells will migrate through the vessels and be hosted in the infarcted area) or directly into the infarcted area either by intramyocardial or endocardial injection [36], as shown in figure 1 a. The advantage of injecting them directly into the infarcted area is that this will ensure that the cells are delivered in the site of interest.

Related Problematic

Many different cell types have been employed in the numerous studies that have been done. Autologous cell sources are interesting because they do not require immunosuppression treatment of the patient and there is no risk of illness transmission. On the contrary, allogenic cells could be ready to use whenever a patient needs them, but would require immunosuppressive therapy after their implantation, and there is always a remaining risk of illness transmission. Another disadvantage is that prior to implantation cells need to be extracted and expanded. This whole process in some cases may take several weeks, limiting its application in the acute state. Besides, autologous cells coming from patients that suffer other conditions like diabetes or are simply aged, may have limited proliferation and attachment [37].

An important aspect of this technique is the low engraftment into the heart tissue of the supplied cells. The retention of the cells in the heart seems to be determined by the cell type and delivery route [38]. It has been estimated that in humans 50-75 min after intracoronary injection of bone marrow cells only 1,3-2,6% of the injected cells remain in the myocardium [39]; after 2 hours less than 10% of the injected cells survive [32]. Many causes can be advanced: the heart beats, so cells can easily be pumped out of the heart; the solution in which cells are injected has a low viscosity, so cells can be washed away; the mechanical loss of the cells through the injection hole left by the needle, etc [40]. A different contributing cause to the low cell engraftment is that the injured heart is not a cell-friendly environment, type I collagen fibers have been substituted by type III, which has worse properties in terms of adhesion and promoting angiogenesis, what can induce anoikis [4]. Another problem is cell survival itself. The conditions in the infarcted myocardium are very hostile for the cells: hypoxic conditions (studies show that the survival of injected cells decreases towards the center of the scar), cytokines, inflammatory factors, etc., are present in the damaged myocardium, and can negatively affect the survival of the injected cells. Immunological rejection can be another cause reducing cell survival [41].

An interesting approach is to train cells prior to their implantation for them to resist the hostile conditions they will find in the implantation site. For instance, the resistance to hypoxic conditions is key and needs to be improved even for skeletal myoblasts (which are the cells that have better resistance to lack of oxygen). Privation of glutamine reduces the oxygen consumption rate, what has been proved to improve survival of myoblasts when implanted [42].

The fact that most of the cells did not graft into the host myocardium in the studies performed to date, that there is a very limited transdifferentiation of implanted cells into beating cardiomyocytes (the differentiation reported in animals may have been fusion events between native cardiomyocytes and injected cells [41]), and that a wide range of non-myogenic cells also induce an improvement of the ventricular function [36], suggests that the mechanism leading to this enhancement cannot be only myogenesis regenerating the myocardium. The pathways through which cell implantation induces improvements in cardiac function remain to be elucidated, but different events that can take place simultaneously have been proposed. The most remarkable are the induction of angiogenesis (formation of new vessels) and the improvement in the myocardial perfusion, the reduction of the wall stress because of the increase in cell mass [43] and the paracrine effect of the injected cells [32].

Cell Types Investigated

As previously said, many cell types from different origins have been employed: embryonic stem cells, mesenchymal stem cells, bone marrow cells, induced pluripotent stem cells, cardiac stem cells, skeletal myoblasts, umbilical cord blood cells and amniotic fluid stem cells, among others. In what follows the use of these cell types is discussed, with the advantages and disadvantages that each one presents for its application in heart regeneration.

Embryonic Stem Cells (ESC)

ESC can be obtained from the inner mass of an embryo in the blastocyst stage. These cells have the capacity of growing undifferentiated indefinitely, and when they differentiate they can form any cell from the three germ layers. But the use of ESC raises ethical issues, requires immunosuppression, and has the risk to form theratomes. Their use in clinical trials has been limited because of these ethical considerations and risks [36, 44].

A protocol for ESC differentiation into cardiomyocytes and improving their survival when implanted has been established; when these differentiated cells were implanted in rodent models the heart function was improved [45]. In another study in mice, ESC-derived cardiomyocytes implantation reduced the reactive collagen deposition in the ventricular septum, which is one of the remodeling process hallmarks. Nevertheless, the implanted cells were isolated from the host myocardium by scar tissue, although the implanted cardiomyocytes were able to couple functionally to each other [46].

Induced Pluripotent Stem Cells (IPS)

Induced pluripotent stem cells are fibroblasts treated with viral factors to recover their pluripotency. Therefore, IPS do not raise the ethical concerns of the ESC. IPS are very interesting because they can be autologous pluripotent cells. However, their application in clinical trials has been limited precisely for the use of viral vectors that may promote malignancy and act as oncogenes [43], as well as for the intrinsic risk of theratomes inherent to their pluripotency [44].

Adult Stem Cells

These cells have the advantage of being autologous and can be obtained from different sources like bone marrow or adipose tissue. In addition, they can be expanded *in vitro* and do not raise ethical or immunologic problems [47, 48].

Bone marrow cells (BMC) are easily accessible, can be obtained rapidly and have been reported to have certain plasticity. This property allows them to differentiate *in vivo* into cardiomyocytes [26] (although this fact remains controversial [42]). They can also differentiate into cardiomyocytes *in vitro* by supplementing the medium [49]. Studies in animal models demonstrate that the injection of these cells increases neovasculature improving heart function [42]. But the use of BMC is not exempt of risks: intracoronary administration of them can cause microinfarctions due to their big size and irregular shape, making necessary the use of an alternative way of delivery [50]. In clinical trials, results indicated only temporary benefits or no improvement after cell administration [38, 51]. A strategy to enhance the therapeutic efficacy of BMC is to precondition them: BMC treated with growth factors improve the therapeutic effect when implanted and show greater survival rate [52].

Adipose derived stem cells (ASC) can be obtained in great quantity without culturing them. These cells have been implanted in small animal models of AMI and left ventricular function was improved [48]. The underlying mechanisms are unclear, although the hypothesis of a paracrine effect is considered [53]. Clinical trials are ongoing for the implantation of ASCs: PRECISE and APOLLO [54]. These cells are also are under study at the moment in the RECATABI project [55] as part of a strategy that combines them within a three-dimensional polymer scaffold with a peptide gel filling, to lengthen their positive effect and serve as a mechanical support for the dilated ventricle.

Cardiac Stem Cells (CSC)

CSC are undifferentiated cells found in the heart that can become endothelial cells, smooth muscle cells, and functional cardiomyocytes [36]. In undamaged hearts, these cells seem to contribute to the normal self-renewal of the tissue. CSC can be isolated from biopsies and can be expanded *in vitro* [56], although there is a lack of availability from human origin as they are obtained from biopsies. Human CSC injected in mice hearts after infarction led to functional improvement and to support myocardial regeneration [57]. Currently, autologous cardiosphere-derived cells are being evaluated in the CADUCEUS clinical trial [58].

Skeletal Myoblasts (SM)

SM are cells present in the basal membrane, where they remain in a quiescent state while there is no damage. These cells have better resistance to hypoxic conditions than many other cell types, and can be from autologous origin, but 2 to 3 weeks are necessary to establish and expand myoblasts from skeletal muscle biopsies [36]. These cells are capable to contract; that is the reason why they were expected to attach to the beating cardiomyocytes and contribute to the effective beating by integrating in the working syncytium muscle. Nevertheless, there is no electro-mechanical coupling between the implanted cells and the native cardiomyocytes. This absence of coupling turns the implanted cells into a pro-arrhythmic substrate [44]. The cause for this uncoupling is the lack of the gap junctional protein connexin 43. Therefore, the implantation of a pacemaker or a defibrillator to avoid malignant arrhythmias and sudden death would be necessary when implanting these cells, to obtain a synchronous beating of the heart and the grafted cells [26, 59]. Despite the lack of electro-mechanical coupling of the myoblasts with the host cardiac cells, improvements in the ventricular performance have been observed in animal models, even with a reduced number of grafted cells, suggesting a cytokine-mediated effect [46].

The encouraging preliminary results and its autologous origin made this cell type the first to reach clinical trials. Initial clinical trials carried out with these cells showed symptomatic improvements in the patients, but some of them experienced arrhythmias, making necessary the use of implantable defibrillators [36]. For instance, in the phase II randomized placebo controlled trial MAGIC [60], skeletal myoblasts and a cardioverter defibrillator were implanted during a coronary artery by-pass graft surgery.

Umbilical Cord Blood Cells (UCBC)

UCBC can be easily obtained from the umbilical cord and do not present ethical concerns [42]. These cells have certain plasticity and reduced risk of rejection because they show low immunogenicity [25]. Their injection in animal models has been found to improve their left ventricular function [61].

Amniotic Fluid Stem Cells (AFSC)

Amniotic fluid is extracted for prenatal diagnosis and AFSC are isolated from it. They have many characteristics of ESC and seem to be in an intermediate stage between embryonic and adult stem cells in terms of versatility. Interestingly, these cells do not present ethical concerns and do not present risk of tumorogenicity [62].

Human AFSC have been successfully differentiated into endothelial or cardiac lineages *in vitro*. When these cells were implanted in an immunosupressed rat model, they contributed to attenuate its left ventricular remodeling, to preserve the thickness of the ventricle and to improve cardiac function [63].

CELL SHEETS

The use of cell sheets is based on the fact that when cells are cultured in normal flasks and enzymatically digested to detach them, the adhesive proteins and membrane receptors are disrupted leaving the cell damaged [64]. The alternative is to grow cell sheets and then detach them from the culture surface in a way that keeps the electromechanical connections between the cells and benefits from the fact that cells are kept together by their own deposited ECM, as figure 1 b displays. In that way, cells maintain the adhesion and membrane proteins, as well as the natural pro-survival and maturation environmental cues that the ECM provides [65]. Altogether, this is expected to help them to survive when implanted onto the infarcted myocardium.

Cells can be cultured, for instance, on temperature-responsive poly(N-isopropylacrylamide) (PnIPAAm)-coated plates. PnIPAAm is a hydrophobic polymer at 37°C, and cells can attach to its surface. When the temperature is lowered, PnIPAAm suffers a transition to a hydrophilic state and this change causes the attachments of the cell monolayer to the surface to disrupt, and the entire cells sheet detaches from the surface [65]. Other materials, such as a thermo-responsive methylcellulose hydrogel, have been used to successfully obtain cell sheets fragments of human amniotic fluid stem cells (hAFSCs) [66]. Results obtained with these cell sheet fragments were superior to those with dissociated cells in terms of heart function, cell retention, proliferation and vascular density. Moreover, cardiomyocyte sheets were found to functionally integrate with the host tissue in a rat myocardial infarct model [67]. New techniques based on patterning with a gelatin stamp the thermo-responsive substrates allow obtaining complex tissue structures with cells having a determined orientation [68].

The muscle mass loss following an infarction is significant, up to 50 g [69], so the amount of cells needed to overcome this loss is obviously not covered with a single sheet of cells. On the other hand, when several layers of cell sheets are superimposed, they are easier to handle. Some groups have tried to obtain thicker grafts by overlapping several monolayer cardiomyocyte sheets, which adhere one to another forming gap junctions and intercellular adhesions within minutes [70]. But this approach poses a problem: as cell sheets lack of vascularization, the maximum thickness that can be achieved by overlapping them is limited to the depth at which diffusion of oxygen and nutrients can take place (a maximum of three cardiomyocyte sheets can be piled up). To try to overcome this problem, three-layer thick cardiomyocyte sheets were implanted in rats at 1-, 2- and 3-day intervals [71]; in the time between transplantations it was assumed that there is enough time for the cell sheet to be vascularized. With this approach constructs of 1 mm were obtained successfully. But anyway, this option is very invasive, so its application in patients might be limited.

A different approach based on the same idea of providing cell-cell connections and ECM to the implanted cells to improve their retention and survival is to implant them as spherical cell-bodies. Human amniotic fluid stem cells (hAFSC) cultured in a methylcellulose hydrogel to form cell aggregates were implanted in immunosuppressed rats as cell-bodies, and cell retention and engraftment were enhanced as compared with disaggregated cells. This enhancement led to functional improvement and limited the progression of heart failure [72].

INJECTABLE GELS

Rationale

As previously stated, cell cardiomyoplasty presents problems in terms of cell attachment and survival. Cells usually reside in a determined microenvironment which regulates their fate and function. The surrounding ECM with its chemical and biophysical cues is a key element, so the lack of cell-ECM interaction limits their survival [73]. To try to overcome the problems of cells supply, alternative approaches are considered in current studies. The use of natural or synthetic materials in an injectable format, alone or together with cells (figure 1 b), has been investigated to limit remodeling and improve both cell attachment and survival upon implantation in the heart. Ideally, they should be tailored to be amenable to delivery with minimally invasive catheter based procedures [69]. The injectable materials have to cure or self-assemble rapidly (without the need or the release of toxic components) once delivered in the site of interest. As injected, they adopt the shape of the cavity, and may increase the stiffness and thickness of the ventricular wall [74]. Simulations showed that the injection of non-contractile materials with proper mechanical properties can contribute to limit the stress the ventricular wall withstands, thus helping to limit the remodeling [75].

These materials can help to keep the cells in the site of interest, provide them a 3D environment and also protect them from the hostile environment represented by the cytokines and hypoxic conditions, reactive oxygen species, etc., consequence of the infarcted condition of the site [41]. The injected gels can provide a cell friendly environment that will prevent anoikis [69]; they can also include adhesion motifs and then actively contribute to cell attachment. Moreover, they can be used as a controlled release system providing in a sustained way drugs or growth factors to improve cells survival, integration and proliferation [32]. And in the case of bioactive materials, their degradation products may provide additional chemicals that stimulate cells.

Among others, the ideal injectable material should be biodegradable, have a low immunogenity, be no cytotoxic, non-adhesive and have antithrombogenic properties, adequate mechanical properties, provide stiffness to the scar but at the same time being compliant with the heart beating and transmit properly the mechanical stimuli to the cells, induce angiogenesis or at least not disturb the angiogenic activity after incorporation, be capable of delivering cells and or bioactive molecules [76]. Next, some of the materials investigated for their potential use as injectable ones are described.

In Situ Gelling Biomaterials Employed

Natural Materials

Fibrin

Fibrin is a natural biopolymer that forms the natural provisory matrix for wound healing. It is FDA approved for many applications and there are different preparations commercially available, but it can also be obtained from autologous origin [77]; it is biocompatible, not toxic, or inflammatory [78]. Besides, some of the degradation products of fibrin have interesting properties, like improving healing promotion or a protective effect against myocardial reperfusion injury [79]. Fibrin contains arginine-glycine-asparagine (RGD), which are known cell adhesion motifs [77]; it is cytoprotective for anoxia and provides a favorable microenvironment for cardiomyogenic differentiation of marrow-derived cardiac stem cells [77]. It can also be used as a controlled release system [80]. In sum, fibrin as a gel is a potential candidate to enhance cell adhesion and survival. To obtain the fibrin, fibrinogen monomers in saline solution are mixed with thrombin and they polymerize forming a 3D net by mechanisms similar to normal clotting *in vivo* [81]. The properties of the network can be tailored by modifying the polymerization process.

A concern about translating the fibrin glue for cardiac tissue engineering into the clinic is the risk of inducing intravascular thrombosis [79]. The concentrations of fibrin amenable to delivery through current percutaneous catheters have been studied, demonstrating the feasibility of using fibrin in a non-invasive injectable application [81]. The injection of fibrin alone was proved to preserve left ventricular geometry and cardiac function in a rat acute MI model [82]. But it has also been combined with many types of cells. As an example, it was employed to deliver bone-marrow derived mesenchymal stem cells, which enhanced cell retention and prevented their redistribution in other organs, improving the beneficial effects of the treatment [81]. Injection of fibrin combined with myoblasts [82], bone marrow stem cells [83] or with autologous endothelial cells [84], improved the results obtained with cells alone.

Chitosan

Chitosan (CHT) is a natural cationic polysaccharide, obtained from the deacetylation of chitin of the mollusks, crustaceans and insects. It is soluble in acidic aqueous solution but after neutralization forms a gel-like precipitate [85]. CHT exhibits numerous positive biological and physicochemical properties: biocompatibility, non immunogenicity, and can be conjugated with various molecules thanks to the amino groups on the polysaccharide backbone [86]. A thermally responsive chitosan-based polymer was capable of scavenging the reactive oxygen species produced by the ischemic conditions and recruit key chemokines for stem cell homing such as SDF-1. As a cell delivery system with adipose-derived mesenchymal stem cells, this material was capable of improving the microenvironment for the cells when injected in the infarcted myocardium of rats, improving their survival and engraftment [87]. Chitosan mixed with collagen has been conjugated with QHREDGS (peptide thought to mediate attachment and survival responses of cardiomyocytes) in the format of a thermoresponsive hydrogel to improve maturation and metabolic activity of cardiomyocytes [86]. Alginate-chitosan nanoparticles have been loaded with placental growth factor (PlGF) to increase the left-ventricular function and vascular density in rats [88].

Matrigel

Matrigel is a commercial ECM proteins mixture that undergoes a temperature mediated sol-gel transition, and is obtained from the ECM of mouse sarcoma cells [27]; its clinical application is limited precisely by the source from which it is obtained. It has been implanted alone and in combination with mouse ESC [89] or neonatal cardiomyocytes [90] into a mice model of infarcted myocardium. The gel prevented worsening of the cardiac function, but animals receiving both Matrigel and cells maintained more wall thickness and preserved better cardiac function in terms of fractional shortening and regional contractility [91].

Hair Keratin

Keratin materials can be obtained from hair, importantly from autologous source. More than 30 growth factors are involved in hair morphogenesis, and the residual of them remains in the keratin, what can be beneficial for cardiac repair. Lyophilized keratin powders have the ability to self-assemble upon addition of water, and form gels. Keratin has been implanted onto infarcted rat hearts, and native cardiomyocytes as well as endothelial cells were able to infiltrate the keratin gel, promoting angiogenesis without inducing inflammation; after 2 months animals exhibited preservation of cardiac function and limited ventricular remodeling [92]. These improvements were attributed to the biomaterial's contribution to the mechanical support to the ventricular wall and the presence of cell binding motifs in it.

Alginate

Alginate is a linear block co-polymer of (1-4)-linked β-D-mannuronate and α-L-guluronate residues obtained from seaweed. It is a negatively charged polysaccharide that gels by the presence of calcium ions and is non-thrombogenic [4] The properties of this material can be tuned either by changing the concentration of the solutions or by controlling the molecular weight. Greater concentrations will increase mechanical strength but also will increase the solution viscosity and the degradation time of the gel [27].

Alginate has been used as an injectable material in recent and old infarcts in rats, and it was observed that its injection augmented the scar thickness and limited systolic and diastolic dysfunction [93]. It has also been proposed as a controlled delivery system: based on the different binding affinity of alginate to insulin-like growth factor-1 IGF-1 and hepatocyte growth factor HGF, a dual delivery system of these factors was developed [94]. The hydrogel beads protected the proteins from degradation maintaining their bioactivity and increasing the therapeutic effect of the system.

Alginate sustains very low protein adsorption and it does not support mammalian cells attachment [95], but it can be combined with adhesion motifs to improve its attachment properties. Its conjugation with RGD increased the arteriole density in a rodent model of chronic ischemic cardiomyopathy [96]. However, the combination of alginate with RGD and tyrosine–isoleucine–glycine–serine–arginine (YIGSR) reduced the therapeutic effects of the hydrogel in terms of scar thickness, left ventricular dilation and function [97]. Another modification of alginate has been the addition of the electrical conducting polymer polypyrrole [98], which increases arteriogenesis and promotes myofibroblasts infiltration.

Hyaluronic Acid

Hyaluronic acid (HA) is a non-sulfated glycosaminoglycan prevalent in the extracellular matrix of many tissues. HA plays an important role in homeostasis, transport of nutrients and also mediates the inflammation and repair processes. It is biocompatible, non-immunogenic, biodegradable and has different biological activities depending on its molecular weight. Precisely the low molecular weight degradation products of HA stimulate angiogenesis and endothelial cell proliferation and migration [99]. It can be functionalized to improve its biological development, for example with PEG-SH$_4$ [100]. Moreover, it is a FDA-approved material for its use in humans in certain applications like dermal and intra-articular injection.

There are already commercially available *in situ* crosslinkable HA-derived hydrogels. Different types of HA hydrogels have been compared with commercial fibrin, poly(vinyl alcohol)-chitosan and elastin hydrogels, in terms of *in vitro* degradation rates and cytotoxicity and *in vivo* degradation, immune response and angiogenic potential [76]. Traut's grafted HA hydrogel and periodate oxidated HA hydrogel, especially the first one, demonstrated to be the most suitable for new artery formation in ischemic myocardium because they were both digested within 2 weeks with low immune response and strong angiogenesis compared with the other examined hydrogels.

HA alone does not support cell adhesion. Cardiosphere-derived cells were delivered using a thiolated hyaluronan-based hydrogel crosslinked with thiol-reactive poly(ethylene glycol) diacrylate and covalently linked or not with thiolated denatured collagen. It was observed that the retention rate achieved with the hydrogel without collagen was similar to that of cells delivered in phosphate buffer saline (PBS), either by a low physical retention or poor cell survival and adhesion of HA [101]. In the *in vivo* study in a mouse model of myocardial infarction, some functional benefits were observed though.

Collagen

Collagen supports growth and survival of cardiomyocytes *in vitro*, and is one of the main components of the ECM in the adult heart [102]. Commercial collagen alone has been implanted in animal models showing improvements in ventricular cardiac function and geometry [103]. In another study in a myocardial infarction model in rats (with ischemia-reperfusion model this time) increased capillarity density and myofibroblasts infiltration after 5 weeks were reported [104].

The therapeutic potential of injectable collagen has been evaluated in combination with different cell types. Bone marrow stem cells were injected via catheter in a swine model in combination with collagen, demonstrating the feasibility of a non-invasive delivery of this system [105]. Collagen was also used as a carrier for mesenchymal stem cells (MSC) transplantation to improve the retention of the cells in the infarcted myocardium [106]. 4 weeks after implantation, rats receiving cells in saline suspension, had the implanted cells in remote organs, whereas in animals receiving the cells with collagen, were detected to a lesser extent in remote organs. However, cardiac function was improved in animals receiving cells in saline and collagen alone but not in the combined collagen MSC group. The mechanisms underlying this negative interaction (controverted in other works) are unknown, but is suggested that collagen may limit oxygen and nutrients diffusion, and compromise cell-cell interactions. In another study, collagen combined with chondroitin 6-sulfate was employed to deliver CD-133+ progenitor cells derived from peripherial blood after expansion *in vitro* [107]. It was expected that the material would improve cell adhesion and survival into ischemic hind limb athymic rats. The collagen increased two-fold the number of cells retained when implanted alone; the implanted material was vascularized and the injected cells added into vascular structures.

Gelatin

It is a non-immunogenic partially degraded product of collagen [108]. It has been injected as a hydrogel in rat infarcted hearts bare or loaded with basic fibroblast growth factor; adding the factor improved arteriogenesis, ventricular remodeling and function [109]. Basic fibroblast growth factor has also been delivered with gelatin microspheres [110], inducing angiogenesis and improving cardiac function. The loaded nanoparticles induced an increase in the blood flow in the infarct border (thanks to stimulated angiogenesis), and as a result left ventricular function was improved.

ECM-derived Materials

A different approach is based on decellularized tissues, their digestion and injection. This type of materials has the advantage of containing a physiological proportion of the native components of the ECM [102] and cues for cell-matrix interactions. ECM coming from different tissues has been studied, and apparently the ECM of each tissue has its unique combination of proteins and proteoglycans. This makes of myocardial decellularized matrix, among all other tissues matrices, the best candidate for myocardial repair when it is available [111]. Decellularized porcine myocardial tissue able to self-assemble into a nanofibrous structure similar to collagen *in vitro* at 37°C and deliverable *in vivo* upon catheter injection was tested in rats. It induced endothelial cells and smooth muscle cells migration increasing the arteriole formation at 11 days post-injection [111].

Small intestinal submucosa (SIS) is a dense sheet of acellular extracellular matrix. This material is used in the clinic for accelerated wound healing. SIS supports proliferation, attachment and migration of various cell types and stimulates angiogenesis thanks to the growth factors and binding motifs embedded in the matrix. Two different types of commercial available SIS-derived gels have been studied as an injectable material for cardiac repair in a murine model [112]. The two materials differed in the concentration of basic fibroblast factor, obtaining best result the material richer in this factor. In another work, an emulsion of digested ECM from SIS was injected into infarcted rat hearts, improving cardiac function, increasing neovascularization and promoting cell recruitment [113].

Synthetic Materials

Synthetic materials are made in the laboratory from primary building blocks, so their properties can be tuned to match desired characteristics. Besides, they are free from animal origin components and the risks related therewith.

Thermosensitive Hydrogels

This group of materials has temperature-dependant sol to gel transition. The great advantage of this group of materials is the possibility to tune their properties for them to undergo the gelation transition around body temperature [114]. In this way they can be comfortably manipulated and injected and only when they are inside the body they will undergo the transition.

Some of the materials of this group are based on N-isopropylacrylamide (NiPAAm). It is non biodegradable, but copolymerized with degradable polymers becomes biodegradable. For instance, NiPAAm was copolymerized with acrylic acid (AAc) and hydroxyethyl methacrylate-poly(trimethylene carbonate) (HEMAPTMC) [115]. The ratio of each material was adjusted to obtain a hydrogel at 37°C. It can also be degraded *in vitro* with a mass loss over 85% after 5 months. This material was injected *in vivo* in rats and proved to preserve the area of the left ventricular cavity and contractility. Tissue ingrowth, a thicker left ventricle (LV) wall and greater capillarity density were also found when compared with PBS controls. After 8 weeks, a layer of smooth muscle cells with contractile phenotype was formed next to the remaining material.

Another family of thermoresponsive hydrogels based on polycaprolactone, N-isopropylacrylamide, 2-hydroxyethyl methacrylate and dimethyl-g-butyrolactone acrylate has been developed [116]. Cardiosphere derived cells

(CDC) combined with the hydrogel were suitable for myocardial injection and the solutions formed solid gels within 5 s at 37°C. Hydrogels with different mechanical properties were obtained and it was shown that they influence the fate of the CDC differentiation. Another thermoresponsive material containing biodegradable dextran chain grafted with hydrophobic poly(ε-caprolactone)-2-hydroxylethyl methacrylate (PCL-HEMA) chain and thermoresponsive poly(N isopropylacrylamide) (PNIPAAm) (Dex-PCL-HEMA/PNIPAAm) has been synthesized. It can shift from sol to gel within 30 s and is reversible within the same time frame [117]. It was injected in rabbits, 4-days post-infarction. Histological analyses one month later indicated that the material prevented the scar expansion and thinning of the wall. Left ventricular ejection fraction was increased and it attenuated left ventricular systolic and diastolic dilation.

Poly (Ethylene Glycol) (PEG)

A strategy based on non-biodegradable *in situ* crosslinkable PEG hydrogel has been developed, to provide a permanent support to limit the remodeling [118]. Its therapeutic effects were tested in rat myocardial infarction model at short and long term. Beneficial effects were observed at 4 weeks, but at long term (13 weeks) it was unable to prevent the dilation. Besides, the material injection induced some inflammatory response.

An injectable α-cyclodextrin/poly(ethylene glycol)–b-polycaprolactone-(dodecanedioic acid)-polycaprolactone–poly(ethylene glycol) (MPEG–PCL–MPEG) hydrogel was used to deliver and encapsulate bone marrow stem cells into infarcted myocardium [119]. The CD/MPEG-PCL-MPEG hydrogel alone does not induce angiogenesis, but can serve as a support in the infarcted zone and contribute to inhibit the left ventricular remodeling. One month after the injection of the gel combined with cells, cell retention and survival and the density of vessels were increased when compared with cells injection alone; moreover, the gel was absorbed, ventricular dilation was limited and the ventricular ejection fraction improved. PEG-based temperature-sensitive hydrogels have also been combined with growth factors or other molecules. VEGF was mixed or conjugated with the aliphatic polyester hydrogel poly(δ-valerolactone)-block-poly(ethylene glycol)-block-poly(δ-valerolactone) (PVL-b-PEG-b-PVL); the sustained VEGF release during the degradation time of the hydrogel translated into an improvement of the myocardial and functional recovery, in dependence of the preparation method [120]. In another work, a metalloproteinase-responsive PEG-based hydrogel was synthesized to be a thymosin β4 (a pro-angiogenic and pro-survival factor) delivering scaffold. It was implanted combined with endothelial and smooth muscle cells derived from human embryonic stem cells (hESC) in rats [121]. The gel provides structural organization and when was loaded with cells and thymosin b4 enhanced more contractile performance than when the hydrogel was only loaded with the factor, because of their paracrine effect. Another PEG-based hydrogel, α-cyclodextrin/MPEG–PCL–MPEG, was tested as a delivery system for erythropoietin (EPO) [122], a hormone that plays a protective role in the infarcted myocardium. Rats treated with this system showed limited cell apoptosis and increased neovasculature formation; also infarct size was reduced and cardiac function improved.

PEG in the format of nanoparticles has also been studied. They can be injected intravenously, circulate in the body for long periods and bind only to desired tissues. Nanoparticles targeting the infarcted myocardium were developed based on the overexpression of angiotensin II type 1 (AT1) receptor in the infarcted heart [123]. The system was formed by a vehicle and a targeter, a ligand specific to AT1 that will make the nanoparticles bind specifically. The vehicle was 142 nm diameter PEGylated liposomes, which could carry therapeutic molecules and release them in a controlled way. This system was proved to target the infarcted heart in mice model, but not the healthy.

Self Assembling Peptides (SAPs)

SAPs are short peptides capable of forming hydrogels at physiological pH and osmolarity [124]. When the SAPs solution is placed in contact with ions or pH is changed, the charges are partially neutralized and a hydrophobic packing takes place forming beta-sheet structures, constituting fibers that build a 3D network if the concentration is high enough. Fibers shape is different depending on the nature of the employed peptides. In the particular case of the RAD16 ionic peptides family (R: arginine, A: alanine, D: aspartate) fibers thicknesses are of 5-10 nm.

Peptides can be combined with cells to encapsulate them within the peptide network [125]. RAD16-I (AcN-RADARADARADARADA-CNH$_2$) has proved to be a useful synthetic gel capable of maintaining the cells in the site of interest, and has been used as a delivery system of different types of cells to the heart. On the contrary, when it was implanted alone limited improvements were observed in the infarct area and the remodeling process. RAD16-II (AcN-RARADADARARADADA-CNH2) peptide has been shown to create microenvironments in the infarcted myocardium that are infiltrated with endothelial and smooth muscle cells, suggesting a potential for vascularization [124]. It was also observed that combining RAD16-II with neonatal cardiomyocytes the density of endogenous -sarcomeric actin positive cells increased.

As stated, SAPs gels can be modified to incorporate growth factors or drugs. The self assembling peptide RAD16-II has been used as a drug vehicle to deliver both platelet derived growth factor and fibroblast growth factor (PDGF-BB and FGF-2) [126]. The first is arteriogenic and the second is angiogenic; their combination targets endothelial cells (EC) and vascular smooth muscle cells (VSMC). Infarct size and cardiomyocyte apoptosis were considerably reduced in rats. The capillary and arterial density was recovered, and cardiac function was almost recovered. This system also induced long-lasting vessel formation. RAD16-II combined with IGF-1, a cytokine that protects and promotes cardiomyocytes growth, has also been used as a delivery system for cardiomyocytes [127]. The addition of IGF-1 acted reducing cell apoptosis and improving systolic function.

PREFORMED GELS AND SCAFFOLDS

Rationale

An alternative approach in the field of cardiac tissue engineering involves the use of biomaterials to produce patches *ex vivo* and implant them epicardially onto the infarcted tissue, conveniently adapted to its size and shape. These patches can be pre-loaded with cells (incorporated within their pores in the case of microporous scaffolds, or encapsulated in the case of a gel conformed before implantation, as shown in figure 1 b) and growth factors or drugs, and act as a cell supply, a mechanical reinforcement to the infarct scar to avoid ventricular dilation and a drug release system simultaneously.

Requirements of the Scaffolds

In this strategy a key aspect is to find a material that matches the required properties. The material needs also to be cell-friendly, non-cytotoxic and promote cell attachment and proliferation, and it must also be non-immunogenic [128]. The scaffolds should provide a 3D environment to the cells with a porous structure able to guide cardiomyocytes alignment and promote maturation, also induce the development of a contractile phenotype and the electro-mechanical coupling of the implanted cells among them, and also with the host tissue [129, 32] and need to be easily vascularized [37].

The mechanical properties exhibited by the scaffolds should be adequate to their application in heart tissue engineering. It implies that they should ideally be compliant with contractions and exhibit non-linear elasticity, as well as be capable to adapt to the shape of the heart in all phases of the heart beat. Anisotropy to mimic the directionally-dependent electrical and mechanical properties of the native myocardium is important too [130]. Besides, the stiffness of the material employed affects to a great extent the phenotype and contractile properties of the neonatal cardiomyocytes [131, 132], and has to be carefully tuned to match physiological conditions. During heart development, the ECM on which cardiomyocytes maturation takes place, stiffen 9 times. An interesting approach to mimic it is the development of materials with time dependant mechanical properties [133]. For instance, hyaluronic acid hydrogels that stiffen with time form more contractile units when compared with cultures in hydrogels without such time-dependant stiffness.

Attending to the type of strategy, three groups can be distinguished, in terms of the nature of the matrices: biologically-derived materials, synthetic (either biodegradable or biostable) materials and decellularized tissues. With the use of biodegradable scaffolds, it is expected that the matrix will degrade as the surrounding tissue is regenerated; the degradation products should not be toxic and metabolized by the body. By using permanent scaffolds, the idea is that they will be infiltrated by the host tissue and contribute to the regeneration, but also act as a permanent mechanical restraint to limit ventricular dilation. The approach of scaffolds derived from decellularized tissue is based on the use of tissues whose cells are removed and the remaining ECM maintains the architecture and mechanical properties similar to those of the native tissue. Obtaining a scaffold matching the desired properties is a hard task, as many different properties are required; thus, materials exhibiting different properties have been mixed in more advanced strategies to obtain a composite that combines them.

Related Problematic

As all the approaches described so far, this one also has some advantages, disadvantages and unsolved problematic. An important disadvantage is that the application of a patch in the heart needs a much more invasive technique than a catheter-delivered system, as it requires a surgical procedure to be implanted. As advantage, the fact that the materials are synthesized and conveniently prepared out of the body can be outlined. It implies that there is no limitation in the preparation procedure and in the use of solvents (if they are properly removed at the end of the fabrication process and do not induce cytotoxicity). Therefore, the range of chemistries and techniques available to obtain scaffolds with different architectures is broadening. Besides, cells can be pre-cultured *in vitro* within them prior to implantation if desired. In addition, the mechanical properties of polymer scaffolds may be tuned to match more closely those of the heart muscle than with gelly biomaterials.

Unlike native myocardium, where the greatest distance between capillaries is around 20 microns [69], scaffolds are not vascularized *a priori*. Then, cells seeded in the scaffolds have their oxygen and nutrients supply limited to their molecular diffusion through the thickness of the scaffold. Given the fact that cardiomyocytes have great consumption rates of nutrients and oxygen, diffusion is insufficient supply for thick constructs. Consequently, to obtain a thick engineered tissue with viable cells through all its thickness, pre-vascularization or improved diffusion throughout the scaffold until it is vascularized is key for the implant to succeed. Otherwise, cell density will be concentrated in the external parts and cell viability will be compromised in the center of the scaffold if the distance to the surface is greater than a critical value estimated around 100 microns [134]. For example, the influence of oxygen concentration in cell density and viability in collagen scaffolds has been studied, the former decreasing linearly with the distance to the surface and the latter exponentially [135]. These results indicate that in order to guarantee an appropriate oxygen concentration throughout the scaffold, additional measures need to be taken.

Many attempts have been done in this direction, like the addition of oxygen carriers to the culture medium to simulate the effect of the hemoglobin in the blood. Their addition contributed to improve mass transport and to increase cell density [136]. Another strategy includes the use of scaffolds releasing growth factors to enhance the vascularization process, like basic fibroblast growth factor [137], vascular endothelial growth factor (VEGF) [138] and Thymosin beta-4 [139]. Another approach is the addition of the growth factor platelet derived growth factor BB to the culture medium to protect cardiomyocytes from apoptosis [140]. In a different methodology, channeled scaffolds were produced to simulate the capillary structure of the native tissues and guide endothelial cells growth. The porosity might be adjusted to increase capillary infiltration but it is limited to the maximum size of the pores on which endothelial cells can form vascular structures [141]. An alternative involves the use of decellularized tissues that already provide a native vascular network [142, 143]. The culture of endothelial cells prior to implantation of cardiac myocytes has also been explored [144], and reduced cardiomyocytes apoptosis and necrosis was found. Another possibility is to pre-implant the scaffold to pre-vascularize it prior to its implantation in the final site: alginate scaffolds loaded with angiogenic and pro-survival factors (Matrigel, SDF-1, VEGF and IGF-1) were pre-implanted into the omentum of rats [145]. It proved to be a very interesting *in vivo* "bioreactor", providing to the patch a functional vascular network that maintained the viability of the transplanted cells.

Pre-culturing the scaffolds *in vitro* in bioreactors has also been a considered an option. There are many types of bioreactors (stirring, spinning flasks rotating, perfusion, etc.), but not all of them improve enough the diffusion to lead to uniform cell density and compact tissue formation. As an example, in a study where rotating bioreactors were used to culture polyglycolic acid (PGA) scaffolds [146], functional and interconnected cells only were found in the peripheral parts, where there was a better diffusion of the oxygen. Perfusion bioreactors have been developed to try to reduce diffusional limitations by establishing interstitial flow through the scaffolds in order to allow the formation of thick tissues with uniform cell density throughout them. The effect of culturing scaffolds in perfusion bioreactors was compared with culturing them in spinner flasks [134] or orbital mixed dishes [147]. In both studies results were improved with the perfusion bioreactors; when cultured in the others, high cell density was only found in the outer layers. However, a limitation of perfusion bioreactors is the medium flow rate, because of the hydrodynamic shear the interstitial flow inflicts to the cells, which could maintain them in a rounded morphology or even wash them out if it is too high. This finding led to the combination of the perfusion culture with the use of channeled scaffolds that provided separated compartments for medium flow [148]. Even more, this strategy has been successfully combined and used simultaneously with a selective pre-seeding of the scaffold in the channels with endothelial cells using a perfusion seeding technique, which provides uniform seeding throughout the entire scaffold without the use of cell carriers [149].

Another step was made when the pulsatile perfusion bioreactor [150] was developed. It was expected that the pulsatile interstitial medium flow would provide mechanical conditioning and improved mass transport, intending that all together would lead to a tissue with better contractile properties. Indeed, scaffolds cultured under these conditions had enhanced contractile properties. A different type of bioreactor, with bidirectional slow flow perfusion obtained with an oscillatory system was tested with culture medium loaded or not with Insuline-like growth factor-I [151]. The advantage of the combined strategies was revealed.

However, despite the great efforts put and the improvements achieved, obtaining vascularized constructs is still an unsolved problem.

Preparation Techniques

Many different techniques have been proposed to obtain 3D porous structures with different topographies and porosities, basically based in phase separation procedures or the use porogen templates to create the pores. Now with the introduction of controlled computer assisted systems, new possibilities are open. Next, a brief description of the main techniques employed to prepare scaffolds for heart tissue engineering is outlined.

The electrospinning technique is based in the application of a high voltage to a polymer melted or in a solution that leads to the formation of ultrathin nonwoven fibers [152], which are projected on a collector giving rise to fiber mats with controlled thicknesses. The fibers diameters can be obtained in the range of the ECM proteins. This technique also allows the preparation of aligned fibers, which can be applied to obtain aligned cardiac cells [153].

The particle leaching technique is based on the use of a porogen that is mixed with a polymer solution or a melted polymer. This porogen is removed after the solvent has been eliminated (solvent casting, freeze extraction) or the polymer has solidified after cooling, leaving empty spaces (pores) with the size and shape of the porogen template (and also small pores for the elimination of the solvent, if used). Porosity and pores interconnection can be tuned by changing the porogen-polymer ratio. Gas foaming avoids the use of solvents and high temperatures, because the pores are obtained by exposition to a high pressure gas followed by a pressure decrease with nucleation and growth of pores. The freeze-drying technique consists in freezing a polymeric solution and then lyophilize it to remove the solvent in the frozen state and obtain a solid porous structure [154]. Different morphologies can be obtained by changing the freezing conditions [155].

Microfluidic patterning consists in forcing a polymer solution through a channeled mould previously obtained with the desired geometry. Once the polymer is consistent, the mould is removed and the scaffold or patterned surface is ready. Selective laser sintering is a technique based in the use of a CO_2 laser to sinterize selectively the powder of a material to form the cross section of each layer of a 3D object.

Microcontact printing is a technique that allows cell adhesion guidance [156]. It consists in the use of a stamp, with the pattern to be followed by the cells. The stamp is inked with the solution that is expected to promote the adhesion (laminin, ECM proteins, etc.) and then pressed against the substrate to transfer the solution. By loading the solution with growth factors, cell differentiation can also be induced in patterns [157].

Biomaterials Employed As Scaffolds

Many different types of materials have been considered for cardiac tissue engineering. According to their origin we can distinguish: biologically-derived materials, decellularized tissues and synthetic materials. Natural materials include collagen, gelatin, fibrin, silk and alginate; and synthetic materials include polyurethane (PU), polylactide acid (PLA), polyglycolic acid (PGA), polycaprolactone (PCL), or polyglicerolsebacate (PGS), among others.

Natural Materials

Collagen

There are a number of commercial collagen patches, widely used by clinicians for other purposes, which are now under study as epicardial patches, because it has been reported to be a good substrate for cell attachment and infiltration [158]. They have been combined with different cell types and molecules. Unfortunately, collagen sponges have a great swelling rate and poor mechanical performance in aqueous medium.

Collagen can be used in two formats, as a porous scaffold or as a hydrogel. To obtain the scaffold a collagen solution is lyophilized and then rehydrated and seeded with cells. In the case of hydrogels, a collagen solution is mixed with cells *ex vivo* and then gelled. As a gel entrapping embryonic chick cardiomyocytes [159], it was found to beat and arrange as a highly organized tissue-like when pulses with different frequency were applied.

The potential of collagen scaffolds as an attractant for neovascularization was demonstrated in a study with rats [160]. Collagen sponges implanted in both healthy and cryoinjured hearts were almost absorbed after 2 months, but the remaining structures were populated by new arterioles and capillaries. In another study, collagen has been combined with chondroitin 6-sulfate to obtain porous scaffolds. These scaffolds delivered MSC in the infarcted region in a rat model, promoting neovascularization [161].

The therapeutical potential of collagen as epicardial patch has been compared with injectable approaches. Collagen matrices loaded with mesenchymal stem cells (MSC) [162], and collagen scaffolds loaded with human umbilical cord blood cells (hUCBCs) [25], gave better results than the injection of cells alone in mice. In the MAGNUM phase I clinical trial [163], intrainfarct cell therapy of autologous BMC was combined with collagen scaffolds loaded with BMC. This treatment was found to be safe and contribute to limit left ventricular remodeling by increasing the thickness of the ventricle wall and then reducing the stress of the wall.

Collagen has been modified to incorporate bioactive molecules to improve its biological behavior. Its scaffolds have been modified with RGD [164] and cardiac markers of cardiospheres derived from cardiac progenitor cultured on them were upregulated. Collagen functionalized with interleukin-10 plasmid [165] (an anti-inflammatory plasmid) increased 5 times cell retention and modulated inflammation.

Gelatin

Gelatin is obtained from chemical denatured collagen; it is therefore weaker and degrades faster than it [27]. It has been reported to provoke unspecific inflammatory response upon degrading; at first this can be considered an undesired effect, but for certain applications it might be beneficial for the positive impact that can have on angiogenesis [166]. A commercial gelatin sponge bare or cultured either with fetal or adult rat heart cells was implanted to replace the resected right ventricular outflow tract (ROVT) of rats [167]. After 4 weeks a great inflammation was observed and after 12 weeks the patches had endothelial cells on the endocardial surface. Nonetheless, the authors concluded that a material inducing less inflammatory response is needed.

Fibrin

Fibrin can be used as an injectable gel, but can also be preformed *ex vivo*, which broadens the possibilities of fabrication. For example, SDF-1 (a factor that is up-regulated for a period of time after a myocardial infarction, and contributes to mobilize cells from bone marrow and peripherial blood to the damaged tissue) was covalently bound to a PEGylated fibrin patch [168] and implanted in an AMI mouse model; the SDF-1 loaded patch reduced more significantly the scar area expansion and improved the left ventricular function than the un-loaded patch.

Alginate

Alginate scaffolds obtained by the freeze drying technique have been extensively explored in myocardial regeneration. Loaded with fetal cardiac cells and implanted in infarcted rats, they limited left ventricular dilation [169]. However, cultured with neonatal or fetal cardiomyocytes in static conditions, cell aggregates were formed due to the non-adhesive nature of the alginate [170].

To improve cell adhesion and survival modifications of alginate scaffolds have been investigated. For example, it has been modified to incorporate the adhesion peptide RGD [171], which improved cell adhesion, reduced apoptosis, accelerated tissue regeneration and led to the organization of cardiomyocytes in myofibers *in vitro*, and also with a combination of RGD and the heparin-binding peptide G4SPPRRARVTY (HBP) [172], with better results.

Polysaccharides

Polysaccharide-based scaffolds have also been investigated with myocardial regeneration purposes. The effectiveness of freeze-dried pullulan and dextran patches was compared to mesenchymal stem cells endocardial delivery alone in a rat myocardial infarction model [173], the scaffolds improving the cell engraftment and survival at 1 and 2 months.

Silk

Because of silk fibroin good mechanical properties, biological performance, and its easy processing to obtain different morphologies, it has generated interest in the tissue engineering field. Silk is produced by some insects like spiders or silkworms, and is considered a non-degradable material by the FDA [174]. Silk fibroin has been combined by chitosan and hyaluronic acid to produce microparticles that were pressed and crosslinked with genipin to obtain cardiac patches [175]. MSC cultured on the composite patches exhibited greater proliferation and cardiomyogenic differentiation than in silk patches.

Recently, non-mulberry silk fibroin from Antheraea mylitta has been investigated as a material for cardiac tissue engineering [176]. It has better mechanical properties than mulberry silk, contains RGD sequences, is non-cytotoxic and induces low level of inflammatory response. When neonatal rat cardiomyocytes were seeded in an Antherea mylitta silk lyophilized scaffold, the results were better than those obtained with a mulberry silk.

Decellularized-tissue Derived Scaffolds

Decellularized extracellular matrices have been used as scaffolds in many studies and also in preclinical and human clinical applications [177]. The decellularization process consists in a set of washes to remove the cells but maintain as much as possible the architecture, proteins and adhesion molecules. The more aggressive the washes and treatments are, the lower the risk of allogenic immune reaction is, but undesired washout of adhesion proteins and architecture damage can be associated [65].

Decellularized sheets have been tested in combination with fibrin, TGF-beta, and MSC and tested in a nude rat model of infarction with positive results [178]. A patch of urinary bladder-derived extracellular matrix (UBM) was implanted in pigs, as a left ventricular wall replacement after infarction, and compared with a polytetrafluoroethlyene (ePTFE) [177] one. At three months, the results were better with the UBM: it was reabsorbed and a cellularized and vascularized tissue rich in collagen was formed.

Sliced decellularized porous scaffolds of acellular bovine pericardia have been combined with cell sheets from bone marrow stem cells, cultured and implanted in rats replacing the resected infarcted myocardium [179]. The patch pores were filled by cells, new vessels and new muscle fibers, indicating that the graft was integrating. Cardiac function was improved and the dilated left ventricle was restored after implantation. In a revolutionary study entire rat hearts were decellularized, and then re-cellularized with neonatal cardiac cells [180]. The architecture was conserved and the preserved vasculature was perfusable. Seeded cardiomyocytes coupled electromechanically and after 8 days under external electrodes stimulation the re-cellularized heart beat and was capable to pump blood.

Synthetic Materials

Synthetic materials are prepared in the laboratory, allowing precise control over their mechanical properties, degradation, morphology and porosity that can be tuned as desired [181]. However, they may not have as good biological performance as biologically derived materials [4].

Polylactic Acid and Polyglycolic Acid (PLA and PGA)

Polylactic acid is a biocompatible, biodegradable and FDA-approved polymer; it degrades into lactic acid (non-cytotoxic), and has been widely used in patients, for example as sutures. However, its degradation products can induce a slight, undesired, acidification of the microenvironment [65]. Polyglycolic acid is a thermoplastic too; it has also been used in the clinic and degrades into non-toxic products. However, neither PLLA nor PGA exhibit the desired elasticity to match that of native heart tissue. In many studies PLA and PGA have been combined as poly(lactic–co-glycolic acid) (PLGA), or other polyesters, to modify their properties as desired. Electrospun PLGA fibrous membranes with different compositions (having different hydrophobicity and degradation rates) [4] were found to align cardiomyocytes in the direction of the nanofibers, the best results being those of the slightly hydrophobic copolymers. Porous beads of PLGA seeded with human amniotic fluid stem cells (hAFSCs) have been tested as a cell delivery vehicle or "cellularized microscaffold" [182]; after implantation by intramyocardial injection in a rat infarct model, they showed good retention of the cells in the site of interest. PLGA has been treated with laminin [183] to improve its biological development and combined with carbon nanofibers (CNF) to increase its conductivity and cytocompatibility [184]. PLLA-PLGA scaffolds loaded with Matrigel have been co-cultured with endothelial cells, cardiomyocytes and embryonic fibroblasts simultaneously [185], for EC to provide vasculature and act synergically with cardiomyocytes to improve cell survival and proliferation.

Poly (Epsilon-caprolactone) (PCL)

Poly(epsilon-caprolactone) is a FDA-approved biocompatible polyester, as PLA and PGA. It is more elastic because of its lower glass transition temperature, and behaves as a rubber at body temperature. Its degradation does not produce acidification because it occurs more slowly [158]. It has been proposed for myocardial regeneration for example in 3D constructs obtained by overlapping electrospun PCL nanofibrous mats (up to 5 layers) on which neonatal cardiomyocytes were cultured [186]. The layers established morphologic and electrical connections between them and exhibited synchronized beating, and no ischemia was found in the center of the constructs.

It is usually combined with PLA, PGA or its copolymer. Poly-glycolide-co-caprolactone (PGCL) biodegradable porous scaffolds have been studied as cell vehicles for bone marrow-derived mononuclear cells (BMMNC) in rat myocardial infarction models [187]. BMNC migrated from the scaffold and neovasculature over the implant was detected; left ventricular function improvement and limitation of the progression of the left ventricular dilation was also observed. Scaffolds made of poly(DL-lactide-*co*-caprolactone) (PLACL), PLGA, and type I collagen [158], cultured with neonatal rat heart cells, have been compared. The composite scaffolds gave better results than controls (collagen and PLGA sponges) in terms of cellularity, contractility and cardiac markers expression (Tn-I and Cx-43). Perfusion culture improved cell density distribution.

Polyurethanes (PU)

Polyurethanes are synthetic biocompatible materials widely used in the biomedical field. Their mechanical properties and biodegradability can be tuned by changing their composition. PU degrades *in vivo* through hydrolytic chain scission, which is accelerated by the enzymes action and loads, among other factors [188], but with the appropriate composition non-biodegradable polyurethanes can be obtained [189]. This family of polymers can be used to obtain fibrous scaffolds by electrospinning with different mechanical properties depending on the fibers orientation [190] or porous elastic scaffolds [191]. Polyester urethane urea (PEUU) elastic porous scaffolds have been implanted in sub-acute infarctions in rats and were found to promote the formation of smooth muscle bundles, to increase the ventricle thickness and to improve contractile function [192]. Cell attachment on polyurethane-based porous scaffolds can be improved by pre-treating them with laminin [193].

Poly(Glycerol Sebacate) (PGS)

Poly(glycerol sebacate) is a biocompatible and biodegradable elastomer capable of recovering from deformation. It can be obtained by polycondensation of glycerol and sebacic acid. By changing the synthesis temperature, the properties of the resulting material can be tuned to match the desired mechanical properties. The degradation rates can also be adjusted from fast degradation to nearly inert [194].

By the use of excimer laser microablation, 3D porous PGS scaffolds with anisotropic structural and mechanical properties were obtained [195, 130]. These scaffolds induced neonatal cardiac cells alignment in the absence of external stimuli and matched the mechanical properties of adult rat right ventricle. Moreover, they allowed cell contractility when stimulated. For its interesting mechanical properties, PGS has been coaxially electrospun with gelatin to form a nanofibrous mat with PGS in the core and gelatin in the shell [196] to enhance cell adhesion and proliferation. PGS has been modified to incorporate acrylic groups in different number (to modify its mechanical properties and degradation) and electrospun in combination with gelatin [197].

Acrylate Based Materials

Acrylate based materials have not been widely exploited for cardiac tissue engineering yet but the interest on them is increasing, for their versatility of processing and variety of properties obtained. For example, scaffolds made of poly(2-hydroxyethyl methacrylate-co-methacrylic acid) (P(HEMA-co-MAA) hydrogel have been obtained by fibers and microspheres templating to obtain spherical pores and parallel channels [198], which allow simultaneously mass transfer and guidance of the cardiomyocyte bundles. Mechanical properties were adjusted intentionally for the elastic modulus to be lower than that of native myocardium in order to make possible the mechanical stimulation of the cells when implanted *in vivo*. In [199], poly(ethyl acrylate) (PEA) scaffolds are filled with HA gel; the scaffolds provide the three-dimensional environment and mechanical properties and the gel may act as an encapsulating medium for the cells and may be also used as a medium for drug or growth factors release. RAD16-I gel may also be used as a filler in PEA scaffolds, where it acts as a diffusion medium and improves cell seeding efficiency (figure 2).

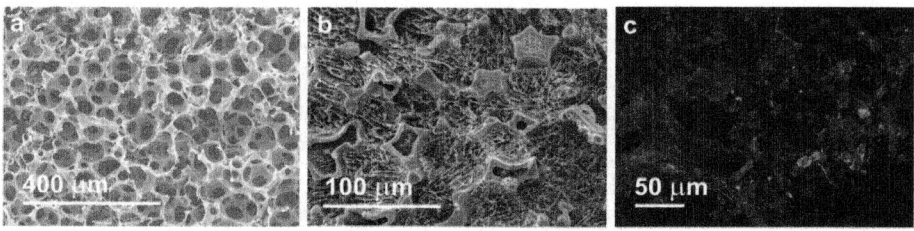

Figure 2. (a) Scanning electron microscopy (SEM) image of poly(ethyl acrylate), PEA, elastomeric membranes with interconnected spherical pores. (b) CryoSEM image (cross section) of a PEA scaffold whose pores are filled with the self-assembling peptide (SAP) gel RAD16-I. (c) Adipose stem cells (nuclei stained in blue and actin cytoskeleton stained in green) seeded in a PEA scaffold with a SAP gel filling. Confocal laser scanning microscopy image of a 50 μm thick internal slice.

Electrical and Mechanical Stimulation

Electrical Stimulation

External electrical fields have been shown to contribute to the differentiation towards cardiomyocytes of different cell types, such as embryonic stem cells (ESC) [200] or BMSC [201] seeded in collagen scaffolds, and to the development of conductive and contractile properties of neonatal cardiac cells, in this case seeded with Matrigel in a collagen porous scaffold [202]. It has been proposed that the intracellular endogenous reactive oxygen species (ROS) produced when an electric field is applied contribute to the hESC differentiation [203].

In an attempt of optimizing the electrical stimulation parameters [204], it has been determined that the electrode material is very important, and best results have been obtained for carbon electrodes. Amplitude and frequency of the stimulation have also a great influence in the cultured cardiac tissue. Micropatterned electrodes can be of interest as they allow spatial control of the electric field [205].

Polymeric scaffolds limit cardiomyocytes electric communication, what restricts the synchronous beating of the engineered tissue. To improve it, gold nanowires were incorporated to a porous alginate scaffold [206]. Another approach to obtain elastic and electrical conductive scaffolds consisted in impregnating thiol-HEMA/HEMA scaffolds with gold nanoparticles [207]. In both cases even without electrical stimulation the improvement in the scaffold conductivity had positive physiological effects.

Mechanical Stimulation

Mechanical stress has a great impact on cell proliferation, ECM formation and hypertrophy (increased cell size), and has been intensively studied in the field of cardiac tissue engineering. Embryonic chick and neonatal rat cardiac myocytes mixed with collagen and mechanically stimulated exhibited hypertrophy and improvement of contractile function [208]. Cardiac myocytes from neonatal rats mixed with collagen I and Matrigel and casted in rings subjected to mechanical stretch [209] showed histological characteristics of adult cardiac tissue. Action potential measurements indicated electrophysiological behavior akin to cardiac tissue. Constructs produced by simultaneously electrospinning PU and electrospraying mesenchymal stem cells [210] were cultured in spinner flasks with stretching, which led to cells alignment, cardiac markers increase and ion channels development. Similarly, cells isolated from neonatal rat hearts seeded in chitosan-collagen I channeled porous scaffolds [211] and cultured under high mechanical stimulation induced cell alignment, elongation and the presence of gap junctions connecting the cells. Mechanical stress applied to human cardiac cells cultured in a gelatin scaffold improved cell distribution and proliferation within the scaffold, increased the production of the ECM, and the structure and organization was similar to normal myocardium, likely because the stretching of the scaffold favors nutrients and oxygen exchange improving cell microenvironment [212].

VENTRICULAR RESTRAINTS

After Chachques and Carpentier work [213], it was found that wrapping the heart even with a passive muscle flap had beneficial effects; this finding led to the development of the ventricular restraint therapy [214]. In this approach the aim is not to regenerate the ischemic tissue, but to avoid the progress of the adverse remodeling following a myocardial infarction. It is based on the application of a mechanical restraint (schematized in figure 1 c), which should limit or revert ventricular dilation. A variety of synthetic meshes have been proposed to achieve this goal.

A bilayer membrane with polypropylene in one side to promote tissue ingrowth (or at least limit the ventricular dilation) and with polytetrafluoroethylene in the other side to prevent pericardial adhesions was studied in a chronic infarction model of pig as a restraint [215]. The use of this patch induced improvements once the remodeling process following an infarction had started. The use of a non-biodegradable material is intentional as authors considered that a permanent mechanical reinforcement would be necessary to limit the remodeling.

To determine the extent at which a mechanical restraint is beneficial, a comparative study of two types of restrain was carried out in sheep: a patch over the infarct (non-biodegradable Marlex mesh) or a wrap (non-biodegradable Merseline mesh) [216]. The use of the mesh wrapping the ventricle reduced the remodeling whereas the patch applied over the infarct did not yield considerable improvements when compared with controls (untreated infarcted animals).

Paracor heartnet is a nitinol mesh proposed as a restrain device that is under clinical study in patients with severe dilated cardiomyopathy. In a study, six months after the implantation in 51 patients, results obtained suggested clinical benefits tending to reverse remodeling and that it could consequently be reliably implanted [217]. The PEERLESS-HF trial is the last carried out with this device so far [218]. It proved to be safe and improved patient's quality of life and ventricular dilation; however, no improvement in the peak of VO_2 was produced (which was an end-point of the trial), what led to stop enrollment in the trial. Nevertheless, a new clinical trial is planned. In another study in an animal model, it was shown that the heartnet can alter myocardial blood flow patterns in dilated cardiomyopathy, although it remains unclear if these changes are clinically relevant [219].

Another left ventricular restraint proposed is Acorn Corcap, a polyester mesh that is also being assessed in clinical trials after the positive results obtained in animal models [220]. 5 years after implantation it exhibited safety, a sustained reverse remodeling with a significant reduction in the left ventricular end diastolic volume and a slight increase in the sphericity index [221]. However, in an echocardiographic study using tissue velocity imaging, no improvement in cardiac output was achieved [222].

Limited results obtained with the ventricular restraint therapy can be, among other reasons, because of the absence of tissue regeneration. A more advanced approach combines the ventricular restraint therapy with a regenerative strategy such as patches or scaffolds loaded with cells. For instance, the Acorn Corcap and a collagen matrix loaded with MSC has been implanted in sheeps, and the combination was found to limit the fibrosis produced as foreign body reaction against the Corcap and improve the systolic and diastolic function [223].

CONCLUDING REMARKS

Several therapeutic strategies have been proposed in the last decade to limit the adverse spread of the ischemic tissue and ventricle dilation or even to generate new myocardial tissue. These treatments consist in cellular therapy (so-called cellular cardiomyoplasty) where cells of different origin are implanted by different techniques onto the infarcted ventricle with the hope that cells will contribute to the generation of new contractile tissue to replace the scar, electrically coupled with the host myocardium. But despite the intense efforts and work put in the field, attempts so far have failed. Most of the implanted cells die soon after transplantation due to the fact that the cells cannot withstand the mechanical forces they experience in the host tissue. Mechanisms underlying the slight improvements observed are still undetermined; the paracrine effect is usually considered the way through which cells act, but the precise mechanisms are not completely understood yet. Besides, for this therapeutic approach to evolve to a realistic alternative to conventional treatments, some critical issues are still to be clarified: the way of delivery to maximize cell engraftment and minimize cell loss and death, the ideal cell type to be used, and the optimal time of cell administration (if they are implanted too soon, the inflammatory process kills the implanted cells, but if it is too late, the presence of the fibrotic scar limits their beneficial effects). New strategies already under study envision to improve cell survival by pre-conditioning the cells, pre-treating the host tissue or combining cells with other elements.

A possible way of localizing the appropriate cells in the target diseased tissue is to entrap them in a cell-friendly gelling biomaterial. Besides, gels can incorporate bioactive molecules for their controlled supply, and their preparation procedure (in the case of *in situ* gelling materials) avoids any invasive surgery. The injection of gelly materials alone onto the infarcted myocardium has shown some beneficial effects by itself and contributes somehow to limit the ventricular remodeling, for their slight role as mechanical support. Combining cells with gelly materials contributes, to some extent, to increase the cells residence time in the site of interest, and enhances cells adhesion and survival by providing them a better microenvironment. However, the consistency of these materials is generally too weak to withstand the synchronous contraction of the heart muscle without spreading from their target location, and their mechanical properties are too low to reach significant improvements in terms of containment of the dilated ventricle and post-infarct ventricular dysfunction.

Alternative tissue engineering strategies combine cells with three-dimensional scaffolds or patches to host them and improve their survival, induce the formation of new blood vessels and extracellular matrix and at the same time support the native tissue mechanically. The advantages of using myocardial patches or scaffolds are not only their usually superior mechanical properties, but also their wide versatility in terms of chemistries and morphology. There are many fabrication techniques for the preparation of scaffolds, leading to very different architectures, and these options are broadening with the computer-assisted techniques. Generally, positive results have been obtained by using scaffolds. In studies in which the therapeutic efficiency of a material was compared when used as an injectable gel or as a pre-fabricated scaffold or patch, the scaffold gave better results. When the scaffolds were loaded with growth factors or adhesion motives, in most of the cases the outcome was better. Mechanical and electrical stimulation are of help for cardiomyocytes to mature within the scaffolds and develop the characteristics and structures typical of cardiac tissue. Unfortunately, the implantation of epicardiac patches is much more invasive than that of injectable gels, and they need to be vascularized to ensure the success of the graft. Many attempts have addressed these questions but a satisfying solution has not been found yet.

ACKNOWLEDGEMENTS

The authors acknowledge the support of the FP7 NMP3-SL-2009-229239 project "Regeneration of cardiac tissue assisted by bioactive implants (RECATABI)".

REFERENCES

1.   Roger VL et al. Heart Disease and Stroke Statistics - 2012 Update A Report From the American Heart Association. Circulation 2012; 125: 2-220.

2.   Vasan SV, Benjamin EJ, Sullivan LM, D'agostino RB. The burden of increasing worldwide cardiovascular disease. In: Fuster V, Walsh RA, O'Rourke RA, Poole-Wilson P (ed.) Hurst the Heart. 12th edition McGraw-Hill Professional; 2010 p17-46.

3.   World Hearth Organitation. WHO: Programes and projects: Cardiovascular disease: The Atlas of Heart Disease and Stroke; 2004. http://www.who. int/cardiovascular_diseases/resources/atlas/en/ (accessed 03 June 2012)

4.   Venugopal JR, Prabhakaran MP, Mukherjee S, Ravichandran R, Dan K, Ramakrishna S. Biomaterial Strategies for Alleviation of Myocardial Infarction. Journal of the Royal Society Interface 2012; 9(66): 1-19. doi:10.1098/rsif.2011.0301.

5.   Walker CA, Spinale FG. The Structure and Function of the Cardiac Myocite: a Review of Fundamental Concepts. The Journal of Thoracic and Cardiovascular Surgery 1999; 118: 375-82.

6.   Di Donato M, Toso A, Dor V, Sabatier M, Barletta G, Menicanti L, Fantini F and the RESTORE Group. Surgical Ventricular Restoration Improves Mechanical Intraventricular Dyssynchrony in Ischemic Cardiomyopathy. Circulation 2004; 109: 2536-43.

7. Smaill BH, LeGrice IJ, Hooks DA, Pullan AJ, Caldwell BJ, Hunter PJ. Cardiac Structure and Electrical Activation: Models and Measurement. Clinical and Experimental Pharmacology and Physiology 2004; 31 (12): 913-9.

8. Kocica MJ, Corno AF, Carreras-Costa F, Ballester-Rodes M, Moghbel MC, Cueva CNC, Lackovic V, Kanjuh V, Torrent-Guasp F. The Helical Ventricular Myocardial Band: Global, Three-Dimensional, Functional Architecture of the Ventricular Myocardium. European Journal Cardio-Thoracic Surgery 2006; 29: 21-40. DOI: 10.1016/j.ejcts.2006.03.011

9. LeGrice IJ, Smaill BH, Chai LZ, Edgar SG, Gavin JB, Hunter PJ. Laminar Structure of the Heart: Ventricular Myocyte Arrangement and Connective Tissue Architecture in the Dog. American Journal of Physiology 1995; 269: H571-82.

10. Chen FY, Cohn LH. The Surgical Treatment of Heart Failure. A New Frontier: Nontransplant Surgical Alternatives in Heart Failure. Cardiology in Review 2002; 10(6): 326-33.

11. Hoyt RH, Cohen ML, Saffitz JE. Distribution and Three-Dimensional Structure of Intercellular Junctions in Canine Myocardium. Circulation Research 1989; 64: 563-74.

12. Spach MS, Heidlage JF. The Stochastic Nature of Cardiac Propagation at a Microscopic Level. Electrical Description of Myocardial Architecture and its Application to Conduction. Circulation Research 1995; 76: 366-80.

13. Severs NJ. The Cardiac Muscle Cell. BioEssays 2000; 22: 188-199.

14. Burke AP, Virmani R. Pathology of myocardial ischemia, infarction, reperfusion and sudden death. In: Fuster V, Walsh RA, O'Rourke RA, Poole-Wilson P (ed.) Hurst the Heart. 12th edition McGraw-Hill Professional; 2010. p1321-1338.

15. Baig MK, Mahon N, McKenna WJ, Caforio ALP, Bonow RO, Francis GS, Gheorghiade M. The Pathophysiology of Advanced Heart Failure. Heart & Lung 1999; 28(2): 87-101.

16. Ferrero JM Jr, Trénor B, Montilla F, Saiz J, Ferrero Á, Rodriguez B. Ischemia. In: Wiley Encyclopedia of Biomedical Engineering. (ed.) John Wiley & Sons, Inc; 2006. p1-17.

17. Douglas JS Jr, King SB III.Percutaneous coronary intervention. In:. Fuster V, Walsh RA, O›Rourke RA, Poole-Wilson P (ed.) Hurst the Heart. 12th edition McGraw-Hill Professional; 2010. p1427-1457.

18. Lally C. Kelly DJ, Prendergast PJ. Stents. In: Wiley Encyclopedia of Biomedical Engineering. (ed.) John Wiley & Sons, Inc; 2006. p1-10.

19. Stefanini GG, Kalesan B, Serruys PW, Heg D, Buszman P, Linke A, Ischinger T, Klauss V, Eberli F, Wijns W, Morice MC, Di Mario C, Corti R, Antoni D, Sohn HY, Eerdmans P, van Es GA, Meier B, Windecker S, Jüni P. Long-term clinical outcomes of biodegradable polymer biolimus-eluting stents versus durable polymer sirolimus-eluting stents in patients with coronary artery disease (LEADERS): 4 year follow-up of a randomised non-inferiority trial. Lancet 2011; 378: 1940-8.

20. Ruwende C, Visovatti S, Pinsky DJ. Molecular and cellular mechanisms of myocardial ischemia-reperfusion injury. In: Fuster V, Walsh RA, O›Rourke RA, Poole-Wilson P (ed.) Hurst the Heart. 12th edition McGraw-Hill Professional; 2010. p1339-1350.

21. Nian M, Lee P, Khaper N, Liu P. Inflammatory Cytokines and Postmyocardial Infarction Remodeling. Circulation Research 2004; 94: 1543-1553.

22. Sun Y, Kiani MF, Postlethwaite AE, Weber KT. Infarct Scar as Living Tissue. Basic Research in Cardiology 2002; 97: 343-347. doi: 10.1007/s00395-002-0365-8.

23. Christman KL, Lee RJ. Biomaterials For the Treatment of Myocardial Infarction. Journal American College of Cardiology 2006; 48: 907-13.

24. Mann DL. Mechanisms and Models in Heart Failure: a Combinatorial Approach. Circulation 1999; 100: 999-1008. DOI: 10.1161/01. CIR.100.9.999.

25. Cortes-Morichetti M, Frati G, Schussler O, Duong Van Huyen JP, Lauret E, Genovese JA, Carpentier AF, Chachques JC. Association Between a Cell-Seeded Collagen Matrix and Cellular Cardiomyoplasty for Myocardial Support and Regeneration. Tissue engineering 2007; 13(11): 2681-2687. doi: 10.1089/ten.2006.0447.

26. Jawad H, Ali NN, Lyon AR, Chen QZ, Harding SE, Boccaccini AR. Myocardial Tissue Engineering: a Review. Journal of Tissue Engineering and Regenerative Medicine 2007; 1: 327–342.

27. Nelson DM, Mab Z, Fujimoto KL, Hashizume R, Wagner WR. Intra-Myocardial Biomaterial Injection Therapy in the Treatment of Heart Failure: Materials, Outcomes and Challenges. Acta Biomaterialia 2011; 7: 1-15.

28. Chachques JC, Salanson-Lajos C, Lajos P, Shafy A, Alshamry A, Carpentier A. Cellular Cardiomyoplasty for Myocardial Regeneration. Asian Cardiovascular & Thoracic Annals 2005; 13: 287-296.

29. Chen QZ, Harding SE, Ali NN, Lyon AR, Boccaccini AR. Biomaterials in Cardiac Tissue Engineering: Ten Years of Research Survey. Materials Science and Engineering 2008; 59: 1-37.

30. Anversa P, Leri A, Kajstura J, Nadal-Ginard B. Myocyte Growth and Cardiac Repair. Journal of Molecular and Cellular Cardiology 2002; 34: 91-105.

31. Bergmann O, Bhardwaj RD, Bernard S, Zdunek S, Barnabe-Heider F, Walsh S, Zupicich J, Alkass K, Buchholz BA, Druid H, Jovinge S, Frisén J. Evidence for Cardiomyocyte Renewal in Humans. Science 2009; 324(5923): 98-102.

32. Wang F, Guan J. Cellular Cardiomyoplasty and Cardiac Tissue Engineering for Myocardial Therapy. Advanced Drug Delivery Reviews 2010; 62: 784–797.

33. Chachques JC, Grandjean PA, Tommasi JJ, Perier P, Chauvaud S, Bourgeois I, Carpentier A. Dynamic Cardiomyoplasty: A New Approach to Assist Chronic Myocardial Failure. Life Support System 1987; 5(4): 323-7.

34. Chachques JC. Development of Bioartificial Myocardium Using Stem Cells and Nanobiotechnology Templates. Cardiology Research and Practice 2011; 2011: 806795. doi:10.4061/2011/806795.

35. Wu J, Zeng F, Weisel RD, Li RK. Stem Cells for Cardiac Regeneration by Cell Therapy and Myocardial Tissue Engineering. Advances in Biochemical Engineering/Biotechnology 2009; 114: 107-128. doi: 10.1007/10_2008_37.

36. Pendyala L, Goodchild T, Gadesam RR, Chen J, Robinson K, Chronos N, Hou D. Cellular cardiomyoplasty and cardiac regeneration. Current Cardiology Reviews 2008; 4: 72-80.

37. Leor J, Amsalem Y, Cohen S. Cells, scaffolds, and molecules for myocardial tissue engineering. Pharmacology and Therapeutics 2005; 105(2): 151-63.

38. Zhou R, Acton PD, Ferrari VA. Imaging stem cells implanted in infarcted myocardium. Journal American college of cardiology 2006; 48(10): 2094-2106.

39. Hofmann M, Wollert KC, Meyer GP, Menke A, Arseniev L, Hertenstein B, Ganser A, Knapp WH, Drexler H. Monitoring of Bone Marrow Cell Homing into the Infarcted Human Myocardium. Circulation 2005; 111: 2198-202.

40. Teng CJ, Luo J, Chiu RC, Shum-Tim D. Massive Mechanical Loss of

Microspheres with Direct Intramyocardial Injection in the Beating Heart: Implications for Cellular Cardiomyoplasty. Journal of Thoracic and Cardiovascular Surgery 2006; 132(3): 628-32. doi: 10.1016/j.jtcvs.2006.05.034.

41. Schussler O, Chachques JC, Mesana TG, Suuronen EJ, Lecarpentier Y, Ruel M. 3-Dimensional structures to enhance cell therapy and engineer contractile tissue. Asian Cardiovascular & thoracic annals 2010; 18(2): 188-198.

42. Zenovich AG, Davis BH, Taylor DA. Comparison of Intracardiac Cell Transplantation: Autologous Skeletal Myoblasts Versus Bone Marrow Cells. Handbook of Experimental Pharmacology 2007; 180: 117–165.

43. Forte E, Chimenti I, Barile L, Gaetani R, Angelini F, Ionta V, Messina E, Giacomello A. Cardiac Cell Therapy: The Next (Re)Generation. Stem Cell Reviews and Reports 2011; 7(4): 1018-1030. doi:10.1007/s12015-011-9252-8.

44. Qian H, Yang Y, Huang J, Dou K, Yang G. Cellular cardiomyoplasty by catheter-based infusion of stem cells in clinical settings. Transplant Immunology 2006; 16: 135-147.

45. Laflamme MA, Chen KY, Naumova AV, Muskheli V, Fugate JA, Dupras SK, Reinecke H, Xu C, Hassanipour M, Police S, O›Sullivan C, Collins L, Chen Y, Minami E, Gill EA, Ueno S, Yuan C, Gold J, Murry CE. Cardiomyocytes derived from human embryonic stem cells in pro-survival factors enhance function of infarcted rat hearts. Nature Biotechnology 2007; 25(9): 1015-24. doi:10.1038/nbt1327.

46. Ebelt H, Jungblut M, Zhang Y, Kubin T, Kostin S, Technau A, Oustanina S, Niebrügge S, Lechmann J, Werdan K, Braun T. Cellular cardiomyoplasty: improvement of left ventricular function correlates with the release of cardioactive cytokines. Stem cells 2007; 25(1): 236-244.

47. Zimmet JM, Hare JM. Emerging role for bone marrow derived mesenchymal stem cells in myocardial regenerative therapy. Basic Research in Cardiology 2005; 100(6): 471-481. doi: 10.1007/s00395-005-0553-4.

48. Madonna R, Geng YJ, De Caterina R. Adipose tissue-derived stem cells: characterization and potential for cardiovascular repair. Arteriosclerosis, Thrombosis and Vascular Biology 2009; 29(11): 1723-9.

49. Heng BC, Haider HK, Sim EK, Cao T, Ng SC. Strategies for Directing the Differentiation of Stem Cells into the Cardiomyogenic Lineage in Vitro. Cardiovascular Research 2004; 62(1): 34–42.

50. Vulliet PR, Greeley M, Halloran SM, MacDonald KA, Kittleson MD.

Intra-Coronary Arterial Injection of Mesenchymal Stromal Cells and Microinfarction in Dogs. The Lancet 2004; 363(9411): 783-4.

51. Meyer GP, Wollert KC, Lotz J, Steffens J, Lippolt P, Fichtner S, Hecker H, Schaefer A, Arseniev L, Hertenstein B, Ganser A, Drexler H. Intracoronary Bone Marrow Cell Transfer After Myocardial Infarction: Eighteen Months Follow-up Data from the Randomized, Controlled BOOST (BOne marrOw transfer to enhance ST-elevation infarct regeneration) Trial. Circulation 2006; 113: 1287–94, doi: 10.1161/CIRCULATIONAHA.105.575118.

52. Hahn JY, Cho HJ, Kang HJ, Kim TS, Kim MH, Chung JH, Bae JW, Oh BH, Park YB, Kim HS. Pre-treatment of Mesenchymal Stem Cells with a Combination of Growth Factors Enhances Gap Junction Formation, Cytoprotective Effect on Cardiomyocytes, and Therapeutic Efficacy for Myocardial Infarction. Journal of the American College of Cardiology 2008; 51(9): 933-43.

53. Miyahara Y, Nagaya N, Kataoka M, Yanagawa B, Tanaka K, Hao H, Ishino K, Ishida H, Shimizu T, Kangawa K, Sano S, Okano T, Kitamura S, Mori H. Monolayered mesenchymal stem cells repair scarred myocardium after myocardial infarction. Nature Medicine 2006; 12(4): 459-465.

54. www.clinicaltrials.gov (accessed 13 November 2012).

55. REgeneration of CArdiac Tissue Assisted by Bioactive Implants. funded by the European Comission under the 7th FP, www.recatabi.com.

56. Messina E, De Angelis L, Frati G, Morrone S, Chimenti S, Fiordaliso F, Salio M, Battaglia M, Latronico MV, Coletta M, Vivarelli E, Frati L, Cossu G, Giacomello A. Isolation and Expansion of Adult Cardiac Stem Cells From Human and Murine Heart. Circulation Research 2004; 95: 911-921.

57. Smith RR, Barile L, Cho HC, Leppo MK, Hare JM, Messina E, Giacomello A, Abraham MR, Marbán E. Regenerative potential of cardiosphere-derived cells expanded from percutaneous endomyocardial biopsy specimens. Circulation 2007; 115(7): 896-908.

58. Makkar RR, Smith RR, Cheng K, Malliaras K, Thomson LEJ, Berman D, Czer LSC, Marbán L, Mendizabal A, Johnston PV, Russell SD, Schuleri KH, Lardo AC, Gerstenblith G, Marbán E. Intracoronary cardiosphere-derived cells for heart regeneration after myocardial infarction (CADUCEUS): a prospective, randomised phase 1 trial. The Lancet 2012; 379: 895-904. doi: 10.1016/S0140- 6736(12)60195-0.

59. Shafy A, Lavergne T, Latremouille C, Cortes-Morichetti M, Carpentier A, Chachques JC. Association of electrostimulation with cell transplantation

in ischemic heart disease. Journal of Thoracic and Cardiovascular Surgery 2009; 138(4): 994-1001.

60. Cleland JG, Coletta AP, Abdellah AT, Nasirb M, Hobsonb N, Freemantlec N, Clarka AL. Clinical Trials Update from the American Heart Association 2006: OAT, SALT 1 and 2, MAGIC, ABCD, PABA-CHF, IMPROVECHF, and Percutaneous Mitral Annuloplasty. European Journal of Heart Failure 2007; 9: 92-7.

61. Hirata Y, Sata M, Motomura N, Takanashi M, Suematsu Y, Ono M, Takamoto S. Human umbilical cord blood cells improve cardiac function after myocardial infarction. Biochemical and Biophysical Research Communications 2005; 327(2): 609-14. doi:10.1016/j.bbrc.2004.12.044.

62. Walther G, Gekas J, Bertrand OF. Amniotic Stem Cells for Cellular Cardiomyoplasty: Promises and Premises. Catheterization and Cardiovascular Interventions 2009; 73(7): 917–924.

63. Yeh YC, Wei HJ, Lee WY, Yu CL, Chang Y, Hsu LW, Chung MF, Tsai MS, Hwang SM, Sung HW. Cellular Cardiomyoplasty with Human Amniotic Fluid Stem Cells: In Vitro and In Vivo Studies. Tissue Engineering Part A 2010; 16(6): 1925-36.

64. Shimizu T, Yamato M, Kikuchi A, Okano T. Cell sheet engineering for myocardial tissue reconstruction. Biomaterials 2003; 24(13): 2309-2316.

65. Alcon A, Cagavi Bozkulak E, Qyang Y. Regenerating functional heart tissue for myocardial repair. Cellular and Molecular Life Sciences 2012; 69(16): 2635-56. doi:10.1007/s00018-012-0942.

66. Yeh YC, Lee WY, Yu CL, Hwang SM, Chung MF, Hsu LW, Chang Y, Lin WW, Tsai MS, Wei HJ, Sung HW. Cardiac repair with injectable cell sheet fragments of human amniotic fluid stem cells in an immune-suppressed rat model. Biomaterials 2010; 31(25): 6444-53.

67. Furuta A, Miyoshi S, Itabashi Y, Shimizu T, Kira S, Hayakawa K, Nishiyama N, Tanimoto K, Hagiwara Y, Satoh T, Fukuda K, Okano T, Ogawa S. Pulsatile cardiac tissue grafts using a novel three-dimensional cell sheet manipulation technique functionally integrates with the host heart, in vivo. Circulation Research 2006; 98(5): 705–712.

68. Williams C, Xie AW, Yamato M, Okano T, Wong JY. Stacking of aligned cell sheets for layer-by-layer control of complex tissue Structure. Biomaterials 2011; 32(24): 5625-32.

69. Vunjak-Novakovic G, Lui KO, Tandon N, Chien KR. Bioengineering Heart Muscle: A Paradigm for Regenerative Medicine. Annual Reviewof Biomedical Engineering 2011; 13: 245–67. doi: 10.1146/annurev-bioeng-071910-124701.

70. Haraguchi Y, Shimizu T, Yamato M, Kikuchi A, Okano T. Electrical coupling of cardiomyocyte sheets occurs rapidly via functional gap junction formation. Biomaterials 2006; 27(27): 4765–4774.

71. Shimizu T, Sekine H, Yang J, Isoi Y, Yamato M, Kikuchi A, Kobayashi E, Okano T. Polysurgery of cell sheet grafts overcomes diffusion limits to produce thick, vascularized myocardial tissues. The Journal of the Federation of American Societies for Experimental Biology 2006; 20(6): 708–710.

72. Lee WY, Wei HJ, Lin WW, Yeh YC, Hwang SM, Wang JJ, Tsai MS, Chang Y, Sung HW. Enhancement of cell retention and functional benefits in myocardial infarction using human amniotic-fluid stem-cell bodies enriched with endogenous ECM. Biomaterials 2011; 32(24): 5558-67.

73. Ye Z, Zhou Y, Cai H, Tan W. Myocardial regeneration: Roles of stem cells and hydrogels. Advanced Drug Delivery Reviews 2011; 63(8): 688-97.

74. Habib M, Shapira-Schweitzer K, Caspi O, Gepstein A, Arbel G, Aronson D, Seliktar D, Gepstein L. A combined cell therapy and in-situ tissue-engineering approach for myocardial repair. Biomaterials 2011; 32(30): 7514-23.

75. Wall ST, Walker JC, Healy KE, Ratcliffe MB, Guccione JM. Theoretical impact of the injection of material into the myocardium: a finite element model simulation. Circulation 2006; 114(24): 2627-35.

76. Shen X, Tanaka K, Takamori A. Coronary Arteries Angiogenesis in Ischemic Myocardium: Biocompatibility and Biodegradability of Various Hydrogels. Artificial Organs 2009; 33(10): 781-7. doi: 10.1111/j.1525-1594.2009.00815.x.

77. Guo HD, Wang HJ, Tan YZ, Wu JH. Transplantation of marrow derived cardiac stem cells carried in fibrin improves cardiac function after myocardial infarction. Tissue Engineering Part A 2011; 17(1-2): 45-58.

78. Christman KL, Vardanian AJ, Fang Q, Sievers RE, Fok HH, Lee RJ. Injectable fibrin scaffold improves cell transplant survival, reduces infarct expansion, and induces neovasculature formation in ischemic myocardium. Journal of the American College of Cardiology 2004; 44(3): 654-60.

79. Barsotti MC, Felice F, Balbarini A, Di Stefano R. Fibrin as a scaffold for cardiac tissue Engineering. Biotechnology and Applied Biochemistry 2011; 58(5): 301-10. doi: 10.1002/bab.49.

80. Christman KL, Fang Q, Yee MS, Johnson KR, Sievers RE, Lee RJ. Enhanced neovasculature formation in ischemic myocardium following

delivery of pleiotrophin plasmid in a biopolymer. Biomaterials 2005; 26(10): 1139-44.

81. Martens TP, Godier AF, Parks JJ, Wan LQ, Koeckert MS, Eng GM, Hudson BI, Sherman W, Vunjak-Novakovic G. Percutaneous cell delivery into the heart using hydrogels polymerizing in situ. Cell Transplantation 2009; 18(3): 297-304.

82. Christman KL, Fok HH, Sievers RE, Fang Q, Lee RJ. Fibrin glue alone and skeletal myoblasts in a fibrin scaffold preserve cardiac function after myocardial infarction. Tissue Engineering 2004; 10 (3-4): 403-9.

83. Ryu JH, Kim IK, Cho SW, Cho MC, Hwang KK, Piao H, Piao S, Lim SH, Hong YS, Choi CY, Yoo KJ, Kim BS. Implantation of bone marrow mononuclear cells using injectable fibrin matrix enhances neovascularization in infarcted myocardium. Biomaterials 2005; 26(3): 319–326.

84. Chekanov V, Akhtar M, Tchekanov G, Dangas G, Shehzad MZ, Tio F, Adamian M, Colombo A, Roubin G, Leon MB, Moses JW, Kipshidze NN. Transplantation of autologous endothelial cells induces angiogenesis. Pacing and Clinical Electrophysiology 2003; 26(1 Pt 2): 496-9.

85. Chenite A, Chaput C, Wang D, Combes C, Buschmann MD, Hoemann CD, Leroux JC, Atkinson BL, Binette F, Selmani A. Novel injectable neutral solutions of chitosan form biodegradable gels in situ. Biomaterials 2000; 21(21): 2155-61.

86. Reis LA, Chiu LL, Liang Y, Hyunh K, Momen A, Radisic M. A peptide-modified chitosan–collagen hydrogel for cardiac cell culture and delivery. Acta Biomaterialia 2012; 8(3): 1022-36.

87. Liu Z, Wang H, Wang Y, Lin Q, Yao A, Cao F, Li D, Zhou J, Duan C, Du Z, Wang Y, Wang C. The influence of chitosan hydrogel on stem cell engraftment, survival and homing in the ischemic myocardial microenvironment. Biomaterials 2012; 33(11): 3093-106.

88. Binsalamah ZM, Paul A, Khan AA, Prakash S, Shum-Tim D. Intramyocardial sustained delivery of placental growth factor using nanoparticles as a vehicle for delivery in the rat infarct model. International Journal of Nanomedicine 2011; 6: 2667-78.

89. Kofidis T, Lebl DR, Martinez EC, Hoyt G, Tanaka M, Robbins RC. Novel injectable bioartificial tissue facilitates targeted, less invasive, large-scale tissue restoration on the beating heart after myocardial injury. Circulation 2005; 112(9 Suppl): I173-7.

90. Zhang P, Zhang H, Wang H, Wei Y, Hu S. Artificial matrix helps neonatal cardiomyocytes restore injured myocardium in rats. Artificial Organs

2006; 30(2): 86-93.

91. Kofidis T, de Bruin JL, Hoyt G, Lebl DR, Tanaka M, Yamane T, Chang CP, Robbins RC. Injectable bioartificial myocardial tissue for large-scale intramural cell transfer and functional recovery of injured heart muscle. The Journal of Thoracic and Cardiovascular Surgery 2004; 128(4): 571-8.

92. Shen D, Wang X, Zhang L, Zhao X, Li J, Cheng K, Zhang J. The amelioration of cardiac dysfunction after myocardial infarction by the injection of keratin biomaterials derived from human hair. Biomaterials 2011; 32(35): 9290-9.

93. Landa N, Miller L, Feinberg MS, Holbova R, Shachar M, Freeman I, Cohen S, Leor J. Effect of injectable alginate implant on cardiac remodeling and function after recent and old infarcts in rat. Circulation 2008; 117(11): 1388-96.

94. Ruvinov E, Leor J, Cohen S. The promotion of myocardial repair by the sequential delivery of IGF-1 and HGF from an injectable alginate biomaterial in a model of acute myocardial infarction. Biomaterials 2011; 32(2): 565-78.

95. Rowley JA, Madlambayan G, Mooney DJ. Alginate hydrogels as synthetic extracellular matrix materials. Biomaterials 1999; 20(1): 45-53.

96. Yu J, Gu Y, Du KT, Mihardja S, Sievers RE, Lee RJ. The effect of injected RGD modified alginate on angiogenesis and left ventricular function in a chronic rat infarct model. Biomaterials 2009; 30(5): 751-6.

97. Tsur-Gang O, Ruvinov E, Landa N, Holbova R, Feinberg MS, Leor J, Cohen S. The effects of peptide-based modification of alginate on left ventricular remodeling and function after myocardial infarction. Biomaterials 2009; 30(2): 189-95.

98. Mihardja SS, Sievers RE, Lee RJ. The effect of polypyrrole on arteriogenesis in an acute rat infarct model. Biomaterials 2008; 29(31): 4205–10.

99. Gaffney J, Matou-Nasri S, Grau-Olivares M, Slevin M. Therapeutic applications of hyaluronan. Molecular BioSystems 2010; 6(3): 437–443. doi: 10.1039/b910552m.

100. Yoon SJ, Fang YH, Lim CH, Kim BS, Son HS, Park Y, Sun K. Regeneration of ischemic heart using hyaluronic acid-based injectable hydrogel. Journal of Biomedical Materials Research Part B: Applied Biomaterials 2009; 91(1): 163-71.

101. Cheng K, Blusztajn A, Shen D, Li TS, Sun B, Galang G, Zarembinski TI,

Prestwich GD, Marbán E, Smith RR, Marbán L. Functional performance of human cardiosphere-derived cells delivered in an in situ polymerizable hyaluronan-gelatin hydrogel. Biomaterials 2012; 33(21): 5317-24.

102. Duan Y, Liu Z, O›Neill J, Wan LQ, Freytes DO, Vunjak-Novakovic G. Hybrid gel composed of native heart matrix and collagen induces cardiac differentiation of human embryonic stem cells without supplemental growth factors. Journal of Cardiovascular Translational Research 2011; 4(5): 605-15.

103. Dai W, Wold LE, Dow JS, Kloner RA. Thickening of the infarcted wall by collagen injection improves left ventricular function in rats: a novel approach to preserve cardiac function after myocardial infarction. Journal of the American College of Cardiology 2005; 46(4): 714-9.

104. Huang NF, Yu J, Sievers R, Li S, Lee RJ. Injectable biopolymers enhance angiogenesis after myocardial infarction. Tissue Engineering 2005; 11(11-12): 1860-6.

105. Thompson CA, Nasseri BA, Makower J, Houser S, McGarry M, Lamson T, Pomerantseva I, Chang JY, Gold HK, Vacanti JP, Oesterle SN. Percutaneous transvenous cellular cardiomyoplasty. A novel nonsurgical approach for myocardial cell transplantation. Journal of the American College of Cardiology 2003; 41(11): 1964-71.

106. Dai W, Hale SL, Kay GL, Jyrala AJ, Kloner RA. Delivering stem cells to the heart in a collagen matrix reduces relocation of cells to other organs as assessed by nanoparticle technology. Regenerative Medicine 2009; 4(3): 387-95.

107. Suuronen EJ, Veinot JP, Wong S, Kapila V, Price J, Griffith M, Mesana TG, Ruel M. Tissue-engineered injectable collagen-based matrices for improved cell delivery and vascularization of ischemic tissue using CD133+ progenitors expanded from the peripheral blood. Circulation 2006; 114(1 Suppl): I138-44.

108. Zhang F, He C, Cao L, Feng W, Wang H, Mo X, Wang J. Fabrication of gelatin–hyaluronic acid hybrid scaffolds with tunable porous structures for soft tissue engineering. International Journal of Biological Macromolecules 2011; 48(3): 474-81.

109. Shao ZQ, Takaji K, Katayama Y, Kunitomo R, Sakaguchi H, Lai ZF, Kawasuji M. Effects of intramyocardial administration of slow-release basic fibroblast growth factor on angiogenesis and ventricular remodeling in a rat infarct model. Circulation Journal 2006; 70(4): 471-7.

110. Iwakura A, Fujita M, Kataoka K, Tambara K, Sakakibara Y, Komeda M, Tabata Y. Intramyocardial sustained delivery basic fibroblast growth

factor improves angiogenesis and ventricular function in a rat infarct model. Heart Vessels 2003; 18: 93–9.

111. Singelyn JM, DeQuach JA, Seif-Naraghi SB, Littlefield RB, Schup-Magoffin PJ, Christman KL. Naturally derived myocardial matrix as an injectable scaffold for cardiac tissue engineering. Biomaterials 2009; 30(29): 5409-16.

112. Okada M, Payne TR, Oshima H, Momoi N, Tobita K, Huard J. Differential efficacy of gels derived from small intestinal submucosa as an injectable biomaterial for myocardial infarct repair. Biomaterials 2010; 31(30): 7678-83.

113. Zhao ZQ, Puskas JD, Xu D, Wang NP, Mosunjac M, Guyton RA, Vinten-Johansen J, Matheny R. Improvement in cardiac function with small intestine extracellular matrix is associated with recruitment of C-kit cells, myofibroblasts, and macrophages after myocardial infarction. Journal of the American College of Cardiology 2010; 55(12): 1250-61.

114. Jeong B, Kim SW, Bae YH. Thermosensitive sol-gel reversible hydrogels. Advanced Drug Delivery Reviews 2002; 54(1): 37-51.

115. Fujimoto KL, Ma Z, Nelson DM, Hashizume R, Guan J, Tobita K, Wagner WR. Synthesis, characterization and therapeutic efficacy of a biodegradable, thermoresponsive hydrogel designed for application in chronic infarcted myocardium. Biomaterials 2009; 30(26): 4357-68.

116. Li Z, Guo X, Matsushita S, Guan J. Differentiation of cardiosphere-derived cells into a mature cardiac lineage using biodegradable poly(N-isopropylacrylamide) hydrogels. Biomaterials 2011; 32(12): 3220-32.

117. Wang T, Wu DQ, Jiang XJ, Zhang XZ, Li XY, Zhang JF, Zheng ZB, Zhuo R, Jiang H, Huang C. Novel thermosensitive hydrogel injection inhibits post-infarct ventricle remodelling. European Journal of Heart Failure 2009; 11(1): 14-9.

118. Dobner S, Bezuidenhout D, Govender P, Zilla P, Davies N. Asynthetic nondegradable polyethylene glycol hydrogel retards adverse post-infarct left ventricular remodeling. Journal of Cardiac Failure 2009; 15(7): 629-36.

119. Wang T, Jiang XJ, Tang QZ, Li XY, Lin T, Wu DQ, Zhang XZ, Okello E. Bone marrow stem cells implantation with a-cyclodextrin/MPEG– PCL–MPEG hydrogel improves cardiac function after myocardial infarction. Acta Biomaterialia 2009; 5(8): 2939-44.

120. Wu J, Zeng F, Huang XP, Chung JC, Konecny F, Weisel RD, Li RK. Infarct stabilization and cardiac repair with a VEGF-conjugated, injectable Hydrogel. Biomaterials 2011; 32(2): 579-86.

121. Kraehenbuehl TP, Ferreira LS, Hayward AM, Nahrendorf M, van der Vlies AJ, Vasile E, Weissleder R, Langer R, Hubbell JA. Human embryonic stem cell-derived microvascular grafts for cardiac tissue preservation after myocardial infarction. Biomaterials 2011; 32(4): 1102-9.

122. Wang T, Jiang XJ, Lin T, Ren S, Li XY, Zhang XZ, Tang QZ. The inhibition of postinfarct ventricle remodeling without polycythaemia following local sustained intramyocardial delivery of erythropoietin within a supramolecular hydrogel. Biomaterials 2009; 30(25): 4161-7.

123. Dvir T, Bauer M, Schroeder A, Tsui JH, Anderson DG, Langer R, Liao R, Kohane DS. Nanoparticles targeting the infarcted heart. Nano Letters 2011; 11(10): 4411-4. doi: 10.1021/nl2025882.

124. Davis ME, Motion JP, Narmoneva DA, Takahashi T, Hakuno D, Kamm RD, Zhang S, Lee RT. Injectable self-assembling peptide nanofibers create intramyocardial microenvironments for endothelial cells.Circulation 2005; 111(4): 442-50.

125. Tokunaga M, Liu ML, Nagai T, Iwanaga K, Matsuura K, Takahashi T, Kanda M, Kondo N, Wang P, Naito AT, Komuro I. Implantation of cardiac progenitor cells using self-assembling peptide improves cardiac function after myocardial infarction. Journal of Molecular and Cellular Cardiology 2010; 49(6): 972-83.

126. Kim JH, Jung Y, Kim SH, Sun K, Choi J, Kim HC, Park Y, Kim SH. The enhancement of mature vessel formation and cardiac function in infarcted hearts using dual growth factor delivery with self-assembling peptides. Biomaterials 2011; 32(26): 6080-8.

127. Davis ME, Hsieh PC, Takahashi T, Song Q, Zhang S, Kamm RD, Grodzinsky AJ, Anversa P, Lee RT. Local myocardial insulin-like growth factor 1 (IGF-1) delivery with biotinylated peptide nanofibers improves cell therapy for myocardial infarction. Proceedings of the National Academy of Sciences of the United States of America 2006; 103(21): 8155-60.

128. Nerem RM. The challenge of imitating nature. In Lanza R, Langer R, Vacanti J.. Principles of tissue engineering. San Diego (Ca) USA: Academic press; 1997 p.9-15.

129. Jawad H, Lyon AR, Harding SE, Ali NN, Boccaccini AR. Myocardial tissue engineering. British Medical Bulletin 2008; 87: 31-47.

130. Engelmayr GC Jr, Cheng M, Bettinger CJ, Borenstein JT, Langer R, Freed LE. Accordion-like honeycombs for tissue engineering of cardiac anisotropy. Nature Materials 2008; 7: 1003–10.

131. Bhana B, Iyer RK, Chen WL, Zhao R, Sider KL, Likhitpanichkul M,

Simmons CA, Radisic M. Influence of substrate stiffness on the phenotype of heart cells. Biotechnology and Bioengineering 2010; 105(6): 1148-60.

132. Marsano A, Maidhof R, Wan LQ, Wang Y, Gao J, Tandon N, Vunjak-Novakovic G. Scaffold stiffness affects the contractile function of three-dimensional engineered cardiac constructs. Biotechnology Progress 2010; 26(5): 1382-90.

133. Young JL, Engler AJ. Hydrogels with time-dependent material properties enhance cardiomyocyte differentiation in vitro. Biomaterials 2011; 32(4): 1002-9.

134. Carrier RL, Rupnick M, Langer R, Schoen FJ, Freed LE, Vunjak-Novakovic G. Perfusion Improves Tissue Architecture of Engineered Cardiac Muscle. Tissue Engineering 2002; 8(2): 175-88.

135. Radisic M, Malda J, Epping E, Geng W, Langer R, Vunjak-Novakovic G. Oxygen gradients correlate with cell density and cell viability in engineered cardiac tissue. Biotechnology and Bioengineering 2006; 93(2): 332-43.

136. Radisic M, Park H, Chen F, Salazar-Lazzaro JE, Wang Y, Dennis R, Langer R, Freed LE, Vunjak-Novakovic G. Biomimetic approach to cardiac tissue engineering: oxygen carriers and channeled scaffolds. Tissue Engineering 2006; 12(8): 2077-91.

137. Perets A, Baruch Y, Weisbuch F, Shoshany G, Neufeld G, Cohen S. Enhancing the vascularization of three-dimensional porous alginate scaffolds by incorporating controlled release basic fibroblast growth factor microspheres. Journal of Biomedical Materials Research Part A 2003; 65(4): 489-97.

138. Miyagi Y, Chiu LL, Cimini M, Weisel RD, Radisic M, Li RK. Biodegradable collagen patch with covalently immobilized VEGF for myocardial repair. Biomaterials 2011; 32(5): 1280-90.

139. Chiu LL, Radisic M. Controlled release of thymosin β4 using collagen–chitosan composite hydrogels promotes epicardial cell migration and angiogenesis. Journal of Controlled Release 2011; 155(3): 376-85. doi: 10.1016/j.jconrel.2011.05.026.

140. Vantler M, Karikkineth BC, Naito H, Tiburcy M, Didié M, Nose M, Rosenkranz S, Zimmermann WH. PDGF-BB protects cardiomyocytes from apoptosis and improves contractile function of engineered heart tissue. Journal of Molecular and Cellular Cardiology 2010; 48(6): 1316-23.

141. Davis ME, Hsieh PC, Grodzinsky AJ, Lee RT. Custom design of the cardiac microenvironment with biomaterials. Circulation Research 2005;

97(1): 8-15.

142. Kaully T, Kaufman-Francis K, Lesman A, Levenberg S. Vascularization--the conduit to viable engineered tissues. Tissue Engineering Part B Reviews 2009; 15(2): 159-69.

143. Bar A, Haverich A, Hilfiker A. Cardiac tissue engineering: "Reconstructing the motor of life". Scandinavian Journal of surgery 2007; 96 (2): 154-8.

144. Narmoneva DA, Vukmirovic R, Davis ME, Kamm RD, Lee RT. Endothelial cells promote cardiacmyocyte survival and spatial reorganization: implications for cardiac regeneration. Circulation 2004; 110(8): 962-8.

145. Dvir T, Kedem A, Ruvinov E, Levy O, Freeman I, Landa N, Holbova R, Feinberg MS, Dror S, Etzion Y, Leor J, Cohen S. Prevascularization of cardiac patch on the omentum improves its therapeutic outcome. Proceedings of the National Academy of Sciences from the United States of America 2009; 106 (35): 14990-5.

146. Bursac N, Papadaki M, White JA, Eisenberg SR, Vunjak-Novakovic G, Freed LE. Cultivation in rotating bioreactors promotes maintenance of cardiac myocyte electrophysiology and molecular properties. Tissue Engineering 2003; 9(6): 1243-53.

147. Radisic M, Yang L, Boublik J, Cohen RJ, Langer R, Freed LE, Vunjak-Novakovic G. Medium perfusion enables engineering of compact and contractile cardiac tissue. American Journal of Physiology Heart and Circulatory Physiology 2004; 286(2): H507-16.

148. Radisic M, Marsano A, Maidhof R, Wang Y, Vunjak-Novakovic G. Cardiac tissue engineering using perfusion bioreactor systems. Nature Protocols 2008; 3(4): 719-38.

149. Maidhof R, Marsano A, Lee EJ, Vunjak-Novakovic G. Perfusion Seeding of Channeled Elastomeric Scaffolds with Myocytes and Endothelial Cells for Cardiac Tissue Engineering. Biotechnology Progress 2010; 26(2): 565-72.

150. Brown MA, Iyer RK, Radisic M. Pulsatile perfusion bioreactor for cardiac tissue engineering. Biotechnology Progress 2008; 24(4): 907-20.

151. Cheng M, Moretti M, Engelmayr GC, Freed LE. Insulin-like Growth Factor-I and Slow, Bi-directional Perfusion Enhance the Formation of Tissue-Engineered Cardiac Grafts. Tissue Engineering Part A 2009; 15(3): 645-53.

152. Li D, Xia Y. Electrospinning of nanofibers: reinventing the wheel? Advanced Materials 2004; 16(14): 1151–1170. doi: 10.1002/adma.200400719.

153. Orlova Y, Magome N, Liu L, Chen Y, Agladze K. Electrospun nanofibers as a tool for architecture control in engineered cardiac tissue. Biomaterials 2011; 32(24): 5615-24.

154. Blan NR, Birla RK. Design and fabrication of heart muscle using scaffold-based tissue engineering. Journal of Biomedical Materials Research Part A 2008; 86(1): 195-208.

155. Madihally SV, Matthew HW. Porous chitosan scaffolds for tissue engineering. Biomaterials 1999; 20(12): 1133-42.

156. Cimetta E, Pizzato S, Bollini S, Serena E, De Coppi P, Elvassore N. Production of arrays of cardiac and skeletal muscle myofibers by micropatterning techniques on a soft substrate. Biomedical Microdevices 2009; 11(2): 389-400.

157. Chiang CK, Chowdhury MF, Iyer RK, Stanford WL, Radisic M. Engineering surfaces for site-specific vascular differentiation of mouse embryonic stem cells. Acta Biomaterialia 2010; 6(6): 1904-16.

158. Park H, Radisic M, Lim JO, Chang BH, Vunjak-Novakovic G. A novel composite scaffold for cardiac tissue engineering. In Vitro Cellular and Developmental Biology Animal 2005; 41(7): 188-96.

159. Eschenhagen T, Fink C, Remmers U, Scholz H, Wattchow J, Weil J, Zimmermann W, Dohmen HH, Schäfer H, Bishopric N, Wakatsuki T, Elson EL. Three-dimensional reconstitution of embryonic cardiomyocytes in a collagen matrix: a new heart muscle model system. The Journal of the Federation of American Societies for Experimental Biology 1997; 11(8): 683-94.

160. Callegari A, Bollini S, Iop L, Chiavegato A, Torregrossa G, Pozzobon M, Gerosa G, De Coppi P, Elvassore N, Sartore S. Neovascularization induced by porous collagen scaffold implanted on intact and cryoinjured rat hearts. Biomaterials 2007; 28(36): 5449-61.

161. Xiang Z, Liao R, Kelly MS, Spector M. Collagen-GAG scaffolds grafted onto myocardial infarcts in a rat model: a delivery vehicle for mesenchymal stem cells. Tissue Engineering 2006; 12(9): 2467-78.

162. Simpson DL, Dudley SC Jr. Modulation of human mesenchymal stem cell function in a three-dimensional matrix promotes attenuation of adverse remodelling after myocardial infarction. Journal of Tissue Engineering and Regenerative Medicine 2011 Nov 18. doi: 10.1002/term.511.

163. Chachques JC, Trainini JC, Lago N, Masoli OH, Barisani JL, Cortes-Morichetti M, Schussler O, Carpentier A. Myocardial assistance by grafting a new bioartificial upgraded myocardium (MAGNUM clinical trial): one year follow-up. Cell Transplantation 2007; 16(9): 927-34.

164. Chimenti I, Rizzitelli G, Gaetani R, Angelini F, Ionta V, Forte E, Frati G, Schussler O, Barbetta A, Messina E, Dentini M, Giacomello A. Human cardiosphere-seeded gelatin and collagen scaffolds as cardiogenic engineered bioconstructs. Biomaterials 2011; 32(35): 9271-81.

165. Holladay CA, Duffy AM, Chen X, Sefton MV, O›Brien TD, Pandit AS. Recovery of cardiac function mediated by MSC and interleukin-10 plasmid functionalised scaffold. Biomaterials 2012; 33(5): 1303-14.

166. Akhyari P, Kamiya H, Haverich A, Karck M, Lichtenberg A. Myocardial tissue engineering: the extracellular matrix. Journal of Cardio-thoracic Surgery 2008; 34: 229-241.

167. Sakai T, Li RK, Weisel RD, Mickle DA, Kim ET, Jia ZQ, Yau TM. The fate of a tissue-engineered cardiac graft in the right ventricular outflow tract of the rat. Journal of Thoracic and Cardiovascular Surgery 2001; 121(5): 932-42.

168. Zhang G, Nakamura Y, Wang X, Hu Q, Suggs LJ, Zhang J. Controlled release of stromal cell-derived factor-1 alpha in situ increases c-kit+ cell homing to the infarcted heart. Tissue Engineering 2007; 13(8): 2063-71.

169. Leor J, Aboulafia-Etzion S, Dar A, Shapiro L, Barbash IM, Battler A, Granot Y, Cohen S. Bioengineered cardiac grafts: A new approach to repair the infarcted myocardium? Circulation 2000; 102(19 Suppl 3): III56-61.

170. Dar A, Shachar M, Leor J, Cohen S. Optimization of cardiac cell seeding and distribution in 3D porous alginate scaffolds. Biotechnology and Bioengineering 2002; 80(3): 305-12.

171. Shachar M, Tsur-Gang O, Dvir T, Leor J, Cohen S. The effect of immobilized RGD peptide in alginate scaffolds on cardiac tissue engineering. Acta Biomaterialia 2011; 7(1): 152-62.

172. Sapir Y, Kryukov O, Cohen S. Integration of multiple cell-matrix interactions into alginate scaffolds for promoting cardiac tissue regeneration. Biomaterials 2011; 32(7): 1838-47.

173. Le Visage C, Gournay O, Benguirat N, Hamidi S, Chaussumier L, Mougenot N, Flanders JA, Isnard R, Michel JB, Hatem S, Letourneur D, Norol F. Mesenchymal stem cell delivery into rat infarcted myocardium using a porous polysaccharide-based scaffold: a quantitative comparison with endocardial injection. Tissue Engineering Part A 2012; 18(1-2): 35-44.

174. Cao Y, Wang B. Biodegradation of Silk Biomaterials. International Journal of Molecular Sciences 2009; 10(4): 1514-1524.

175. Yang MC, Wang SS, Chou NK, Chi NH, Huang YY, Chang YL, Shieh MJ, Chung TW. The cardiomyogenic differentiation of rat mesenchymal stem cells on silk fibroin–polysaccharide cardiac patches in vitro. Biomaterials 2009; 30(22): 3757-65.

176. Patra C, Talukdar S, Novoyatleva T, Velagala SR, Mühlfeld C, Kundu B, Kundu SC, Engel FB. Silk protein fibroin for cardiac tissue engineering. Biomaterials 2012; 33(9): 2673-80.

177. Robinson KA, Li J, Mathison M, Redkar A, Cui J, Chronos NA, Matheny RG, Badylak SF. Extracellular matrix scaffold for cardiac repair. Circulation 2005; 112(9 Suppl): I135-43.

178. Godier-Furnémont AF, Martens TP, Koeckert MS, Wan L, Parks J, Arai K, Zhang G, Hudson B, Homma S, Vunjak-Novakovic G. Composite scaffold provides a cell delivery platform for cardiovascular repair. Proceedings of the National Academy of Sciences of the United States of America 2011; 108(19): 7974-9.

179. Wei HJ, Chen CH, Lee WY, Chiu I, Hwang SM, Lin WW, Huang CC, Yeh YC, Chang Y, Sung HW. Bioengineered cardiac patch constructed from multilayered mesenchymal stem cells for myocardial repair. Biomaterials 2008; 29(26): 3547-56.

180. Ott HC, Matthiesen TS, Goh SK, Black LD, Kren SM, Netoff TI, Taylor DA. Perfusion-decellularized matrix: using nature's platform to engineer a bioartificial heart. Nature Medicine 2008; 14(2): 213–221.

181. Giraud MN, Armbruster C, Carrel T, Tevaearai HT. Current state of the art in myocardial tissue engineering. Tissue Engineering 2007; 13(8): 1825-36.

182. Huang CC, Wei HJ, Yeh YC, Wang JJ, Lin WW, Lee TY, Hwang SM, Choi SW, Xia Y, Chang Y, Sung HW. Injectable PLGA porous beads cellularized by hAFSCs for cellular cardiomyoplasty. Biomaterials 2012; 33(16): 4069-77.

183. McDevitt TC, Angello JC, Whitney ML, Reinecke H, Hauschka SD, Murry CE, Stayton PS. In vitro generation of differentiated cardiac myofibers on micropatterned laminin surfaces. Journal of Biomedical Materials Research 2002; 60(3): 472-9.

184. Stout DA, Basu B, Webster TJ. Poly(lactic–co-glycolic acid): Carbon nanofiber composites for myocardial tissue engineering applications. Acta Biomaterialia 2011; 7(8): 3101-12. doi:10.1016/j.actbio.2011.04.028 4.

185. Caspi O, Lesman A, Basevitch Y, Gepstein A, Arbel G, Habib IH, Gepstein L, Levenberg S. Tissue engineering of vascularized cardiac muscle from human embryonic stem cells. Circulation Research 2007;

100(2): 263-72.

186. Ishii O, Shin M, Sueda T, Vacanti JP. In vitro tissue engineering of a cardiac graft using a degradable scaffold with an extracellular matrix–like topography. Journal of Thoracic and Cardiovascular Surgery 2005; 130(5): 1358-63.

187. Piao H, Kwon JS, Piao S, Sohn JH, Lee YS, Bae JW, Hwang KK, Kim DW, Jeon O, Kim BS, Park YB, Cho MC. Effects of cardiac patches engineered with bone marrow-derived mononuclear cells and PGCL scaffolds in a rat myocardial infarction model. Biomaterials 2007; 28(4): 641-9.

188. Gorna K, Gogolewski S. Biodegradable polyurethanes for implants. II. In vitro degradation and calcification of materials from poly(epsilon-caprolactone)-poly(ethylene oxide) diols and various chain extenders. Journal of Biomedical Materials Research 2002; 60(4): 592-606.

189. Zhang JY, Beckman EJ, Piesco NP, Agarwal S. A new peptide-based urethane polymer: synthesis, biodegradation, and potential to support cell growth in vitro. Biomaterials 2000; 21(12): 1247-1258.

190. Rockwood DN, Akins RE Jr, Parrag IC, Woodhouse KA, Rabolt JF. Culture on electrospun polyurethane scaffolds decreases atrial natriuretic peptide expression by cardiomyocytes in vitro. Biomaterials 2008; 29(36): 4783-91. doi:10.1016/j.biomaterials.2008.08.034.

191. Guan J, Fujimoto KL, Sacks MS, Wagner WR. Preparation and characterization of highly porous, biodegradable polyurethane scaffolds for soft tissue applications. Biomaterials 2005; 26(18): 3961-3971. doi:10.1016/j.biomaterials.2004.10.018.

192. Fujimoto KL, Tobita K, Merryman WD, Guan J, Momoi N, Stolz DB, Sacks MS, Keller BB, Wagner WR. An elastic, biodegradable cardiac patch induces contractile smooth muscle and improves cardiac remodeling and function in subacute myocardial infarction. Journal of the American College of Cardiology 2007; 49(23): 2292-300. doi: 10.1016/j.jacc.2007.02.050.

193. Siepe M, Giraud MN, Liljensten E, Nydegger U, Menasche P, Carrel T, Tevaearai HT. Construction of skeletal myoblast-based polyurethane scaffolds for myocardial repair. Artificial Organs 2007; 31(6): 425-33.

194. Chen QZ, Bismarck A, Hansen U, Junaid S, Tran MQ, Harding SE, Ali NN, Boccaccini AR. Characterisation of a soft elastomer poly(glycerol sebacate) designed to match the mechanical properties of myocardial tissue. Biomaterials 2008; 29(1): 47-57.

195. Jean A, Engelmayr GC Jr. Finite element analysis of an accordion-like honeycomb scaffold for cardiac tissue engineering. Journal of Biomechanics 2010; 43(15): 3035-43.

196. Ravichandran R, Venugopal JR, Sundarrajan S, Mukherjee S, Ramakrishna S. Poly(glycerol sebacate)/gelatin core/shell fibrous structure for regeneration of myocardial infarction. Tissue Engineering Part A 2011; 17(9-10): 1363-73. doi: 10.1089/ten.tea.2010.0441.

197. Ifkovits JL, Devlin JJ, Eng G, Martens TP, Vunjak-Novakovic G, Burdick JA. Biodegradable fibrous scaffolds with tunable properties formed from photo-cross-linkable poly(glycerol sebacate). ACS Applied Materials and Interfaces 2009; 1(9): 1878-86.

198. Madden LR, Mortisen DJ, Sussman EM, Dupras SK, Fugate JA, Cuy JL, Hauch KD, Laflamme MA, Murry CE, Ratner BD. Proangiogenic scaffolds as functional templates for cardiac tissue engineering. Proceedings of the National Academy of Sciences of the United States of America 2010; 107(34): 15211-6. doi: 10.1073/pnas.1006442107.

199. Arnal-Pastor M, Vallés-Lluch A, Keicher M, Pradas MM. Coating typologies and constrained swelling of hyaluronic acid gels within scaffold pores. Journal of Colloid and Interface Science 2011; 361(1): 361-9.

200. Sauer H, Rahimi G, Hescheler J, Wartenberg M. Effects of electrical fields on cardiomyocyte differentiation of embryonic stem cells. Journal of Cellular Biochemistry 1999; 75(4): 710–723.

201. Haneef K, Lila N, Benadda S, Legrand F, Carpentier A, Chachques JC. Development of bioartificial myocardium by electrostimulation of 3D collagen scaffolds seeded with stem cells. Heart International 2012; 7(2): e14.

202. Radisic M, Park H, Shing H, Consi T, Schoen FJ, Langer R, Freed LE, Vunjak-Novakovic G. Functional assembly of engineered myocardium by electrical stimulation of cardiac myocytes cultured on scaffolds. Proceedings of the National Academy of Sciences of the United States of America 2004; 101(52): 18129-34.

203. Serena E, Figallo E, Tandon N, Cannizzaro C, Gerecht S, Elvassore N, Vunjak-Novakovic G. Electrical stimulation of human embryonic stem cells: Cardiac differentiation and the generation of reactive oxygen species. Experimental Cell Research 2009; 315(20): 3611-9.

204. Tandon N, Marsanno A, Maidhof R, Wan L. Park H, Vunjak-Novakovic G. Optimization of electrical stimulation parameters for cardiac tissue

engineering. Journal of Tissue Engineering and Regenerative Medicine 2011; 5: e115–e125.

205. Tandon N, Marsano A, Maidhof R, Numata K, Montouri-Sorrentino C, Cannizzaro C, Voldmand J, Vunjak-Novakovic G. Surface-patterned electrode bioreactor for electrical stimulation. Lab on a Chip 2010; 10: 692–700.

206. Dvir T, Timko BP, Brigham MD, Naik SR, Karajanagi SS, Levy O, Jin H, Parker KK, Langer R, Kohane DS. Nanowired three-dimensional cardiac patches. Nature Nanotechnology 2011; 6(11): 720-5. doi:10.1038/nnano.2011.160.

207. You J-O, Rafat M, Ye GJC Auguste,DT. Nanoengineering the heart: conductive scaffolds enhance connexin 43 expression. Nano Letters 2011; 11(9): 3643–3648.

208. Fink C, Ergün S, Kralisch D, Remmers U, Weil J, Eschenhagen T. Chronic stretch of engineered heart tissue induces hypertrophy and functional improvement. Federation of American Societies for Experimental Biology Journal 2000; 14(5): 669-79.

209. Zimmermann WH, Schneiderbanger K, Schubert P, Didié M, Münzel M, Heubach F,Kostin S, Neuhuber WL, Eschenhagen T. Tissue engineering of a differentiated cardiac muscle construct. Circulation Research 2002; 90: 223-230.

210. Guan J, Wang F, Li Z, Chen J, Guo X, Liao J, Moldovan NI. The stimulation of the cardiac differentiation of mesenchymal stem cells in tissue constructs that mimic myocardium structure and biomechanics. Biomaterials 2011; 32(24): 5568-80.

211. Zhang T, Wan LQ, Xiong Z, Marsano A, Maidhof R, Park M, Yan Y, Vunjak-Novakovic G. Channelled scaffolds for engineering myocardium with mechanical stimulation. Journal of Tissue Engineering and Regenerative Medicine 2011. doi: 10.1002/term.481.

212. Akhyari P, Fedak PW, Weisel RD, Lee TY, Verma S, Mickle DA, Li RK. Mechanical stretch regimen enhances the formation of bioengineered autologous cardiac muscle grafts. Circulation 2002; 106(12 Suppl 1): I137-42.

213. Chachques JC, Jegaden O, Mesana T, Glock Y, Grandjean PA, Carpentier AF, et al. Cardiac bioassist: results of the French multicenter cardiomyoplasty study. Asian Cardiovascular and Thoracic Annals 2009; 17: 573-80.

214. Kwon MH, Cevasco M, Schmitto JD, Chen FY. Ventricular restraint therapy for heart failure: A review, summary of state of the art, and future directions. Journal of Thoracic and Cardiovascular Surgery 2012; 144(4): 771-777.

215. Liao SY, Siu CW, Liu Y, Zhang Y, Chan WS, Wu EX, Wu Y, Nicholls JM, Li RA, Benser ME, Rosenberg SP, Park E, Lau CP, Tse HF. Attenuation of left ventricular adverse remodeling with epicardial patching after myocardial infarction. Journal of Cardiac Failure 2010; 16 (7): 590-8.

216. Enomoto Y, Gorman JH 3rd, Moainie SL, Jackson BM, Parish LM, Plappert T, Zeeshan A, St John-Sutton MG, Gorman RC. Early ventricular restraint after myocardial infarction: extent of the wrap determines the outcome of remodeling. Annals of Thoracic Surgery 2005; 79(3): 881-7.

217. Klodell CT, Aranda JM, McGiffin DC, Rayburn BK, Sun B, Abraham WT, Pae WE, Boehmer JP, Klein H, Huth C. Worldwide surgical experience with the Paracor HeartNet cardiac restraint device. The Journal of Thoracic and Cardiovascular Surgery 2008; 135(1): 188–195.

218. Costanzo MR, Ivanhoe RJ, Kao A, Anand IS, Bank A, Boehmer J, Demarco T, Hergert CM, Holcomb RG, Maybaum S, Sun B, Vassiliades TA Jr, Rayburn BK, Abraham WT. Prospective evaluation of elastic restraint to lessen the effects of heart failure (PEERLESS-HF) trial. Journal of Cardiac Failure 2012; 18(6): 446-58. doi: 10.1016/j.cardfail.2012.04.004.

219. Dixon JA, Goodman AM, Gaillard WF 2nd, Rivers WT, McKinney RA, Mukherjee R, Baker NL, Ikonomidis JS, Spinale FG. Hemodynamics and myocardial blood flow patterns after placement of a cardiac passive restraint device in a model of dilated cardiomyopathy. Journal of Thoracic and Cardiovascular Surgery 2011; 142: 1038-45.

220. Pilla JJ, Blom AS, Brockman DJ, Ferrari VA, Yuan Q, Acker MA. Passive ventricular constraint to improve left ventricular function and mechanics in an ovine model of heart failure secondary to acute myocardial infarction. Journal of Thoracic and Cardiovascular Surgery 2003; 126(5): 1467-76.

221. Mann DL, Kubo SH, Sabbah HN, Starling RC, Jessup M, Oh JK, Acker MA. Beneficial effects of the CorCap cardiac support device: five-year results from the Acorn Trial. Journal of Thoracic and Cardiovascular Surgery 2012; 143(5): 1036-42.

222. Olsson A, Bredin F, Franco-Cereceda A. Echocardiographic findings using tissue velocity imaging following passive containment surgery with the Acorn CorCap cardiac support device. European Journal of Cardio-Thoracic Surgery 2005; 28: 448-53.

223. Shafy A, Fink T, Zachar V, Lilaa N, Carpentier A, Chachques JC. Development of cardiac support bioprostheses for ventricular restoration and myocardial regeneration. European Journal of Cardio-Thoracic Surgery 2012; 0: 1–9. doi:10.1093/ejcts/ezs480.

Chapter 9

MWCNT USED IN ORTHOPAEDIC BONE CEMENTS

Nicholas Dunne and Ross W. Ormsby

School of Mechanical & Aerospace Engineering, Queen's University of Belfast, Ashby Building, Belfast, UK

INTRODUCTION

This chapter discusses the use of carbon nanotube (CNT) based nanocomposites for biomedical applications, particularly in the area of orthopaedic bone cement used in joint replacement surgery.

The chapter initially introduces total joint replacements and poly methyl methacrylate (PMMA) bone cement. The associated issues and drawbacks with the use of these PMMA bone cements in terms of mechanical and thermal properties are then discussed in detail. The application of various MWCNT types (in terms of chemical functionality) at various weight loadings in augmenting some of the issues described is then presented. The next section of this chapter discusses the biological response to the various nanocomposite bone cements with MWCNT. The chapter concludes by discussing issues of CNT interaction with the body, and outlines the current trends in tagging and tracking the movement of MWCNT.

THE HIP JOINT

The hip joint (Figure 1) is a synovial ball and socket joint allowing for rotation about three perpendicular axes. It is constructed of the femoral head and the acetabulum of the pelvic bone. The femoral head and acetabulum are covered by cartilage. In a healthy hip joint the cartilage acts as a protective cushion to allow smooth movement of the joint, thus reducing friction and to some extent absorb shock. The presence of the synovial membrane secretes synovial fluid into the joint in order to nourish and lubricate the articulating cartilage (Martini and Bartholomew, 2000). The hip joint is responsible for the transfer of weight from the leg to the body, and as such, can be under substantial mechanical stresses.

Potential Problems with the Hip Joint

Problems with the hip joint can arise due to cartilage damage within the joint caused by disease, trauma, or congenital conditions. This can lead to the surrounding tissues becoming inflamed, causing considerable pain. Arthritis (joint inflammation) is the main cause of hip joint degradation (Havelin *et al.* 2003; Malchau*et al.* 2002). There are more than one hundred rheumatic diseases that can cause chronic pain, stiffness, and swelling in the synovial joints. The Arthritis Research Campaign (ARC 2002) reported that in the UK, 206 million working days were lost due to arthritis and joint related conditions. The National Institute of Arthritis and Musculoskeletal and Skin Diseases (NIAMS 2004) stated that two of the most common forms of arthritis are osteoarthritis and rheumatoid arthritis. Primary osteoarthritis is a result of the gradual eroding of the cartilage layer (Figure 2a). It most commonly affects those over the age of 60 (ARC 2002) and remains the most common cause for primary joint surgery (94% of patients in 2005 (NJR 2006)). Congenital conditions such as a deformed joint or defective cartilage can result in osteoarthritis; however obesity, joint fracture, ligament tears, or other injury can damage cartilage, resulting in secondary osteoarthritis. It is noteworthy that while increased occurrences of osteoarthritis are indicative of an aging population, obesity is currently a major risk factor of osteoarthritis (ARC 2002). Overall, it is clear that osteoarthritis is the most common indication for joint replacement irrespective of age (Furnes *et al.* 2005; Karrholm *et al.* 2008; NJR 2006).

Hip Joint

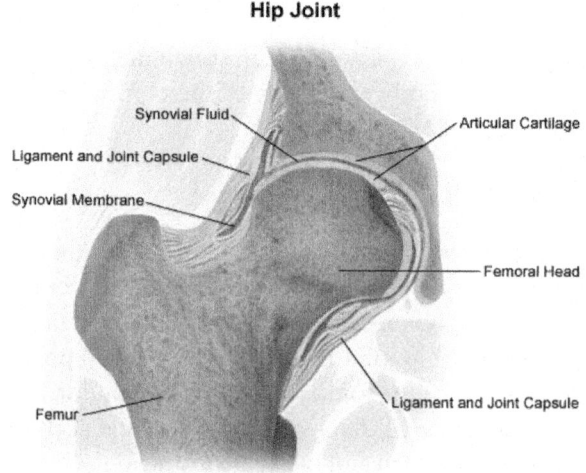

Figure 1. Anatomy of a healthy hip (Martini and Bartholomew, 2000).

Rheumatoid arthritis is a chronic inflammatory disease of the joints whereby the synovium within the joint becomes inflamed. This inflammatory process damages the surrounding bone and cartilage (Figure 2b). Rheumatoid arthritis most commonly occurs during middle age of adulthood; however the disease can affect children and young adults as well. Rheumatoid arthritis usually affects joints symmetrically and most frequently attacks the hands, wrists, elbows, shoulders, knees and elbows.

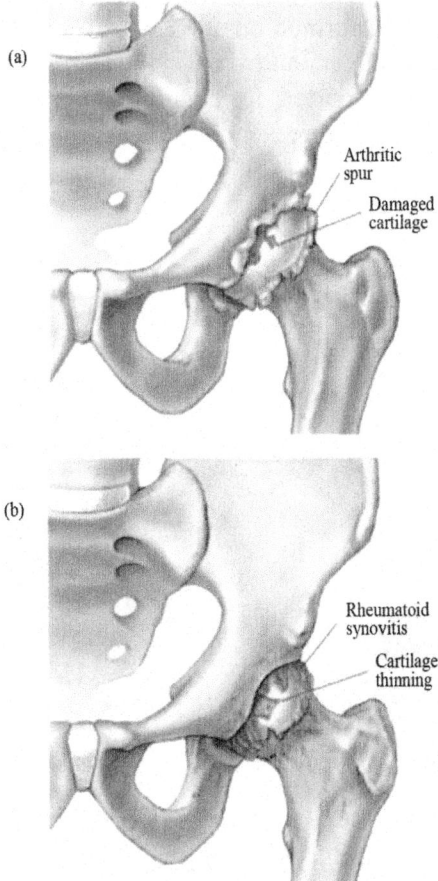

Figure 2. Illustration of (a) Osteoarthritis and (b) Rheumatoid arthritis of the hip (Zimmer Inc., 2010)

Primary Joint Replacement

It is estimated that more than 29% of the population in the UK, are affected by arthritis and joint pain (ARC 2002). If partial damage of the joint has occurred, it may be possible to repair or replace just the damaged areas; if the entire joint is damaged, however, a total joint replacement (TJR) may be necessary to relieve pain and to maintain function of the joint (Prendergast 2001). When replacing a total joint, the diseased or damaged parts are removed and artificial parts, i.e. prostheses or implants, are fitted. Due to the associated risks of surgery, in addition to high financial cost (in 1999-2000, hip and knee replacements alone cost the UK's health and social services £405 million (ARC 2002)), TJR is considered the last resort after failure of non-surgical treatment (Felson *et al.* 2000). TJR may be performed on a variety of joints, including hip, knee, ankle, shoulder, elbow, fingers and wrist. However, hip replacements are by far the most common, as reported, for example, in Norway between 1987 and 2004 (Furnes *et al.* 2005). Figure 3 shows an example of total hip replacement (THR) components.

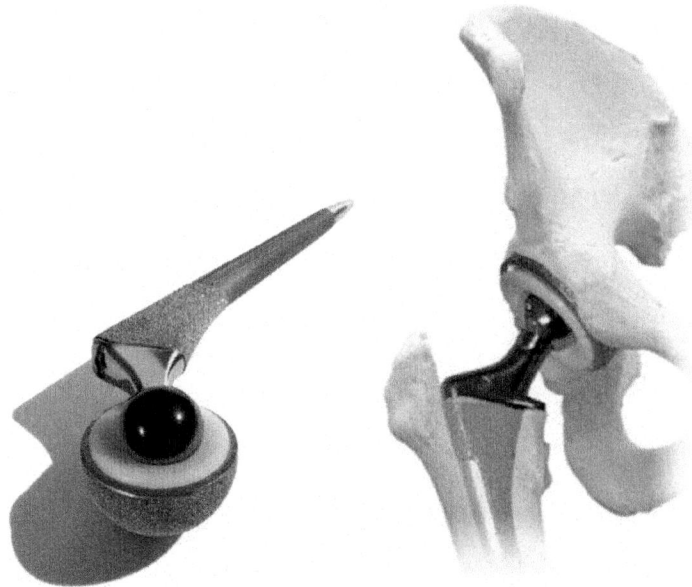

Figure 3. (a) Typical components of a total hip replacement (THR) and (b) the components *in vivo* (Smith and Nephew Inc., 2008)

During TJR, the most commonly used method of implant fixation is with a load transferring grout-like material, typically an acrylic based bone cement. The major advantage of these cemented joint replacements is the reduced operation recovery time: once polymerised the cement is capable of bearing load and offers immediate stability (figure 4).

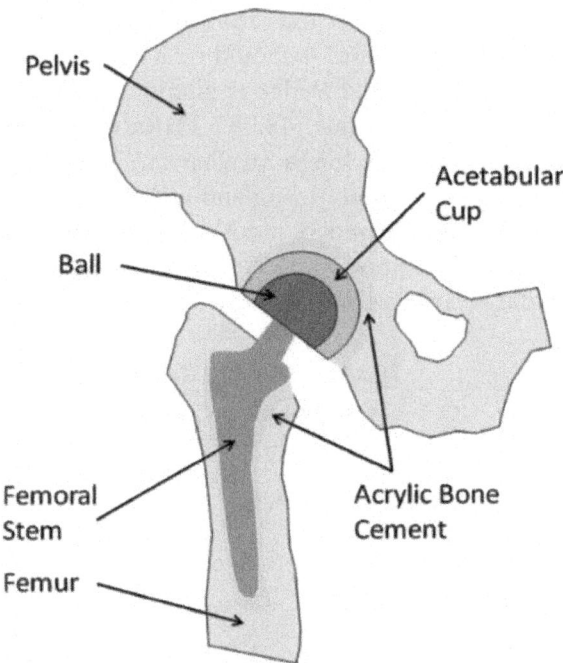

Figure 4. Schematic diagram of a cement TJR.

However, if the cement mantle becomes loose, the surrounding bone may resorb and ultimate failure of the implant may occur. Uncemented implants were introduced to overcome these shortcomings, for example, cement wear particles, in addition to residual monomer and the highly exothermic polymerisation causing cellular necrosis to the surrounding bone. Uncemented implants typically use a roughened porous surface to promote bone growth around the prosthesis (Hungerford and Jones 1988). However, the bone cavity produced during the operation needs to be precise to ensure the implant is initially held in place through an interlocking mechanical fixation between the implant and the bone. It is also essential that the surrounding bone is healthy to enable this technique to be successful. In addition, the recovery time is long as the bone is required to regenerate. A combination of cemented and uncemented implants is also employed and often termed a 'hybrid'. More recently, resurfacing arthroplasty has been introduced, where less of the bone is removed compared with conventional TJR. Resurfacing procedures not only require the removal of less bone, but cause fewer complications during revision surgeries because the femoral canal is retained intact (Amstutz *et al.* 1998). On average, the number of primary arthroplasties in developed nations is increasing each year (Furnes *et al.* 2005; Karrholm *et al.* 2008; NJR 2006). Figure 5 demonstrates the proportion of cemented, uncemented and hybrid replacements. It is obvious from this graph just how much more popular cemented procedures are. It should be noted that the total number of TJRs performed in England and Wales is significantly greater than Sweden and Norway. In 2004, for example, 48,987 THRs were recorded in England and Wales, compared to just 13,366 in Sweden and 7,061 in Norway. It should also be noted that the population of England and Wales (approximately 55m) is significantly greater than Sweden and Norway (approximately 13m). This equates to approximately 1 in every 1100 people in England and Wales, and 1 in every 650 people in Sweden and Norway.

Number of primary THRs
per type of fixation, 1979-2007

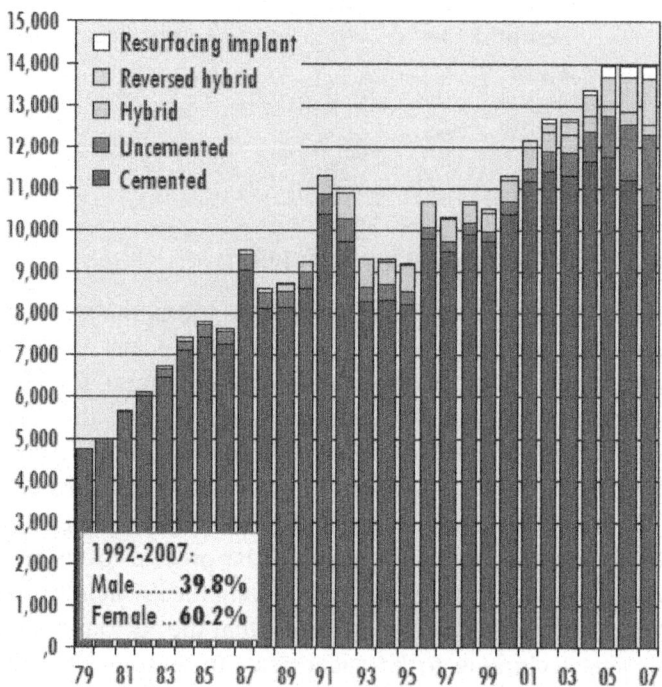

Figure 5. Number and fixation type of primary THRs preformed in Sweden from 1979 to 2007. (Karrholm *et al.* 2008)

Fully cemented TJR remain the most frequently used implant fixation procedure with 51% of primary THR in England and Wales being cemented in 2005, compared with 54% in 2004. In contrast, there was a slight increase in the application of bone cement for other fixation surgical procedures (NJR 2006). Alternative studies have shown that use of primary cemented TJRs over the last 10 years has remained consistent, whilst the application of cementless implants has almost doubled over the same period (Karrholm *et al.* 2008). This may be partly explained by the increase in the number of TJRs required for a younger age group (<60 yrs and <55 yrs for Sweden and England/Wales respectively). This cohort received more surgical procedures involving uncemented and hybrid implants (Karrholm *et al.* 2008; NJR 2006). It is important to note that whilst there is a slight decrease in the use of cemented implants in THR procedures; bone cement is still required for the majority of implant procedures. In 2005, cement was used for the fixation of 73% of femoral stems and 53% of acetabular cups, in England and Wales (NJR 2006).

Acrylic Bone Cement

Poly (methylmethacrylate) (PMMA) has been used in orthopaedics since the early 1960s (Charnley 1960). It was first introduced by Sir John Charnley and Dr Dennis Smith. Also known as acrylic bone cement, it acts as a grouting agent for the fixation of artificial joints as well as the treatment of spinal compression fractures (vertebroplasty). In TJR, bone cement fills the space between prosthesis and bone and acts as an elastic buffer, therefore transferring mechanical load on the implant to the bone. This function of distributing stresses is critical for implant longevity. If the external stresses exceed the ability of the cement to transfer the load, a fracture results (Kuehn *et al.*, 2005).

Acrylic bone cement is a two phase system, consisting of a polymer powder and monomer liquid. The powder phase primarily consists of spherical PMMA beads (82–89 wt. %), in addition to an inorganic radiopacifying agent, usually barium sulphate or zirconium dioxide (10 – 15 wt. %). The powder component also contains benzoyl peroxide (BPO; 0.5–2.6 wt. %), which catalyses polymerisation. The liquid phase is largely MMA monomer (98 wt. %), with 2 wt. % N, N-Dimethyl-*p*-toluidene (DmpT) which accelerates the polymerisation. From a chemical point of view, MMA is an ester of methacrylic acid with a polymerisable double bond. When the liquid and powder phases are mixed, the initiator (BPO) reacts with the accelerator (DmpT) to form free radicals in what is known as the 'initiation reaction'. These free radicals initiate polymerisation of MMA into PMMAby adding to the polymerisable double-bond of the monomer molecule. Temperatures during this reaction can reach up to 110°C. During polymerisation, the bone cement is worked into a 'dough' phase that can be moulded or injected. In a relatively short amount of time (10 – 15 minutes) the bone cement hardens to ca. 90% of its final mechanical properties (Kuehn *et al.*, 2005). Although current revision rates of cemented TJR are low, improved mechanical and thermal properties are required to further reduce subsequent surgeries of cemented arthroplasties, and increase the longevity of the implant. With 88.7% of current cemented implants expected to last at least 14 years (Karrholm *et al.* 2008), this would mean that more physically active patients would have to undergo a number of revision surgeries in their lifetime. Furthermore, younger patient populations are more likely to impose heavier, more complex loadings on the implant, as they would wish to continue pursuing an active lifestyle.

COMPOSITION AND POLYMERISATION REACTION

Composition

Acrylic bone cement, as mentioned is primarily composed of poly methylmethacrylate (PMMA). Most commercial acrylic bone cements comprise of a two part self-curing acrylic polymer, usually formulated as a 2:1 powder to liquid ratio. These components are mixed immediately prior to implantation during surgery and delivered directly to the implant site. The compositions of the main commercial bone cements are summarised in Table 1.0, showing variations in chemical composition. Other cements may also contain antibiotics (e.g. gentamicin sulphate (Lewis 2003; Hendriks *et al.* 2004)) in order to improve the body's response to the implant, reducing risk of subsequent infection and implant rejection.

Table 1. Compositions of six commercial formulations of bone cement (Lewis 1997). The compositions are given in percent (w/w) except where stated otherwise.

Constituent	CMW-1	CMW-3	Palacos R	Simplex P	Zim-mer LVC
POWDER COMPO-NENTS					
Benzoyl peroxide (BPO)	2.60	2.20	0.5-1.6	1.19	0.75
Barium sulphate (BaSO$_4$)	9.10	10.00	-	10.00	10.00
Zirconium dioxide (ZrO$_2$)	-	-	14.85	-	-
Chlorophyll	-	-	200 ppm	-	-
PMMA	88.30	87.80	-	16.55	89.25
PMMA-Methacrylic acid (P(MMA/MA))	-	-	83.55-84.65	-	-
PMMA-styrenecopolymers P(MMA/ST)	-	-	-	82.26	-
LIQUID COMPONENTS					

NN Dimethyl P Toluidine (DmpT)	0.40	0.99	2.13	2.48	2.75
Hydroquinone	15-20 ppm	15-20 ppm	64 ppm	75 ppm	75 ppm
Mehtylmethacrylate (MMA)	98.66	98.07	97.87	97.51	97.25
Ethanol	0.92	0.92	-	-	-
Ascorbic Acid	0.02	0.02	-	-	-
Chlorophyll	-	-	267 ppm	-	-
Gentamicin sulphate	-	-		-	-

Polymerisation Reaction

PMMA is an amorphous polymer, which is plasticised on the addition of the monomer methyl methacrylate (MMA). When bone cement is mixed two processes occur, firstly the monomer is absorbed by the PMMA beads and secondly, a free radical polymerisation reaction occurs (Kuehn *et al.*2005). This reaction is shown schematically in Figure 6 below.

During this reaction the DmpT causes the BPO to decompose leaving a benzoyl radical, and a benzoyl anion (Figure 6a). These benzoyl radicals then initiate the polymerisation of the MMA by combining and forming an active centre (Figure 6b). These active centers then combine with multiple molecules to form a polymer chain (Figure 6c). This reaction forms a viscous fluid allowing the polymerising cement to be moulded as required, i.e. this is the stage when the surgeon would inject the bone cement into the prepared bone canal prior to implanting the stem. As the monomer begins to polymerise, the cement hardens around the stem, holding it in place. This reaction is highly exothermic, an example of a temperature plot of bone cement during polymerisation is shown in Figure 7. The heat energy produced during polymerisation is 57 kJ per mole MMA, resulting in temperatures, which can exceed 100° C. These elevated temperatures can cause cellular bone necrosis which can ultimately contribute to aseptic loosening (Dunne and Orr 2002; Stanczyk and van Rietbergen 2004; Kuehn *et al.* 2005). It should be noted though that the polymerisation temperatures experienced *in vivo* have been much lower (between 40–47° C) at the bone interface (Toksvig-Larsen *et al.*, 1991). This is due to the reduced thicknesses of bone cement mantle, the presence of blood circulation, and the dissipation of heat through the implant and surrounding tissue (Kuehn *et al.* 2005). It has been shown that volumetric shrinkage can occur due to thermal contraction on cooling and the changing density as polymerisation progresses (Gilbert *et al.*2000; Kuehn *et al.* 2005).

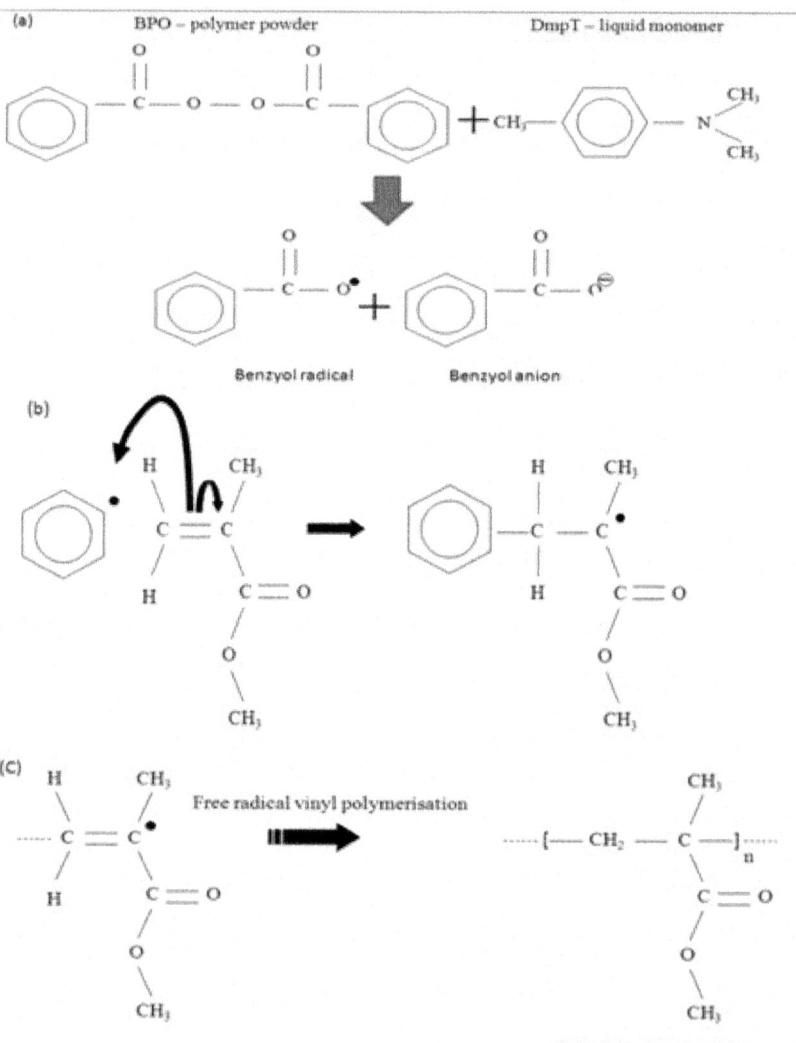

Figure 6. a) Schematic diagram showing the decomposition of BPO leaving a benzoyl radical, and a benzoyl anion; (b) How these benzoyl radicals initiate polymerisation of MMA; (c) formation of a polymer chain.

Gilbert *et al.* (2000) reported that volumetric shrinkage as a result of density variation, due to the exothermic polymerisation was between 5.1 % and 6.5 % depending on mixing method employed and type of cement. Both shrinkage mechanisms have been identified as factors which influence the levels of residual stresses within the cement (Gilbert *et al.* 2000; Orr *et al.* 2003).

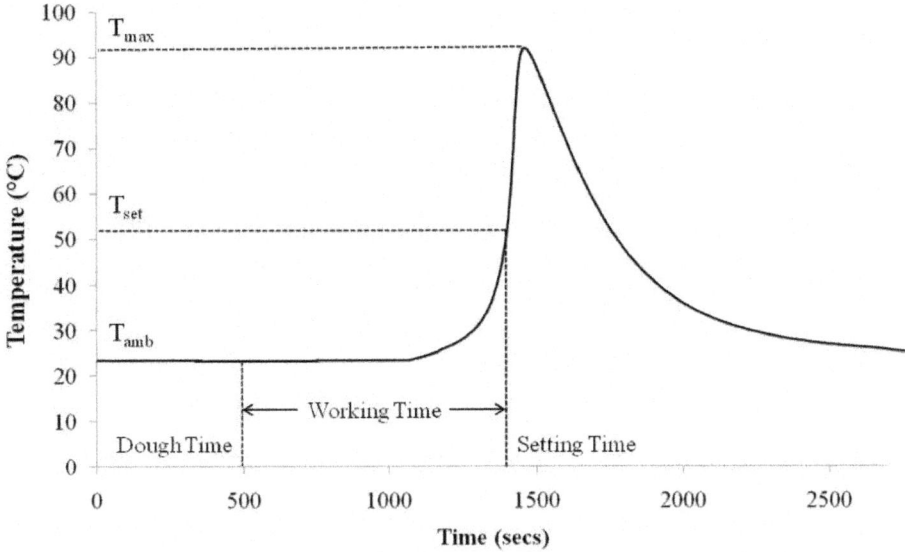

Figure 7. A typical curing curve for acrylic bone cement where T_{max} is the maximum temperature reached, T_{set} is the setting temperature and T_{amb} is the ambient temperature.

As illustrated in Figure 7, the time that has elapsed after initial mixing when the cement takes a homogeneous dough-like state is known as the 'dough time'. This point may be identified with temperature or, average molecular weight of the polymer. However, as specified in the British Standard BS 7253 (ISO 5833:2002), it is the point at which the cement will no longer stick to powderless surgical gloves (typically 2-3 minutes after initial mixing). The time from the end of dough time until the cement can no longer be manipulated, is defined as the working time. During an operation this is the time during which the surgeon must insert the stem and adjust its position. Finally, the setting time is the time from the onset of mixing until the surface temperature reaches one half of the maximum temperature, as described in ISO 5833:2002.

CURRENT ISSUES WITH ACRYLIC BONE CEMENT

Mechanical Properties

The main role of bone cement is to transfer load between bone and the metallic prosthesis. Several studies have shown that the composition of acrylic bone cement significantly influences the mechanical properties of the cement (including Harper and Bonfield 2000; Lewis 2000). It is during the polymerisation process that numerous cement properties, for example viscosity, setting time, maximum cure temperature, and volumetric shrinkage etc, can be determined.

These material characteristics may influence a cemented TJR performance. It has also been shown that the variability in the mechanical static and dynamic properties of commercial bone cements is significant, with greater relative differences reported in fatigue properties (Lewis 1997; Harper and Bonfield 2000). Harper and Bonfield (2000) found that there was some correlation between the static and fatigue strengths, however the ranking of the different cements tested did not match exactly. Mechanical properties are known to be affected by: cement composition, size and morphology of the PMMA beads, molecular weight, cement mixing technique, and the powder-liquid ratio (Harper and Bonfield 2000; Lewis 1997). The variation in tensile strength, for example, is reported to vary between 24–49 MPa for five different commercial bone cement formulations, depending on the mixing technique, specimen age and test conditions (Lewis 1997).

Thermal Properties

As mentioned previously, *in vivo* temperatures during the exothermic polymerisation of bone cement can cause thermal necrosis (tissue death) of the bone cells and impaired local blood circulation, which can lead to early failure through aseptic loosening of the implant (Huang *et al.* 2005). It has been reported that for epithelial cellular death to occur, an exposure time of 1 s is required for temperatures above 70° C, 30 seconds for temperatures greater than 55° C, and approximately five hours for temperatures greater than 45 °C (Starke *et al.* 2001). Collagen protein molecules are denatured at 45° C, and experience irreversible damage at 60° C if held at these temperatures for an hour. It has also been reported that thermal necrosis occurs in bone tissue when exposure is greater than 1 minute for temperatures above 50° C and denaturation of sensory nerves occurs for temperatures above 45° C if exposure exceeds 30 minutes. The amount of heat generated during polymerisation is dependent on the amount of reacting monomer, however the maximum temperature reached is also dependent upon the rate of heat dissipation. *In vitro* testing completed by Stanczyk and van Rietbergen (2004) suggested that the tips of bone trabeculae protruding into setting cement may experience temperatures in excess of 70° C. In the 1960s, upon first use of bone cement in TJR, Charnley believed that while temperatures of ~100° C could be reached during polymerisation, in the presence of a metallic prosthesis, which would act as a heat sink, there was a reduction in the peak temperature experienced *in vivo*. (Charnley 1960). Since then, numerical simulations and *in vitro* studies of thermal necrosis and peak exotherms in TJR, have helped establish two methods which may assist the reduction of thermal necrosis: (a) the use of thin cement mantle layers, and (b) pre-cooling of the bone surface (Chandler *et al.* 2006; Fukushima *et al.* 2002).

An additional potential adverse consequence of using standard acrylic bone cements is the leaching of residual liquid monomer into the surrounding tissue, which may cause inflammation, chemical necrosis and even death. Average levels of residual monomer can be as high as 5%, however local concentrations may be as high as 15 %, increasing the likelihood of chemical necrosis (Stanczyk and van Rietbergen 2004). Vacuum mixing of acrylic bone cement has been associated with reduced levels of residual monomer as mixing bone cement at reduced pressures increases monomer polymerisation (Bettencourt *et al.* 2001).

There is considerable variation in the chemical composition of different brands of cement (Table 2.1). Often this difference involves more than one of the basic constituents, making it difficult to draw any conclusions regarding the effect of composition on mechanical properties of the cement. It is accepted that the intrinsic properties of the monomer units and the high molecular weight dictate their subsequent mechanical properties such as craze strength, creep resistance and fatigue performance (Sauer and Richardson 1980; Hull and Clyne 1996a). Lewis (2003) reviewed the effect of molecular weight on fatigue performance of bone cement, reporting that increasing the molecular weight of either the powder or the fully cured cement improves the fatigue performance of acrylic bone cement, assuming all other parameters remain fixed. Lewis (2003) suggested that this increase in mechanical performance was related to the increase in polymer chain entanglement due to increased molecular weight which in turn, increased the resistance of the bone cement to craze formation and lead to subsequent increased fatigue crack propagation resistance (Sauer and Richardson 1980; Lewis 2000). Deb *et al.* (2003) reported that increasing the quantity of initiator and activator increased the peak temperature reached during polymerisation reaction and, in addition, lowered the setting time. The content of the residual monomer in the cured bone cement specimens was additionally determined, and it was reported that the highest concentrations of initiator and activator provided the lowest content of residual monomer. However, the concentration of these compounds within the cement must be controlled as they have detrimental health implications when released into the patient. It has also been shown that the type of activator used in polymerisation may significantly influence the fatigue life and fracture toughness of bone cement due to changes in the molecular weight of the resulting polymer (Deb *et al.* 2003). Residual MMA can result after incomplete polymerisation, and is known to influence the mechanical properties and fatigue performance of acrylic bone cement by acting as a plasticiser (Vallo *et al.* 1997;Lewis and Janna 2004). Unreacted MMA is also a possible source of toxicity in the surrounding tissue with possible effects such as hypotension, tissue irritation and alveolar lesions. It has been seen that complete polymerisation and therefore minimal residual MMA content, can be ensured by selecting a suitable initiator activator ratio without significantly affecting fracture toughness (Hasenwinkel *et al.*2002). Alternatively, the presence of residual monomer can reduce the amount of shrinkage of the bone cement, assuming no other sources of shrinkage occur (Gilbert *et al.* 2000).

Fatigue Failure of Bone Cement - *in vivo* Analysis

Within a cemented implant femur, four main areas of weakness have been recognized as potential failure initiation sites, and can be identified as the: (1) cement, (2) bone-cement interface, (3) cement-prosthesis interface and (4) host bone. Jasty *et al.* (1991) used fractographic analysis to examine *ex-vivo*femoral components, reporting evidence of de-bonding at the cement-prosthesis interface in the majority of the TJR investigated. Partial or complete fracture of the cement mantle was frequently coupled with de-bonding at the cement-prosthesis interface. In the early stages of failure, micro-cracking was evident at the cement-bone interface, although these micro-cracks were considered to be non-critical events as there was no evidence to suggest they were associated with complete fracture across the cement mantle. Fatigue damage accumulation is therefore common prior to overall loosening of the implant *in vivo*. Cemented hip replacements typically experience final failure after several fracture sites have developed, although single, longitudinal cement fractures causing loosening, and subsequent failure have also been recorded *in vivo* (Jasty *et al.* 1991; Topoleski *et al.* 1990). As mentioned previously, fractographic analysis performed on *ex-vivo* specimens of failed bone cement has allowed *in vivo* failure mechanisms to be observed and, as a result, several groups have demonstrated that *in vitro* testing can replicate the micro-mechanisms of failure *in vivo* (Topoleski *et al.* 1990/1993;Verdonschot and Huiskes 1997a; Murphy and Prendergast 2002).

Typically, fracture surfaces were identified with a stepped or irregular fatigue region, this region then evolved into a flat, rapid fracture region (Topoleski *et al.* 1990). This stepped or irregular surface can be attributed to the coalescence of micro-cracks that have formed ahead of the crack tip during crack propagation. Initiating micro-cracks (Figure 8) were believed to exist as a result of internal defects such as pores, aggregates of the radiopaque agent, inclusions from the bone at the bone-cement interface, residual stress-induced cracks at the cement-prosthesis interface, and implant design (Jasty *et al.* 1991;Bishop *et al.* 1996; McCormack and Prendergast 1996;Orr *et al.* 2003; Prendergast 2001b; Murphy and Prendergast 2002).

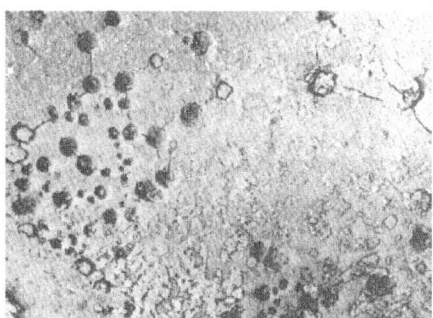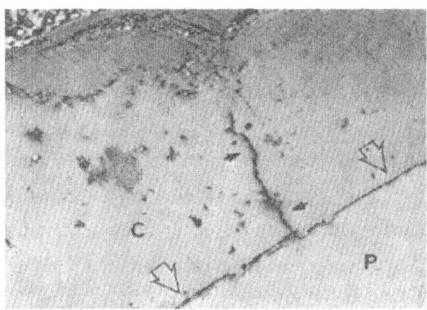

Figure 8. Scanning electron micrographs showing (a) micro fractures through pores near distal end of prosthesis and (b) an incomplete fracture through the cement mantle originating at the cement-prosthesis interface, Jasty *et al.* (1991).

McCormack *et al.* (1998) used experimental and finite element modeling of the cemented construct to complete statistical analysis of micro-crack accumulation. Representation of micro-crack initiation and propagation was achieved for a longitudinal cross-section of the implanted construct. This allowed for the modeling of the bone-cement and cement-prosthesis interactions. The damage accumulation was found to vary significantly over different regions of the cement mantle. It was reported that more significant cracking occurred at the lateral side of the cement mantle compared with the medial side, however an increased rate of crack formation was seen at the distal end (*cf.* proximal), with more cracks initiating from the bulk of the cement (*cf.* the interfaces). It was also noted that a greater incidence of cracks originating from the bone-cement interface was seen to occur compared to the cement-prosthesis interface. Alternative studies have reported that the location at which a fracture initiates depends on the type of loading applied to the specimen. McCormack and Prendergast (1999) reported a greater occurrence of fatigue cracks initiated from pores within the cement mantle when examining cement under bending loads. Under torsional loads, they observed that cracks initiated most often at the interfaces (McCormack *et al.* 1999). Additionally, as previously mentioned in a study by Jasty *et al.* 1991, *ex-vivo* observations reported evidence of cracks initiating from the cement-prosthesis interface and from voids within the bulk of the cement, suggesting both crack growth scenarios may be important. Prendergast (2001b) confirmed the dependence of crack initiation on loading type, and also suggested that in order to reduce this damage accumulation, the volume of cement stressed to a critical degree must be minimised. There is some disagreement as to the predominant source of fatigue damage accumulation; *in vitro* test specimens demonstrate the benefits of a reduced porosity within the cement (Dunne *et al.* 2003).

However, the associated complexity of the *in vivo* cement mantle, in addition to the stress singularities introduced at sharp corners of the implant, and the cement interfaces, may over-shadow the stress amplifying effect of porosity (Janssen *et al.* 2005b). It is however, widely accepted that porosity has a marked influence on damage accumulation, as pores have the potential to act as initiation sites or aid crack coalescence. It should be noted that failure of the cemented construct is not just influenced by damage accumulation and final fracture of the cement mantle. Wear particles associated with the breakdown of cement during de-bonding and fracture, may be transported throughout the implant, leading to an immune-response and the development of osteolysis. Resultant bone degradation will ultimately lead to aseptic loosening of the implant (Anthony *et al.* 1990). A further feature of bone cement is its ability to creep under sustained loading (either static or fatigue), which may contribute to damage development over time. The relationship between creep and damage accumulation is complex. Creep is thought to promote stress relaxation within the cement mantle, reducing the damage accumulation rate (Stolk *et al.* 2004). However, it may also serve to increase levels of implant migration, but the magnitude of this has been shown to be insignificant (Verdonschot and Huiskes 1997b).

Mechanisms of Failure in Bone Cement – *in vitro* analysis

Fatigue Crack Initiation

In vitro strain measurements completed by O›Connor *et al.* (1996) have shown the variation in stresses within the cement mantle. The presence of stress raisers within the cement mantle (e.g. porosity) have the potential to sufficiently raise stresses and cause fatigue crack initiation, and subsequent failure. Whilst extensive research has been conducted on the factors that cause crack initiation, a full understanding of the micromechanics involved is yet to be achieved (Lewis 2003). *In vitro* studies by Orr *et al.* (2003) suggested that cracks may be present prior to the loading of the implant, i.e. once the cement has polymerised. Whether cracks are more likely to occur at the bone-cement interface or at the cement-prosthesis interface is a source of discussion. Bishop *et al.* (1996) reported that pores may be more likely to occur at the cement-prosthesis interface due to the presence of a temperature gradient. If a prosthesis conditioned at room temperature is implanted into bone at body temperature, the polymerisation process will begin at the bone-cement interface, hence the cement-prosthesis interface will polymerise later. Porosity at the cement-prosthesis interface due to cement shrinkage will cause reductions in the static and dynamic properties. In contrast, Orr *et al.* (2003)

reported that voids and micro-cracks are more likely to occur at the cement-bone interface due to the presence of residual stresses caused by thermal shrinkage around the metallic implant, with a small proportion of cracks initiating from pores within the mantle. McCormack and Prendergast (1999) proposed that initial levels of new crack initiation are higher early on in the loading history, due to stress relief occurring at regions of stress intensity. Furthermore, McCormack and Prendergast (1999) suggested that crack growth rate is the same for all types of micro-cracks, whether "pre-loaded" (i.e. cracks formed as a result of stress relief during cement shrinkage or, from regions of high stress concentration) or 'load-initiated' (i.e. cracks formed due to fatigue loading). As a result it is believed that pre-loaded cracks play a critical role in the aseptic loosening process and thus, the overall failure of cement mantle. Any improvement made to the mixing process (reduction in porosity) and to the level of shrinkage during polymerisation, may then, in theory, impede levels of damage accumulation.

Fatigue Crack Growth

Fatigue crack growth can propagate in two different phases and are typically observed as a flat, rapid fracture region proceeded by an irregular, or stepped fatigue region (Topoleski *et al.* 1990). The stepped or irregular region, is representative of the early stages of slow crack growth, and may be accounted for in polymers by a process known as "discontinuous crack growth" (DCG). DCG refers to a single burst of fatigue crack advance after several hundred fatigue cycles (Takemori 1984). At high stress intensity factors (K), striated growth usually occurs at the crack tip. Striations refer to the growth bands visible on a fracture surface whose spacing is equivalent to crack growth rate per stress cycle. Striations are orientated perpendicular to the direction of crack growth. Striations are often confused with DCG bands, with the main differences being that the DCG band spacing is significantly greater than the crack length increment per cycle and these bands arise at low K values. Once crack initiation has occurred, it will be in the DCG regime, and the mechanisms by which the crack develops throughout this regime will ultimately determine the fatigue crack growth resistance of the material (Takemori 1984). Fractographic studies have shown that DCG is of relevance for acrylic bone cement with distinct bands being observed in *ex-vivo* samples (Jasty *et al.* 1991; Topoleski *et al.* 1990). DCG is a function of the testing and specimen preparation conditions, environmental effects and compositional changes, all factors that influence the fracture properties of the polymer (Takemori 1984). Changes to the bone cement that influence these factors must be carefully considered with respect to their affect on the overall structural performance of the cement. During the early stages of fatigue crack propagation, DCG band formation is favoured by the development and growth of crazes ahead of the crack tip (Skibo *et al.* 1977). Crazes are identifiable as dense arrays of fibrils inter-dispersed with elongated voids that appear ahead of the crack tip, effectively reducing the density of the polymer in that region. Crazes are generally perpendicular to the applied stress, which result in inelastic deformation by craze widening in the local principal stress direction. In amorphous glassy polymers (e.g. PMMA) brittle fractures occur through crazing and crack propagation (Scheirs 2000b). Crazing has been reported in detail for PMMA by Pulos and Knauss (1998a/b/c). Pulos and Knauss (1998a/b/c) described how damage (identifiable with crazing) ahead of the fatigue crack tip may occur over many cycles, causing a sudden jump in the crack. As mentioned previously, crazing is prominent in polymers ahead of the crack tip at low K values and DCG may occur within this craze zone once the maximum opening of the craze zone reaches a critical value (Figure 9).

Crazing is a common form of polymer deterioration. Crazing is often a precursor to crack growth and failure, however in thermoplastics the presence of crazing can aid fracture toughening. In these cases, the mechanism of crazing enables polymers to absorb energy through the matrix (in-elastic) deformation. This is possible because the energy used to initiate crazing, and crack growth is large and allows the energy to be dissipated over a large area (Luo *et al.* 2004; Topoleski *et al.* 1990). Alternatively, in thermosetting plastics, crazing may lower the strength of the polymer and lead to premature failure (Scheirs 2000b). Crack propagation through a polymer may also be retarded through crack bridging and, to some extent, micro-cracking; this effect may influence both static and cyclic failure. Previous work in the literature suggests that secondary cracks are present in cement failure (a result of tensile stress relief) (Verdonschot and Huiskes 1997b), therefore consideration of these toughening mechanisms may be appropriate. Non-uniform extension of a crack tip can result in un-cracked ligaments. It should be noted that micro-cracks only act as a toughening mechanism when they are constrained; otherwise they are detrimental to the fracture toughness as they propagate and develop into long cracks (Nalla *et al.* 2004).

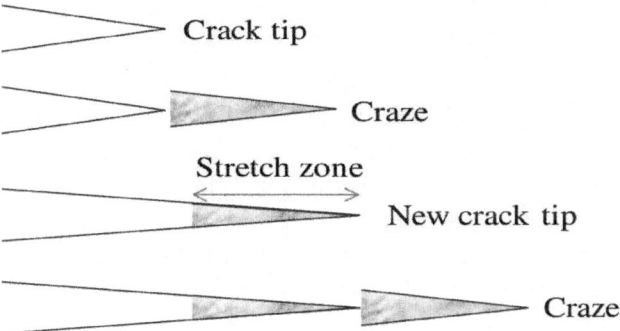

Figure 9. Illustration of discontinuous band growth (DCG) within the craze zone, ahead of a crack tip.

Effect of Residual Stresses and Cement Shrinkage

It is well accepted that residual stresses are generated within the cement mantle following polymerization and have a direct influence on the stress distribution at the cement-prosthesis interface. Knowledge and understanding of these processes may allow a more accurate prediction of load transfer and in-service conditions in the cement mantle (Nuno and Amabili 2002; Nuno and Avanzolini 2002;Orr et al. 2003; Roques *et al.* 2004). Stresses due to shrinkage, exist in cement surrounding the stem in both the longitudinal and the hoop direction (Roques *et al.* 2004). These stresses will be at their greatest immediately post-operatively, with a reduction occurring with time as stress relaxation, and creep occur (Verdonschot and Huiskes 1997a; Nuno and Amabili 2002; Nuno and Avanzolini 2002; Stolk *et al.*2004). This may create more favourable stress distributions at the interfaces between the cement-bone, and cement-prosthesis, as finite element modelling of bonded and un-bonded stems predicts that an increase in compressive stresses at these regions may occur (Verdonschot and Huiskes 1997a). The presence of pores at either interface has been attributed to volume shrinkage of the cement during polymerization. Some polymerization shrinkage will occur while the cement is still viscous and hence can be accommodated by flow (Orr *et al.* 2003). However, as polymerization progresses, this flow may not accommodate shrinkage and cracks can initiate in high stress areas as a mechanism of stress relief. While residual stresses do exist in fully polymerized bone cement, the additional presence of porosity, high stress concentrations or excessive heat generated during polymerization may still be required for large cracks to initiate. As residual stresses alone may not be enough to generate cracks (Lennon and Prendergast 2002). The ultimate tensile strength of various bone cements range between 24 and 49 MPa (Lewis

1997), whereas residual stresses of between 2.5 MPa (Nuno and Avanzolini 2002) and 12.6 MPa (Orr *et al.* 2003) have been reported. The direction in which the cement will shrink is of great significance. Orr *et al.* (2003) reported this has a direct relation to the levels of micro-cracking that may occur as a result of shrinkage stress, although the use of acoustic emission has provided evidence for the shrinkage of the cement onto the femoral implants (Roques *et al.* 2004). Furthermore, shrinkage is known to be affected by the volume fraction of monomer content (Gilbert *et al.* 2000).

The Role of Porosity

Lewis (1997) identified four main reasons why porosity occurs in bone cements;

- The entrapment of air between the polymer powder and monomer liquid as the powder is wetted by the monomer upon mixing,
- Evaporation of the liquid monomer during polymerisation,
- Entrapment of air during mixing,
- Entrapment of air upon transfer of the dough into the cement gun (depending on mixing method).

Materials engineering principles and the relevant literature explain that the presence of pores within the cement mantle act as stress raisers, which may then act as crack initiation sites under applied loads. Many researchers have demonstrated that reduced porosity allows for improved compressive, flexural and fatigue properties of acrylic bone cement (Lewis 1997; Murphy and Prendergast 2000; Dunne and Orr 2002; Dunne *et al.* 2003), therefore the level of porosity (both macro- and micro-pores) should be minimised. Pores of diameter ≥1 mm are deemed macro-pores, and are generally introduced during the mixing process when air is trapped within the cement mixture. These macro-pores are often cited as being the cause of low fatigue life for test specimens as crack initiation is often associated with a single pore. Micro-pores have diameters ≤1 mm, and may be established due to the evaporation of the liquid monomer during the polymerisation process and/or entrapment of air during mixing (Dunne *et al.* 2003). It is often observed that multiple smaller pores (≤1 mm) in close proximity are more detrimental than one larger pore (≥2 mm); this is often a result of the type of mixing method employed (Murphy and Prendergast 2000). A multiple pore arrangement is typically observed for hand mixed specimens (Figure 10) where the combined interaction of the pores produces a stress concentration large enough to cause fatigue crack initiation. In contrast, vacuum mixing (Figure 11) usually generates a smaller distribution of pores. There is evidence to suggest that hand mixed cement reduces the level of shrinkage that cement experiences due to the high level of porosity introduced during mixing, (Dunne *et al.* 2003), as only the cement shrinks during polymerisation and not the voids (Kuehn *et al.* 2005). However, porosity may be beneficial to reduce residual stresses prior to loading; this benefit could be outweighed by the adverse effects observed for fatigue crack initiation and propagation. When the propagating crack tip reaches a pore, failure is considered to occur instantly across the void area, effectively causing the crack propagation rate to increase. Conversely though, there are studies that suggest that pores act as crack "blunters" thereby increasing the fatigue life of the bone cement (Topoleski *et al.* 1993), although crack acceleration into the void must also occur due to the local stress concentration at such a defect.

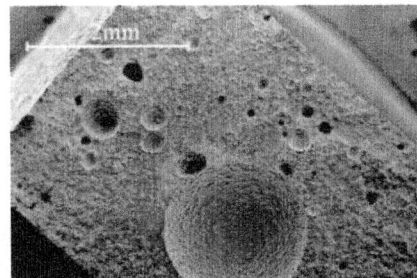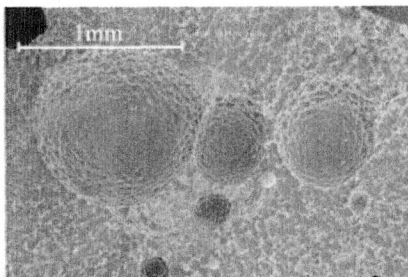

Figure 10. Scanning electron micrograph of a hand-mixed fracture surface for commercial bone cement showing a large pore with a large number of small pores (Murphy and Prendergast 2000).

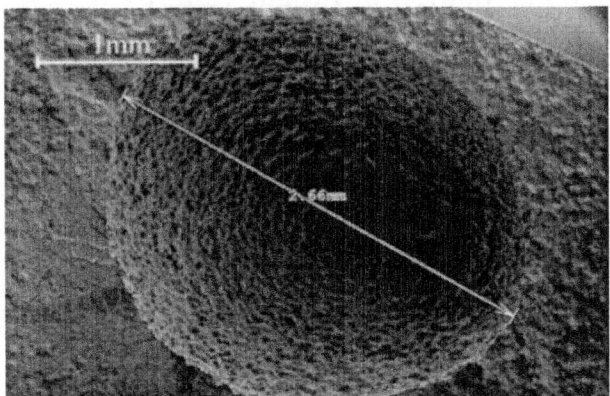

Figure 11. Scanning electron micrograph of a vacuum mixed fracture surface of commercial bone cement, with a larger pore size compared to hand mixed cement (Murphy and Prendergast 2000).

Presence of Radiopaque Agent

Radiopaque agents are included in bone cement formulations (approximately 10-15 % wt.) to allow the cement to be distinguishable from the surrounding body tissues on radiographs. Barium sulphate ($BaSO_4$), Zirconium dioxide (ZrO_2) and iodine-containing copolymers are a few of the possible radiopaque agents used, however $BaSO_4$ is most commonly used. It has been reported that $BaSO_4$ particles do not influence the polymerisation reaction or handling properties of bone cement (Pascual et al. 1996). Additional studies reviewed by Lewis (2003) shown that radiopacifiers may have a positive effect on the fatigue life of acrylic bone cement, although this depended on the particle size and morphology, with the inclusion of "nanoparticles" of $BaSO_4$ (~100 nm in diameter) leading to significant increases in the fatigue life (Ginebra et al. 2002). This improvement in fatigue life was attributed to crack tip blunting, possibly due to the increased number of $BaSO_4$ particles encountered by the crack tip. This is in agreement with Vallo et al. (1997) who proposed that it is the interactions between the crack front and secondary phase particles that account for an increase in toughness; such a mechanism would involve 'crack pinning' and, in effect, an increase in crack length. Conversely, detrimental effects on bending strength, bending modulus and impact strength have been reported after increasing the loading of radiopaque agents (Liu et al. 2001). These reductions have been linked to limited bonding between the $BaSO_4$ particles and the host polymeric matrix (Molino and Topoleski, 1996). Furthermore, it has been observed that large agglomerations of $BaSO_4$ can act as fatigue crack initiation sites with the potential of causing overall failure (Kurtz et al. 2005).

Micromechanical Analysis of Fatigue Failure

When examining the fatigue life of PMMA bone cement, Topoleski et al. (1993) suggested that micro-crack propagation occurred primarily through the inter-bead matrix, in addition to micro-crack formation ahead of the crack tip, as is modeled in Figure 12. Topoleski et al. (1993) also stated that the PMMA beads themselves may experience cleavage or crazing during rapid fracture. Other works by Murphy and Prendergast (2002) suggested that micro-cracks propagate primarily through the inter-bead matrix, but indicated that crack arrest could occur within pre-polymerised beads.

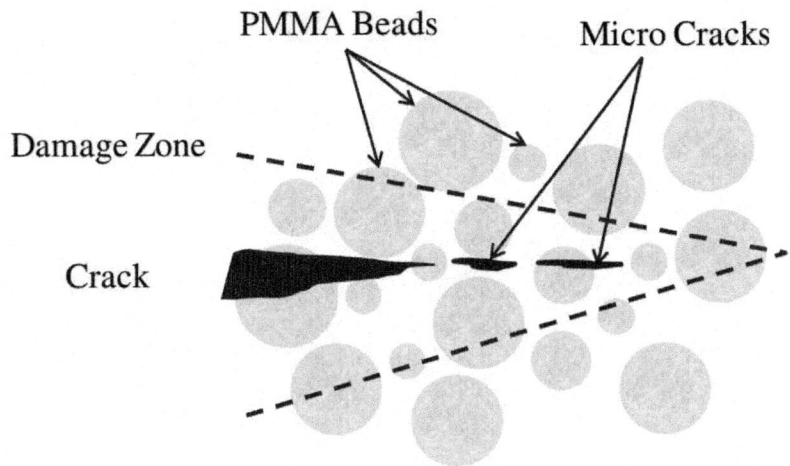

Figure 12. Schematic of the proposed model of fatigue crack propagation and damage formation of Topoleski *et al.* (1993).

In relation to the porosity that remains after mixing, it is well established that thelower the porosity, the better the static and dynamic properties of cement(Dunne and Orr 2002). Murphy and Prendergast (2000/2002) suggested that pore initiatedfractures may be linked to mechanical stress concentration, caused by adjacent PMMAbeads at the pore surface, as seen in Figure 13. Topoleski *et al.* (1993) also suggested that pores situated within the fatigue crack damage zone act as micro-crack nucleation sites (see Figure 14), effectively increasing the area of the fatigue damage zone ahead of the crack tip. Conversely, the presence of porosity promotes levels of micro-crack initiation and could be considered to increase rates of crack propagation. Hence porosity can be seen as being both destructive and constructive. Finite element (FE) analysis showed that pores contributed to both fatigue crack acceleration and deceleration, depending on the location of the pores within the stress field, irrespective of size (Janssen *et al.* 2005a). Crack retardation was prominent when pores existed near to the propagating crack, but not close enough to initiate the crack deviating from its original path. The presence of the pore in this scenario reduced the stress in the cement by causing the formation of secondary cracking initiating at the pore.

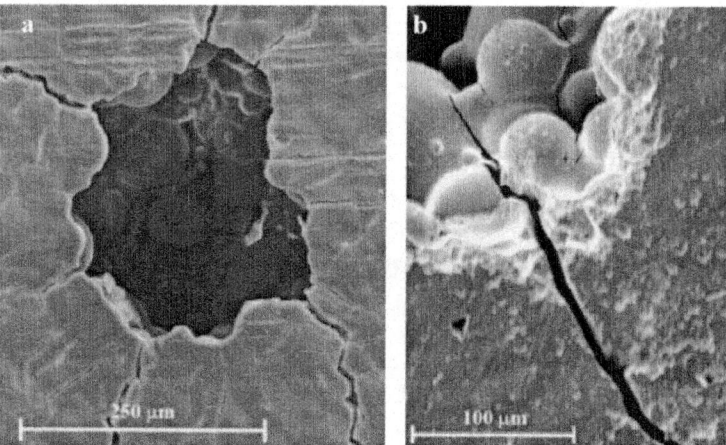

Figure 13. SEM micrograph of (a) microcracks propagating from a pore and (b) a crack initiation site at a stress concentration between PMMA beads (Murphy and Prendergast 2002).

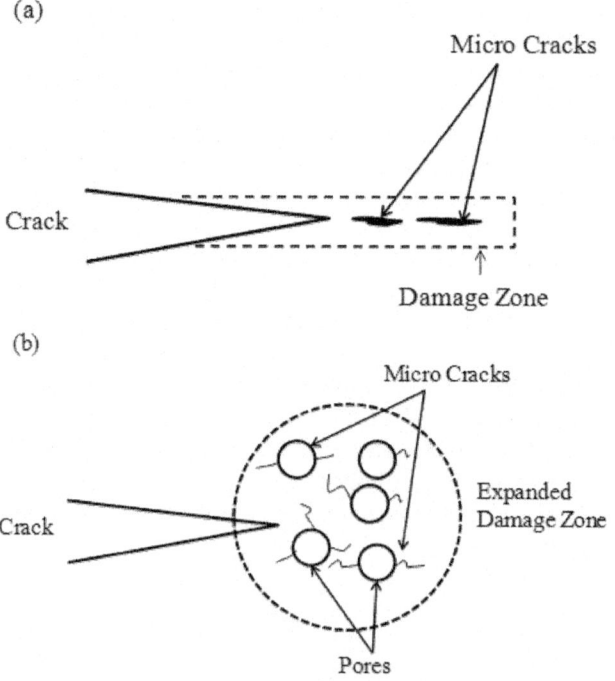

Figure 14. Expansion of the fatigue crack due to porosity at the crack tip, as suggested by Topoleski *et al* (1993). (a) Damage zone remains linear when no pores are at the crack tip. (b) Expansion of damage zone as a result of micro-crack nucleation (i.e. pores).

In general, it is understood that crack propagation characteristics of bone cement at a microstructural level are heavily reliant on whether the failure regime is a fatigue crack or a fast 'impact' fracture (Prendergast 2001b). Fatigue crack propagation is directly influenced by bone cement microstructure, porosity, residual stresses and agglomerations of radiopaque agent. An impact or fast failure however, does not have a dependence on these same parameters. For any polymer, the success in achieving improved mechanical performance remains in the materials' potential to inhibit or delay crack initiation and improve its resistance to crack propagation.

DEVELOPMENTS IN ACRYLIC BONE CEMENT

Mechanical Properties

The intrinsic mechanical properties of acrylic bone cement (such as strength, fracture toughness and fatigue crack propagation resistance) in addition to the presence of extrinsic factors such as porosity, agglomerates of radiopaque agents and other such stress concentrations may limit its long-term survival (Lewis 2003). Within the current literature there have been many attempts to improve the fatigue performance of Acrylic bone cement. Most studies have tried to control the extrinsic factors, in particular porosity (Norman *et al.* 1995; Murphy and Prendergast 2000; Lewis 2003) by means of vacuum mixing or centrifugation. However, this does not address the underlying intrinsic factors which can be broadly categorised into two areas: (a) mechanical studies, focusing on improving mechanical performance, and (b) biological studies where the focus may be on the effect of bioactive inclusions or the addition of antibiotics.

Mechanical Performance

A significant portion of the literature is directed towards discussing the potential to increase mechanical performance of acrylic bone cement *via* reinforcement with fibres or secondary phase particles: for example, carbon (Pilliar *et al.* 1976; Robinson *et al.* 1981; Pal and Saha 1982; Wright and Robinson 1982; Saha and Pal 1986), polyethylene (Yang *et al.* 1997; Narva *et al.* 2005), titanium (Topoleski *et al.*1998; Kotha *et al.* 2006), hydroxyapatite (HA) (Serbetci *et al.* 2004), glass beads (Shinzato *et al.* 2000), glass flake (Franklin *et al.* 2005), glass fibres (Narva *et al.* 2005), and steel fibers (Kotha *et al.* 2004). Mechanical properties that have been reported to improve include: compressive, tensile, and bending strength, elastic modulus, fracture toughness and fatigue resistance, when compared to cement without reinforcement. In addition to the mechanical improvements provided by these fillers, further benefits have been identified with respect to the peak temperature reached during polymerisation. As mentioned previously, high temperatures experienced *in vivo* can cause thermal necrosis of the bone cells surrounding the cement mantle, in addition to the coagulation of blood, which can potentially lead to aseptic loosening of the implant, and ultimately implant failure (Lewis 1997). Reduced *in situ*polymerisation temperatures have been observed for, but not limited to, steel, carbon fibres (CF) and multiwalled carbon nanotube (MWCNT) reinforced bone cement (Pilliar *et al.* 1976; Saha and Pal 1986; Kotha *et al.* 2004, Marrs *et al.*, 2006). A number of researchers have investigated adding CF as a reinforcing agent using clinically applicable cement mixing techniques for both *in vitro* testing (Robinson *et al.* 1981; Pal and Saha 1982; Wright and Robinson 1982; Saha and Pal 1986;) and for *in vivo* applications (Pilliar *et al.* 1976). Pilliar *et al.* (1976) reported that the inclusion of randomly oriented CF (0.6 cm) improved fatigue performance, tensile strength, Young's modulus and impact resistance (i.e. indicative of toughness), compared to cement without reinforcement. The thermal properties were also observed for the two cement types; the dough time and the setting time were unaffected by the addition of CF, whilst the maximum curing temperature was lowered for the cement with added CF (53° C compared to 57° C). Interestingly these research groups found that the addition of CF increased the viscosity of the cement above the required level by ASTM standards (ASTM F451–99a), meaning that use of these cements in a clinical setting would not be ideal. Fractographic analysis identified poor distribution of CF, and evidence of poor CF-PMMA bonding, although fibre pullout was noted. This CF-reinforced cement was used *in vivo* with no detrimental mechanical or biological response observed after 18 months. During the 1980s, problems associated with the high starting viscosity of the cement, and subsequent reduced levels of intrusion, were investigated *in vitro* following the development of low viscosity cement. Robinson *et al.* (1981) confirmed that CF-reinforcement of a commercial cement increased fracture toughness of both regular and low viscosity cements. However, the low viscosity cements (both reinforced and conventional) displayed a reduction in fracture toughness when compared to the equivalent regular viscosity cement. For the reinforced cement, Wright and Robinson (1982) reported a decreased crack growth rate versus theunreinforced cement). Saha and Pal (1986) investigated the effect of mechanically, or hand-mixed CF-reinforced bone cements, and found that mechanical mixing provided superior performance. They attributed this to the improved dispersion of CFs throughout the cement matrix.

Investigations concerning the addition of titanium (Topoleski *et al.* 1998; Kotha *et al.* 2006) or CF (Pilliar *et al.* 1976; Saha and Pal 1986) to bone cement suggested that commercially viable mixing methods are indeed possible. Topoleski *et al.* (1998) used SEM analysis to confirm that before cement failure, a good bond between the fibers and the host matrix existed, although subsequent damage led to evidence of fiber de-bonding, plastic deformation and ductile rupture of the fibers. Topoleski *et al*(1998) also reported that the presence of the fibers prevented crack propagation (Topoleski *et al.* 1998). Additionally, fiber based additives have been shown to dissipate energy associated with static crack propagation, resulting in improved fracture toughness of acrylic bone cement, through crack diversion and crack tip blunting (Gilbert *et al.* 1995). Orientation and dispersion of the fibers, in addition to good interfacial bonding, were all identified to have a positive effect on improving mechanical properties due to reinforcement (Gilbert *et al.* 1995; Yang *et al.* 1997).

Biological Performance

Bone cement is a biologically inert component of the implant construct. Conventional acrylic bone cement does not normally promote bone ingrowth. Several studies however have attempted to improve the biological performance of bone cement. These have included the incorporation of bioactive agents, such as HA based powders, glass ceramic particles or glass beads (Lee *et al.* 1997; Mousa *et al.* 2000; Shinzato *et al.* 2000). Each of these additives has been reported to enhance the biocompatibility of bone cement, thus reducing the formation of fibrous tissue at the bone-bone cement interface. Mousa *et al.*(2000) used apatite-wollastonite glass ceramic (AW-GC) particles to reduce the amount of monomer required for polymerisation, which lead to a reduction in the peak exotherm, and thermally induced bone necrosis as well as decreasing the levels of cement shrinkage. Similar results have been reported for cements containing glass beads, which have also been shown to improve bioactivity (i.e. osteoconductivity) compared with HA powder (Shinzato *et al.* 2000). Additionally, it has been reported that many of these bioactive cement composites exhibited no detrimental influence on mechanical performance, and in some cases improvements were observed (Mousa *et al.* 2000; Shinzato *et al.* 2000).

Concerns regarding biological performance include the use of antibiotics, which are integrated to reduce risk of infection and associated revision (Kuehn *et al.* 2005); many antibiotic-loaded cements are currently commercially available and, for those containing gentamicin sulphate, are believed to not cause any adverse affect on the fatigue performance (Baleani *et al.* 2003).

POLYMER MATRIX COMPOSITES

The mechanical success of any polymer composite is governed by the successful transfer of load between the matrix and the reinforcement. This transfer of load is dependent upon the volume fraction, dispersion, orientation of the reinforcing phase, the host matrix-reinforcement interface and the individual mechanical properties of the phases that are present (Gilbert *et al.* 1995; Hull and Clyne 1996b; Yang *et al.* 1997). Within fibre-reinforced composites four main microstructural regions exist: (1) the matrix, (2) the fibre, (3) the interface, and, in some composite systems, (4) the interphase. An interphase may be present if a mechanical or chemical interaction takes place between the polymer matrix and the reinforcing phase (examples includes adsorption of the polymer onto the surface of the reinforcing agent in particulate-reinforced polymers, inter-diffusion of the components during blending and chemical reactions at the polymer/fibre interface) (Pukanszky 2005).

Fibres aligned in the direction of applied load are particularly effective at reinforcing composites. Corresponding mechanical properties which effect failure performance may be identified, with a complex interaction between individual phase properties, the interface strength between the host polymer and the reinforcing fibres and the composite microstructure. Polymers are the most common form of composite matrix and are often reinforced with a low fraction of fillers such as glass, CF or Aramid. This results in composites of high specific strength and modulus as the low levels of additives allows a more homogeneous dispersion (Callister 2000a). Of these three reinforcements, CF composites often exhibit the best resistance to fatigue failure due to superior mechanical properties as well as the higher thermal conductivity of carbon fibres which assists in the dissipation of heat during cyclic loading (Scheirs 2000a). In compression, the mechanical performance of fibre-reinforced composites is dependent on the interaction between the host polymer matrix and the fibre. For optimum reinforcement, the matrix would provide lateral stabilisation to the fibre preventing subsequent buckling. Alternatively, the tensile behaviour is governed by the tensile strength of the fibre additive (Hull and Clyne 1996a). Fatigue failure in polymer composites is commonly characterised by a gradual reduction in stiffness (Scheirs 2000c). Without reinforcement, fatigue failure typically occurs perpendicular to the applied load; in contrast, the presence of fibres generally results in a diffuse damage zone due to the combination of a number of sub-critical failure modes and crack shielding mechanisms. In general, crack propagation through fibre-reinforced polymers may be considered as a multi-faceted interaction between the polymer matrix, the fibre reinforcement and the associated interface/interphase regions. A combination of mechanisms may occur and subsequently, fibre inclusions may impede crack growth by three main mechanisms (Mandell *et al.* 1980; Sauer and Richardson 1980):

- Debonding of interface/interphase between fibre and matrix – as a crack approaches, failure of the interface occur serving to blunt the crack tip and reduce crack propagation.
- Crack bridging – transferring load across a given matrix crack, reducing the crack.
- Fibre pullout, subsequent to crack bridging, may also absorb energy due to matrix deformation and/or interface friction.

CARBON NANOTUBES

It was in 1980 that Sumio Iijima first recorded an 'onion-shaped particle' in the order of $0.8 - 1$ nm in diameter. It was not until five years later that Iijima realised that this 'onion-like structure' was the fullerene C_{60}, which was believed to be discovered by Kroto, Heath, O'Brien, Curl and Smalley in 1985, (Figure 15).

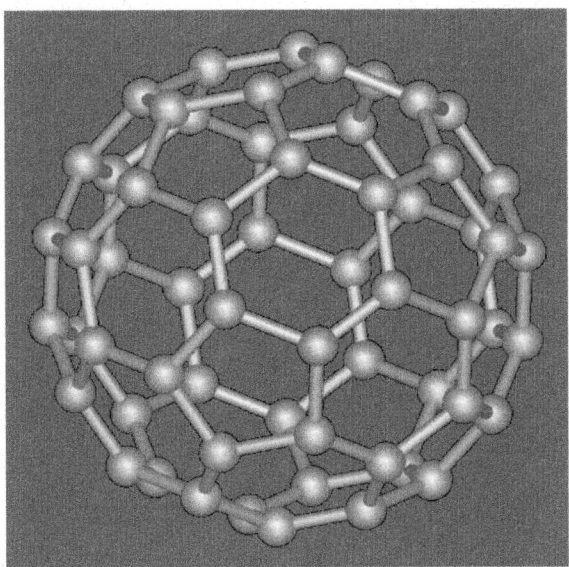

Figure 15. Carbon C_{60} molecule(Iijima, 1991).

Although Curl *et al.* (2001) later confirmed that it was Osawa who first documented the concept in 1970. It was in 1991, whilst working as an electron microscopist that Iijima's study of soot deposited on the cathode during the arc-evaporation synthesis of fullerenes led to the sighting of a needle-shaped material. What was originally described as *"microtubules of graphitic carbon"* is now commonly known as carbon nanotube (CNT). Whilst being considered an accidental discovery, Iijima believes it was the *"power of serendipity"*. Initially, Iijima produced individual tubes of graphitic carbon with diameters of 4-30 nm and a length of up to 1 μm using arc-discharge evaporation methods (Iijima 1991). At present, CNT can be synthesised *via* electric arc discharge (Iijima 1991; Shi *et al.* 2000), laser ablation (Zhang *et al.* 1998; Zhang and Iijima 1998) or, more commonly chemical vapour deposition (Sinnott *et al.* 1999; Andrews *et al.* 2002). Extensive research has been conducted on these processing methods by Andrews *et al.* (2002), and Thostenson *et al.* (2001).

CNT can occur as either single-walled nanotube (SWCNT) or multiwalled nanotube (MWCNT) structures. SWCNT consist of a single graphene sheet rolled up as a seam-free tube. They can be thought of as a linearly extended fullerene (Ajayan 1997; Iijima 1991/2002; Baughman *et al.* 2002). SWCNT usually exist as agglomerations due to the van der Waals forces between each tube, with diameters on average between 0.7-2 nm, whilst their lengths are often 5-30 μm (Ajayan 1997; Colbert 2003).

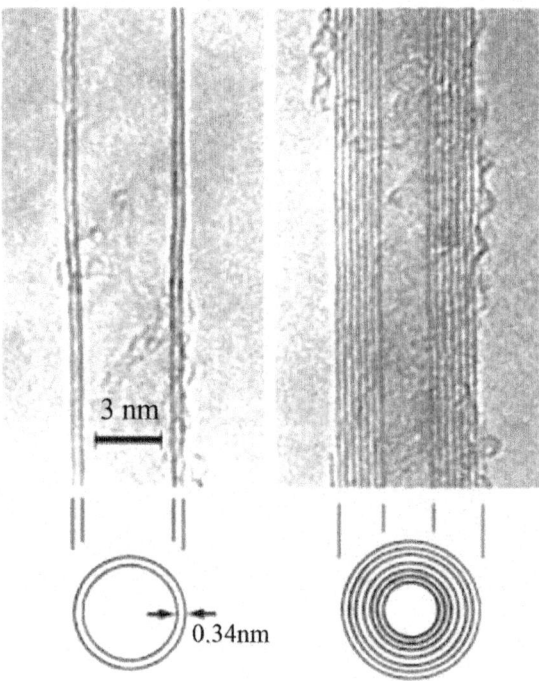

Figure 16. Transmission electron micrograph (TEM) of MWCNT (Iijima 1991).

MWCNT can be described as an array of SWCNT that are concentrically arranged inside one another with an internal diameter as small as 2.2 nm. The distance between the individual SWCNT that constitute MWCNT (or the graphite inter-layer separation) is typically 0.34 nm (Ajayan 1997; Iijima 1991/2002) (Figure 16). Iijima (1991) used electron diffraction to establish that the crystal axis of the graphene tubes consisted of carbon-atom hexagons arranged in a helical manner about the tube axis (Figure 17). The ends of CNT are closed off by the presence of pentagonal carbon rings near the tip regions, whilst deformations and imperfections of the cylinder occur as pentagons or heptagons within the main structure of the tube (Ajayan 1997).

SWCNT, are known to be stiff and exceptionally strong (high Young's modulus and high tensile strength). Furthermore, SWCNT can stretch beyond 20% of their original length and bend over double without kinking (Baughman et al. 2002; Colbert 2003). However, the mechanical properties of individual CNT, whether SWCNT or MWCNT are the subject of much research with a significant variation in recorded properties existing. The use of CNT in various matrices can greatly enhance mechanical properties. Wong et al. (1997) provided an insight into the potential uses of CNT. Atomic force microscopy (AFM) was employed to determine the elasticity, strength and toughness of individual silicon carbide nanorods (SiC NRs) and MWCNT that were attached to molybdenum disulphide surfaces. The average bending strength of the MWCNT was 14.2 ± 8.0 GPa; with the maximum bending strength being substantially smaller than that of the SiC NRs at 53.4 GPa. In contrast, whilst both nanostructures exhibited high values for the Young's modulus (highlighting their suitability as reinforcing agents in ceramic, metal and polymer matrix composites) the Young's modulusfor the MWCNT was almost double that of the SiC NRs (1.28 ± 0.59 TPa and ~600 GPa, respectively). The Young's modulusvalue for the in-plane modulus of highly orientated pyrolytic graphite was recorded at 1.06 TPa (Blakslee et al. 1970) and is believed to be the largest known for a bulk material. Wong et al.(1997) concluded that while the stiffer MWCNT had a lower ultimate strength, the elastic buckling displayed by the MWCNT (i.e. the energy storing capabilities of CNT before failure) showed them to be the "tougher" nanostructure. More recently, Demczyk et al. (2002) investigated the direct failure of individual MWCNT under tension using TEM. While the mode of failure, either ductile or brittle, could not be determined, results confirmed a tendency to fail via a mode now known as 'telescopic failure', with initial failure observed in the outermost walls followed by a 'sword in sheath effect' of the inner cylinders. TEM observations also confirmed the elastic capabilities of MWCNT during deformation in bending, even after being highly distorted.

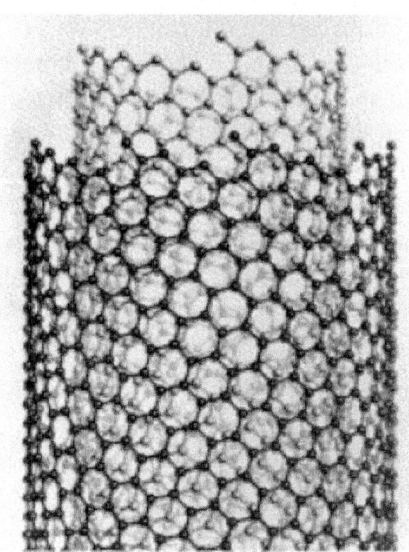

Figure 17. Helical arrangement of carbon atom hexagons that make up a graphene sheet in a MWCNT (Iijima 1991).

It is clear that CNT offer significant potential to improve the properties for many existing materials; the challenge remains for the superior properties exhibited by CNT individually to be successfully applied and optimised in practical applications such as nanocomposites. Not only do the properties of the CNT themselves vary due to impurities during processing (Baughman *et al.* 2002), but on addition of CNT to a matrix, the problem becomes multi-faceted: CNT dimensions, dispersion, alignment, concentration, CNT-matrix interface/adhesion and choice of matrix are some of the many issues that govern the final properties of the composite material. At present, production of high purity SWCNT still remains costly and of a low yield: purification reduces yield further, adds to cost and damages the structure (Andrews*et al.* 2002). Low manufacturing costs and high yields of aligned MWCNT are now possible however, making them the preferred choice in bulk composite material development.

PROPERTIES OF CNT-REINFORCED POLYMERS

Since the discovery of CNT in 1991, research incorporating them into various matrix materials has been plentiful. This increase in research can be attributed to the fact that CNT have extremely high aspect ratios(typically >150:1), modulus and low density. The addition of CNT to polymer composite materialshas enhanced mechanical (Wong *et al.* 1997; Andrews *et al.* 2002),electrical (Baughman *et al.*2002; Colbert 2003) and thermal properties(Kim *et al.* 2001; Baughman *et al.* 2002; Colbert 2003), in matrices including polycarbonate(Ding *et al.* 2003; Eitan *et al.* 2006), polystyrene (Andrews *et al.* 2002;Thostenson and Chou 2003; Park *et al.* 2005) ultrahigh molecular weight polyethylene (Ruan *et al.*2003) andPMMA (Hwang *et al.* 2004; Marrs *et al.* 2005).

Extensive literature has explored the effects of CNT on mechanical propertiesof various polymer matrices. It has been shown that the addition of CNT can increase the toughness ofpolymer matrices due to crack bridging, changes in morphology of the matrix and theadditional energy required for de-bonding and nanotube pullout (Dalton *et al.* 2003; Ruan *et al.* 2003; Andrews and Weisenberger 2004). As with other polymer composites, increases inmodulus may be identified with stress transfer from the matrix to the CNT. It should be noted though that the presence ofagglomerations of CNT can have significant adverse influence on the mechanical properties ofCNT-polymers, acting as stress concentrations and fracture initiation points within the composite microstructure. This effect was recorded by Marrs *et al.* (2005), who incorporated MWCNT at various levels of loading in to PMMA bone cement. They characterised the fatigue, quasi-static tensile and bend properties for these MWCNT-PMMA nanocomposites. They found that the optimal performance was for the addition of 2 wt% MWCNT. They also report that loadings above this resulted in reducedmechanical properties, although results were still superior when compared to pure PMMA (Marrs *et al.* 2005). Cadek *et al.*(2004) reported an increase in Young's modulus by a factor of two after theaddition of 0.6 vol% CNT to poly (vinyl alcohol), an effect which they attributed to nanotubediameter and resultant surface area. Varying levels of reinforcement as a result of a change innanotube diameter suggested that MWCNT of smaller diameter provided optimal reinforcementdue to increased surface area. Whilst the enhancing effects of CNT with respect to tensile strength and modulus have been recorded (Ruan *et al.* 2003), it has been established that theoretical predictive models such as Rule of Mixtures approach or the Halpin-Tsai model predict superior reinforcement capabilities than experimental data provides. Part of this discrepancy may be due to factors such as poor interfacial bonding, inhomogeneous dispersion, and CNT quality (Andrews *et al.* 2002; Fisher *et al.* 2002; Andrews and Weisenberger 2004). Poor adhesion/bonding at the interface between the host polymer and the CNT may have a detrimental effect on the mechanical properties of CNT-composites (Andrews *et al.* 2002). Nanotube pullout experiments, using atomic force microscopy, may be used to determine the force required to separate a single

CNT from a polymer matrix (Barber *et al.* 2003; Baroud *et al.* 2004). It is widely accepted that a strong interfacial adhesion between the reinforcing nanotube and the polymer matrix leads to the effective transfer of load (Cooper *et al.* 2002; Barber *et al.* 2003; Goh *et al.* 2003, Marrs *et al.*, 2007). Barber *et al.* (2003) measured the average interfacial stress required to remove a single MWCNT from a polyethylene-butene matrix as 47 MPa. Comparing this value to the 10 MPa measured for poorly bonded interfaces in other fibre-reinforced polymers, Barber *et al.* (2003) suggested that this enhancement was due to the presence of covalent bonding at the interface between CNT and the host polymer, potentially due to a chemical interaction between the polyethylene-butene matrix and defects on the surface of the nanotube. Moreover, it is believed that the mechanical properties of the polymer immediately surrounding the nanotube may be enhanced when compared to the bulk of the polymer. Nano pullout test results by Barber *et al.* (2003) showed no evidence of the polymer yielding, even at pullout stresses that were ten times higher than average tensile strength of the polymer matrix. This may be explained using differential scanning calorimetry (DSC) measurements to determine the polymer crystallinity. Cadek *et al.* (2004) compared polymer crystallinity for PVA after the addition of 0.6 vol. % CNT and measured a linear increase in crystallinity with increasing volume fraction of CNT, suggesting a crystalline polymer coating is formed at the nanotube surface. Observations of the fracture surface using SEM confirmed that polymer wetting of the nanotube surface was achieved (Figure 18); diameters of the nanotubes in the composite were larger than the as-received CNT (Ding *et al.* 2003).

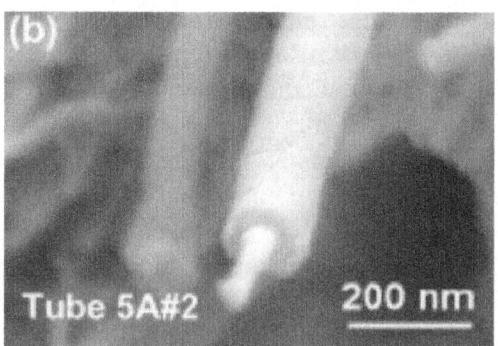

Figure 18. High-resolution SEM image highlighting MWCNT coated with a polymer sheath protruding from a MWCNT-polycarbonate fracture surface, as observed by Ding *et al.* (2003).

The interface between the host matrix and reinforcement phase, in addition to the interphase region may play a pivotal role in optimising the mechanical performance of a polymer composite (Gilbert *et al.*1995; Hull and Clyne 1996b; Yang *et al.* 1997; Eitan *et al.* 2006). When investigating the effect of MWCNT on the crystallinity of PVA and PVA nanocomposites Ryan *et al.* (2006) used dynamic mechanical analysis (DMA) to confirm significant improvements in the Young's modulus. Ryan *et al.*(2006)also confirm the findings reported by Marrs *et al.* (2005), reporting that limits in the amount of CNT added to the polymer exist for achieving optimal mechanical performance. Ryan *et al.* (2006) explained that improvements in mechanical properties are seen for lower fractions of CNT with detrimental effects introduced at higher levels of loadings due to the higher incidence of CNT agglomerations. Of further interest is the degree of crystallinity present at the CNT-polymer interface: reported for CNT-reinforced PVA, the large increases in Young's modulus were attributed to the variations in crystallinity. A consequence of the ability of CNT to act as nucleation sites for crystals in both the solution and melt/solid-state phase (Coleman *et al.* 2004; Ryan *et al.* 2006). It is the presence of a well-bonded crystalline interface between the polymer matrix and the nanotubes that may account for the improved mechanical properties due to the increased levels of stress transfer (Cadek *et al.* 2004; Coleman *et al.* 2004). This would allow for failure/crack deflection to occur at the matrix-crystalline interface rather than at the nanotube interface. It has been highlighted that the presence of CNT agglomerations, particularly seen with the use of SWCNT, limits the ability of PVA to act as crystal nucleation sites and, as result inferior mechanical performance are not seen. Similar findings have been reported for other semi-crystalline polymers (Hull and Clyne 1996a) such as UHMWPE (Ruan *et al.* 2003), polypropylene (Leelapornpisit *et al.* 2005; Seo *et al.* 2005) and polyamide (Chao *et al.* 2006). These reports highlighted the need for careful selection of the processing method that allows for optimal levels of crystallisation at the nanotube-matrix interface (Coleman *et al.* 2004). To date, limited work has been published regarding the crystallisation of PMMA at the nanotube-matrix interface: Coleman *et al.* (1998) proposed that PMMA would be unable to bond to CNT due to the spatial arrangement of the polymer. Alternative mechanisms have been sought to improve the interface and interphase properties of CNT-amorphous polymers. The most commonly employed approach is the covalent attachment of chemically functional groups to the CNT at the defect sites. This is completed in order to achieve similar polymer sheathing effects around the nanotube. In chlorinated polypropylene, Coleman *et al.*(2004) reported that the thickness of the polymer sheath surrounding the nanotubes depends on the volume occupied by the functional groups. Upon failure, fracture was seen to occur away from the CNT-polymer matrix interface. Immobilisation of the polymer chains in the region surrounding the nanotubes was proposed as an additional reinforcement mechanism associated with MWCNT-reinforcement of amorphous polycarbonate. Functionalisation of the MWCNT surface led to an increase in thickness of this interphase region, subsequently improving load transfer capabilities between the matrix and the nanotubes (Eitan *et al.* 2006). This suggestion was highlighted by Jia *et al.* (1999), they reported that PMMA can bond with CNT, although this was dependent on the processing methods utilised. Using *in situ* polymerisation, initiated using the free radical initiator, Azobisisobutyronitrile (AIBN), to form the polymer, additions of MWCNT (both unfunctionalised and carboxyl functionalised) resulted in nanocomposites of improved mechanical properties (in particular, tensile strength, toughness and hardness), with the carboxyl functionalised nanotubes out-performing their unfunctionalised counterparts. High interfacial strengths were associated with bonding between the open π-bonds of the CNT (believed to be initiated by the AIBN) and the open bonds in the PMMA possibly creating a C-C bond between the PMMA and the CNT. Jia *et al.* (1999) also reported that higher loadings of MWCNT led to a more brittle polymer with reduced toughness and tensile strength. Velasco-Santos *et al.* (2003) demonstrated the use of an amorphous polymer matrix is potentially advantageous over semi-crystalline polymers like PVA; clear reasoning behind this is not given although the presence and nature of the interphase region may be an explanation.

MECHANISMS OF FAILURE OF CNT-POLYMERS

Andrews *et al.* (2002) reported that CNT within polymer matrices under tensile stress may align themselves parallel to the direction of the applied load, enabling crack bridging behind a crack tip. Andrews *et al.* (2002) explained that this phenomenon reduced the stress concentration in the region surrounding the crack tip, and ultimately reduced crack propagation. Key reinforcement mechanisms that have been identified in CNT-polymer systems are nanotube pullout, bending of nanotubes (often due to surface defects such as iron oxide catalyst inclusions from the CNT production process) and telescopic fracture of nanotubes (Andrews *et al.* 2002; Cooper *et al.* 2002; Demczyk *et al.* 2002; Ding *et al.* 2003; Hwang *et al.* 2004). Such phenomena are schematically illustrated in Figure 19.

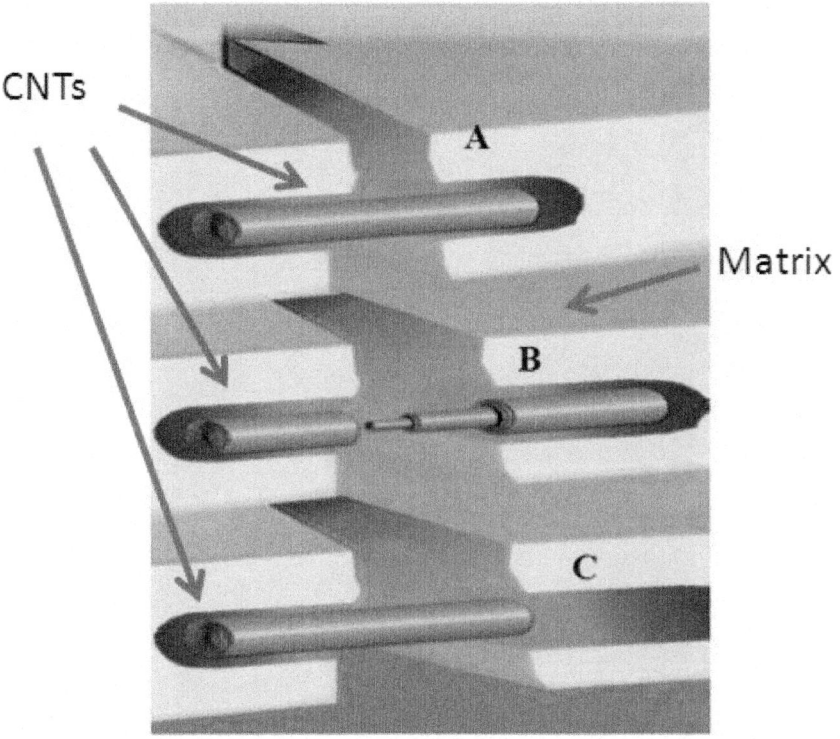

Figure 19. Schematic illustration of (A) a CNT bridging a crack, (B) telescopic failure of a CNT and (C) CNT fibre pullout experienced in CNT-reinforced polymers (Sinnott and Andrews 2001).

Crack bridging of the matrix may arise in CNT-containing polymers. Hwang *et al.* (2004) directly observed nanotube pullout. (Figure 20b) and failure of the graphene layers resulting in telescopic failure (Figure 20c).

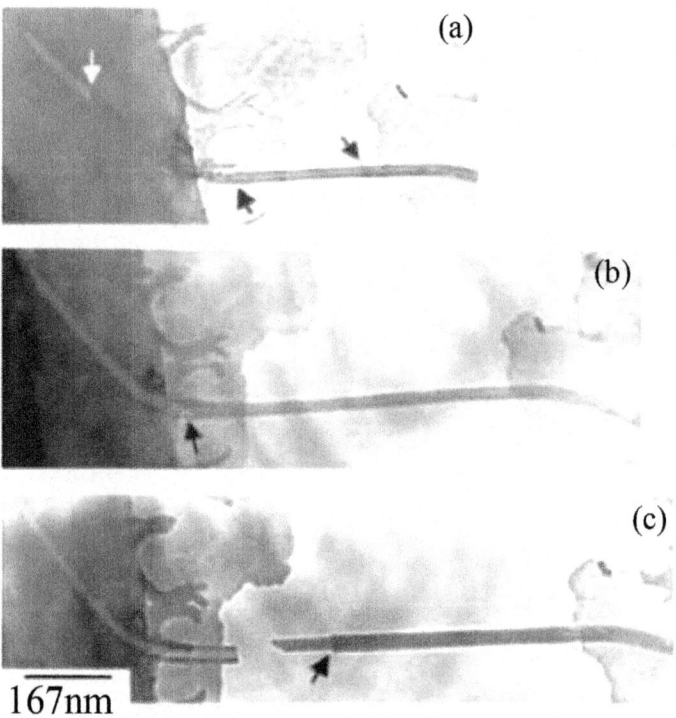

Figure 20. TEM images of MWCNT-containing PMMA showing (a) breaking of graphene layers, (b) MWCNT pullout and (c) final telescopic failure of the MWCNT (Hwang *et al*. 2004).

BIOCOMPATIBILITY OF CNT

The Royal Society and the Royal Academy of Engineering, UK, published a report (2004) discussing the associated ethical, health and safety, and social implications of nanotechnology (The Royal Society and the Royal Academy of Engineering 2004). With an increased interest in the use of nanotechnology, the Government later published its own report (*'Characterising the potentialrisks posed by engineered nanoparticles'*, November 2005) and follow-up studies (*'First quarterly update on the Voluntary Reporting Scheme for engineered nano-scale materials'*, December 2006). The full report addressed many issues concerning the potential use of nanotechnology and CNT. Concerns have been raised that the properties that promote the use of nanoparticles in certain applications may also have health implications, such as their high aspect ratios, surface reactivity and their ability to cross cell membranes (The Royal Society and the Royal Academy of Engineering 2004; Kagan *et al*., 2005; Fadeel *et al.*, 2007). The report highlighted that the main risks associated with CNT stem from their high surface to volume ratio to which a target organ may be exposed, in addition to the chemical reactivity of the surface, the physical dimensions of the nanoparticles and their solubility. Speculation surrounding the use of CNT has equated their effect on health to that of asbestos (due to their similar size and shape). CNT are therefore suspected as being potentially carcinogenic, and additionally, may cause inflammation or functional changes to proteins due to their large surface area. However, it has been argued that no new risks to health have been introduced as a result of the increasing use of nanoparticles as part of composite materials, and that most concerns derive from the possibility of detached, or 'free' nanoparticles and nanotubes from the matrix (The Royal Society and the Royal Academy of Engineering 2004). It is believed that, if airborne, the likelihood of CNT existing as individual fibres is improbable as electrostatic forces cause the CNT to agglomerate which reduces their ability to be inhaled into the deeper areas of the lungs. However, when investigating of the inhalation of stable non-purified SWCNT aerosols in mice, Shvedova *et al.* (2008) reported that the chain of pathological events was realised through an early inflammatory response and oxidative stress culminated in the development of multifocal granulomatous pneumonia and interstitial fibrosis (Figure 21).

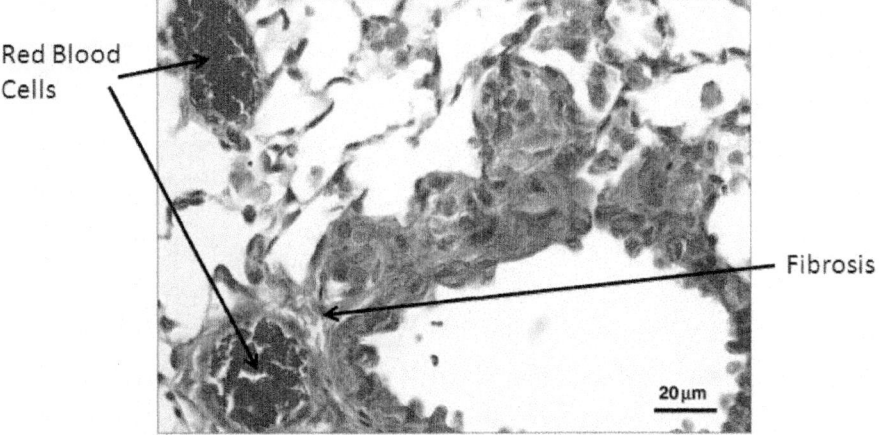

Figure 21. Representative image of lung section from the SWCNT inhalation study depicting granuloma formation on day 28 post treatment. Fibrosis is indicated by blue staining in this Masson's Trichrome stained section of the lung (Shvedova *et al.* 2008).

Smart *et al.* (2006) reviewed the often conflicting findings pertaining to the cytotoxicity and biocompatibility of CNT. They concluded that, as-received (i.e. untreated, or unfunctionalised) CNT exhibited some degree of toxicity (observed both *in vitro* and *in vivo*) with detrimental effects associated with the presence of transition metal ions, used as catalysts in the CNT production. Smart *et al.* (2006) also reported that CNT that have been chemically functionalised have yet to demonstrate toxicity effects. It is highlighted that the tendency for CNT to aggregate may impact the reported results, although quantification of this fact has yet to be investigated. With research into the use of CNT, and nanotechnology ever increasing, the uncertainty regarding toxicity has been brought to public attention. As a result, it has been recommended that further research is necessary regarding the biological impacts of nanoparticles and nanotubes, including their exposure pathways within the body, and that methodologies for *in situ* monitoring should also be developed (The Royal Society and the Royal Academy of Engineering 2004). Recent studies have addressed the issue of CNT uptake by different cell types.

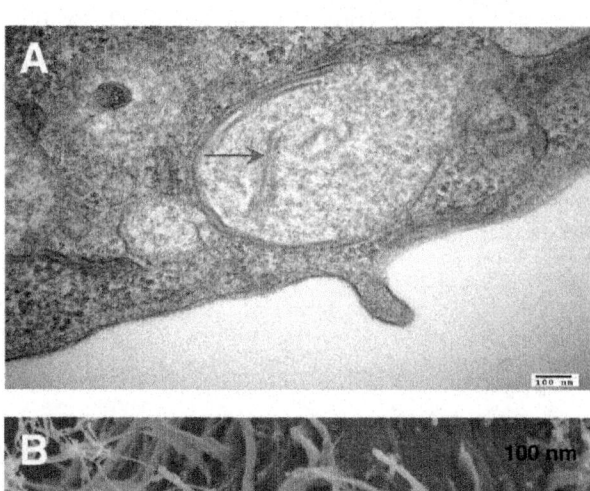

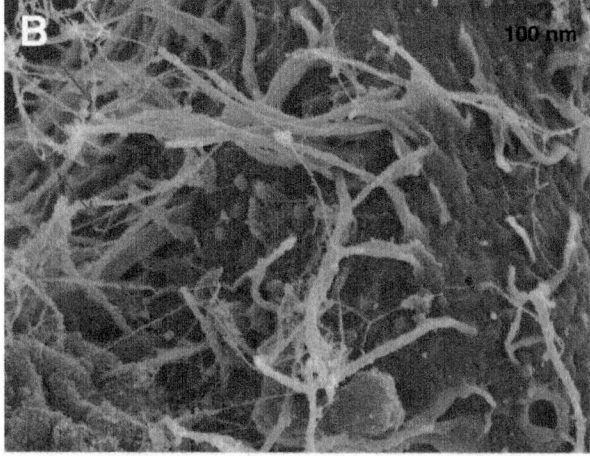

Figure 22. Representative transmission electron micrograph (A) and scanning electron micrograph (B) of RAW264.7 macrophages with engulfed PS-coated SWCNT. Arrows indicate SWCNT. (Shvedova *et al.*, 2009).

While the results seem to be controversial, it is apparent that the presence or absence of specialised signals determined the recognition and subsequent interactions of CNT with cells. Overall, pristine CNT carrying no recognisable signals were poorly taken-up whereas CNT modified chemically (e.g. oxidatively modified and functionalised) or by adsorbed macromolecules (e.g. proteins, lipids) were more readily recognised and engulfed by cells (Shvedova et al., 2010). Several in vitro studies support the concept that pristine CNT are not readily taken up by lung cells.Davoren et al. (2007) reported no measurable uptake of CNT in A549 cells (a human alveolar type II cancer cell line). Likewise, Herzog et al. (2007) reported no uptake of CNT in either A549 cells or BEAS-2B cells (a human bronchial epithelial cell line). Lastly, no evidence of uptake of CNT was reported after electron microscopic evaluation of exposed RAW 264.7 cells (mouse peritoneal macrophage cell line) (Shvedova et al., 2005). In contrast, functionalistion of SWCNT with a phospholipid signal, phosphatidylserine, made CNT recognisable in vitro by different phagocytic cells, including murine RAW264.7 macrophages, primary monocyte-derived human macrophages and dendritic cells, and microglia from rat brain (Figure 22) (Shvedova et al., 2009).

CNT-REINFORCED BIOMATERIALS

Nanotechnology in biomaterials is not a new idea (Hrkach et al., 1997). Nanomaterials have been used as implant coatings, bulk materials, drug delivery, actuators, diagnostic tools and devices (Sinha and Yeow, 2005). When biomaterials incorporating nanomaterials are studied, much of the emphasis is on the interaction between the biological tissue and the biomaterial at a molecular level. Using the interface between bone, and a metallic implant as an example, a positive biological interaction is essential if a good fixation is to be obtained. Chun et al. (2004) examined this interaction by coating titanium (Ti) substrates with helical rosette self-assembled organic nanotubes (HRN). HRN display chemical and structural similarities to various constituents of bone (Figure 23). Chun et al. (2004) found that theHRN-coated titanium displayed enhanced interaction with the naturally-occurring nanostructures' constituents such as collagen fibres and HA; this was measured as a function of the cell adhesion of human fetal osteoblas (hFoBs) cells (Figure 24).

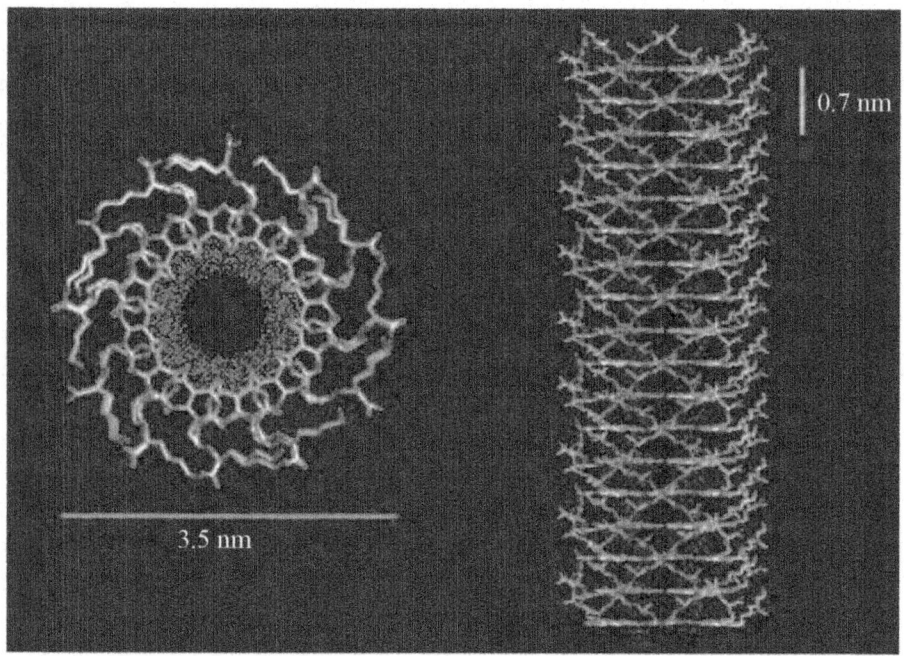

Figure 23. Diagram of helical rosette nanotube (HRN) (Chun *et al.*, 2004).

Webster *et al.* (2004) incorporated carbon nanofibres (CNF) into polycarbonate-urethane (PCU) for neural or orthopaedic prosthetic devices. They reported that this material had the potential to increase neural and osteoblast functions, as cell attachment increased with CNF loading. Additionally they stated that the functions of cells that contributed to glial scar-tissue formation for neural prostheses (astrocytes) and fibrous-tissue encapsulation for bone implants (fibroblasts) decreased on the PCU composites containing increasing amounts of CNFs. In this manner, this study provided the first evidence that CNF formulations may interact with neural and bone cells, which is important for the design of successful neural probes and orthopaedic implants. Furthermore, Webster *et al.* (2004) summarised that using nanotechnology in biological systems may be potentially feasible as biological systems are governed by molecular behaviour at the nanoscale, and therefore the properties of which are accustomed to high levels of interaction at this nanoscale. This study by Webster *et al.* highlighted the potential for CNT to be used in PMMA bone cement to encourage cell growth at the bone-cement interface with the aim of reducing aseptic loosening by enhancing the mechanical interlock in the cancellous bone.

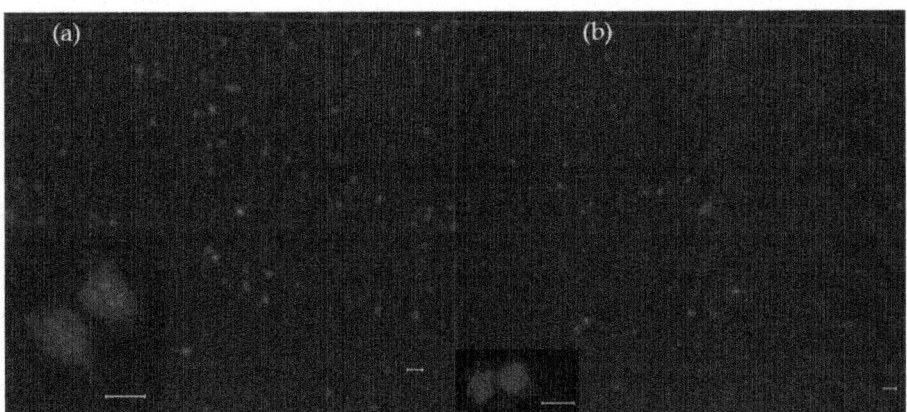

Figure 24. Fluorescently stained cells on Ti substrates. (a) HRN coated Ti. (b) Uncoated Ti. (Magnification: 20×; inset magnification 200×). Scale bars = 60 μm, inset bars = 50 and 100 μm for (a) and (b), respectively (Chun *et al.,* 2004).

CNT exhibit many unique mechanical, thermal, and electrical properties. However, their potential use for bioengineering applications and medical materials is almost wholly dependent on their biocompatibility. Cui *et al.* (2005) investigated the effect of SWCNT on human HEK293 cells (human embryo kidney cells). Results showed that SWCNT can inhibit HEK293 cell proliferation, inducing cell apoptosis (programmed cell death as controlled by the nuclei in normally functioning cells) and decreasing cellular adhesive ability in a dose and time-dependent manner. Their results also showed that HEK293 cells initiated active responses such as secretion of small 'isolation' proteins to isolate the cells attached to the SWCNT from the rest of the cell mass; a response that offers potential for medical chemistry and disease therapy.

Synthetic bone scaffolds is an area where the biocompatibility of materials used, such as polymers or peptide fibers, is still an issue where possible rejection by the body is feasible. CNT offer mechanical advantages over the polymers or peptide fibers currently used in bone scaffolds. Zhao *et al.* (2005), investigated the use of chemically functionalised SWCNT as a scaffold material for the growth of artificial bone, they identified the potential for the self-assembly of HA on the surface of SWCNT. They suggested that this was possibly due to the presence of negatively charged functional groups on the SWCNT that attract the calcium cations present in HA (Zhao *et al.* 2005). The group also proposed that it is the high tensile strength, high degree of flexibility, and low density of CNT that make these materials ideal for the production of bone. The diameters of SWCNT used in the study by Zhao *et al.*(2005) are of similar order and magnitude to the triple helix collagen fibres within bone, and as such can act as scaffolds for the nucleation and growth of HA.

The potential for CNT to be used within bioengineering applications is by no means endless, however while many more applications could be discussed, the following papers offer further information on the use of nanotechnology for biomedical applications: Sinha and Yeow (2005), Webster *et al.* (2004) andBellare *et al.* (2002). Investigations concerning the cytotoxic response of CNT-containing materials have reported encouraging results confirming their potential use in orthopaedic applications (Smart *et al.* 2006); however, many questions remain unanswered and as yet, the understanding of the toxicity and biocompatibility of CNT-reinforced materials is not fully established.

CNT-REINFORCED BONE CEMENT

Mechanical Properties

MWCNT offer the potential to augment mechanical properties of PMMA bone cement due to their strength and aspect ratio. The addition of MWCNT to PMMA bone cement has been shown to significantly improve the static mechanical properties(Marrs *et al.*, 2006 and Marrs, 2007; Ormsby *et al.*, 2010a;Ormsby *et al.*, 2010b), and the fatigue performance of MMA-co-Sty copolymer based bone cement(Marrs *et al.*, 2006). Marrs *et al.*(2006) investigated the influence of unfunctionalised MWCNT in PMMA based bone cements. They reported moderate improvements (13-24 %) in the static properties when 2 wt. % MWCNT was incorporated into PMMA bone cement. Marrs(2007) reported significant improvements (>300 %) in the dynamic properties of methyl methacrylate-styrene copolymer (MMA-co-Sty), a chief component of commercial bone cement when unfunctionalised MWCNT (2 wt. %) were added. However, both studies(Marrs *et al.*, 2006 and Marrs, 2007) used non-clinically relevant methods to ensure optimal dispersion of the MWCNT. The MWCNT were dispersed through a molten matrix of pre-polymerised commercial bone cement powder using stainless steel counter rotating rotors in a mixing chamber at 220° C. The two materials were heated and subjected to high-shear mixing. Once the molten composite had cooled and hardened, it was crushed into pellets and hot pressed under vacuum to form films. These films were subsequently machined into testing specimen. Each specimen was then annealed at 125° C for a minimum of 15 h to alleviate any residual stresses that formed during machining.

The uniform distribution of CNT within the polymer matrix is critical for maximising the interfacial bond between the CNT and polymer matrix and therefore achieving optimal improvements in mechanical properties (Andrews *et al.*, 2002; Marrs, 2007). It has also been reported that alignment and optimum dispersion of the CNT is important in the context of improving the thermal properties of a nanocomposite (Xie *et al.*, 2005). The CNT must create a well dispersed, overlapping network facilitating the transport of electrons, phonons, and heat energy.

Many processing techniques have been employed to uniformly disperse CNT within polymer matrices (Xie *et al.*, 2005; Andrews *et al.*, 2002). The two most commonly used techniques involve (i) *in situ*dispersion (sonication of the CNT in solution) and (ii) high temperature shear mixing. These techniques are primarily used to separate the entanglements and agglomerations of the as-produced CNT, and secondly to disperse the individual CNT throughout the matrix. Andrews *et al.*(2004) stated that these techniques produce more favourable results when small concentrations of CNT are used, however, mixing higher concentrations of CNT (>5 wt. %) increases the viscosity of the mixture irrespective of the state of the polymer. Andrews *et al.* (2002) postulated that an elevated viscosity hinders effective dispersion of the CNT into the polymer matrix, therefore, the energy induced into the mixing process must be increased, but, at the risk of shortening the CNT or irreversibly damaging the matrix material. Moreover, it has been reported that the efficacy of MWCNT reinforcement is largely dependent on the level of loading of MWCNT, the dispersion of these MWCNT and the peak stress of dynamic loading cycle (Marrs *et al.*, 2006; Marrs, 2007).

Ormsby *et al.*(2010a) addressed the limitations of the studies by Marrs *et al.*, (2006; Marrs, 2007) by incorporating unfunctionalised (MWCNT-UNF) and carboxyl (MWCNT-COOH) functionalised MWCNT (0.1 wt. %) into PMMA bone cement using three different preparation techniques. CNT were either added to the liquid MMA component of the cement via magnetic stirring or ultrasonic disintegration, or dry blended with the polymer powder component. A contemporary vacuum mixing system was subsequently used to mix the bone cement following the normal protocol for a joint replacement surgical procedure. Improvements in static mechanical properties and thermal properties of the MWCNT-PMMA nanocomposite cement were observed(Ormsby *et al.*, 2010a). Ormsby *et al.*, (2010a)demonstrated that adding MWCNT (0.1 wt. %) to the polymer powder or liquid monomer components prior to cement mixing with a proprietary mixing system, improved the mechanical properties of the resultant cement, provided the appropriate method for incorporating the MWCNT was used (≈21 %). This was a significant finding because mechanical failure of the bone cement mantle remains a major problem in joint replacement surgery (Topoleski *et al.*, 1990). Like typical fibre-reinforced composites, mechanical failure of PMMA bone cement is believed to take place in three phases, (1) crack initiation due to an initial imperfection in material stability, (2) slow crack growth, and (3) rapid propagation to fracture (Figure 25a) (Topoleski *et al.*, 1995). Although mixing the cement under the application of a vacuum and injecting the cement into the surgical site using a closed delivery system have improved the mechanical performance of the cement, residual material voids and poor surgical technique can contribute to weak or thin regions within the cement mantle causing these regions to be more susceptible to mechanical failure (Marrs *et al.*, 2006).

Ormsby *et al.*, (2010a)reported that adding MWCNT to the liquid monomer by magnetic stirring had an overall negative effect on the mechanical performance of the bone cement. This was largely attributed to the poor dispersion of MWCNT in the liquid monomer and resulting in MWCNT agglomerations within the cement matrix (Figure 25b).

These agglomerations acted as stress concentrations within the cement, providing a mechanism for premature failure of the cement when subjected to load. In contrast, dry blending MWCNT in the polymer powder or disintegrating the MWCNT in the liquid monomer using ultrasonic agitation suitably disentangled the nanotubes and homogenously dispersed the MWCNT in the resulting nanocomposite (Ormsby *et al.*, 2010a). Andrews and Weisenberger (2004) also reported that ultrasonic disintegration was an effective method for dispersion of MWCNT at low levels (<5 wt. %) of concentration (Andrews and Weisenberger, 2004). Marrs *et al.* (2006) stated that care is needed when dispersing MWCNT within a polymer matrix, and reported the adverse effects of sporadic, inadequately dispersed, clumps of MWCNT, particularly at levels of loading greater than 5 wt.%.

The presence of well-dispersed MWCNT in PMMA cement with their anticipated strong nanotube-matrix bonding and high tensile properties, suggests that a percentage of the MWCNT would be orientated with their longitudinal axis perpendicular to the crack wave. Such MWCNT were effective in bridging the initial crack and preventing crack propagation, further enhancing the longevity of the cement mantle (Figures 25c and 25d), by improvement in mechanical properties. These improvements are clinically beneficial for the use of reinforced PMMA bone cement in TJR due to a reduction in the rate of crack propagation. This effect may be most important for improperly placed femoral implants with thinner cement mantle layers, which continues to be cited as a factor that may reduce implant longevity (Morscher and Wirz, 2002). Additionally PMMA dental prostheses (dentures) are also known to fail prematurely through thin connectors due to impact and fatigue loading (Ormsby *et al.*, 2010a). There could be an application for MWCNT inclusion in PMMA dental prostheses, enhancing the functionality of denture-based acrylic materials when subjected to fatigue loading (Polyzois *et al.*, 1996).

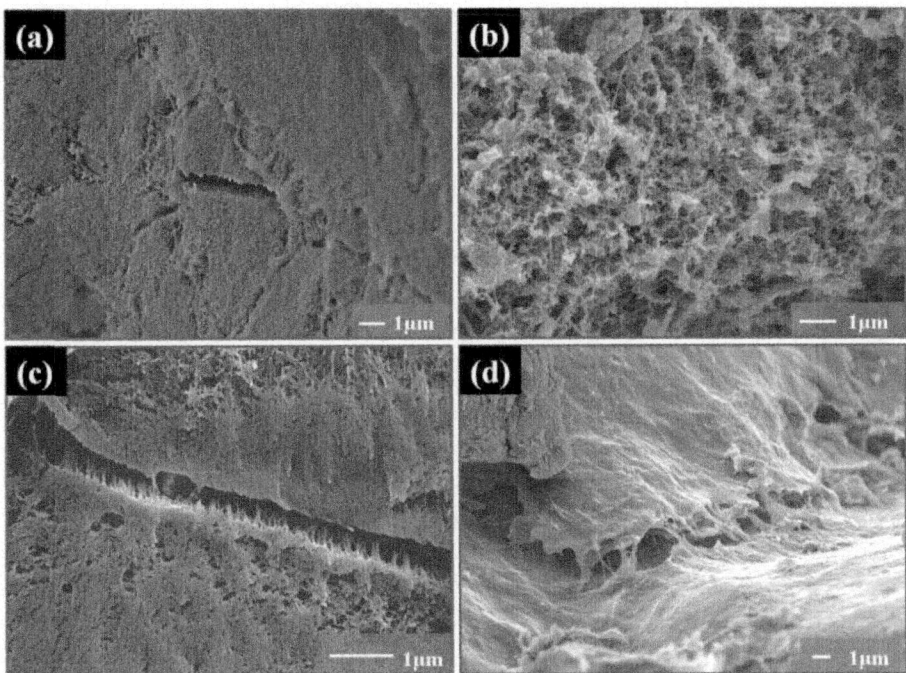

Figure 25. SEM images showing (a) A large pore on the short rod chevron notched fracture surface of the control cement (X 300). (b) Unfunctionalised MWCNT dry blended in the PMMA polymer powder cement showing an agglomeration of barium sulphate, which was the fracture initiation point for this specimen (X 150). (c) Functionalised MWCNT disintegrated in the MMA liquid monomer by ultrasonication, MWCNT can be seen to bridge a micro-crack across the cement surface, X 5,000, (d) Functionalised MWCNT ultrasonically disintegrated within the MMA liquid monomer, MWCNT can be seen to bridge a micro-crack on the cement surface, X15,000 (Ormsby *et al.*, 2010a).

The filler/matrix interface in fibre-reinforced polymer composites is critical in controlling load transfer from the matrix to the fibre, failure mechanisms, and degradation (Ormsby *et al.*, 2010a). Gojny *et al.* (2003) reported that functionalisation of MWCNT led to reduced agglomeration and improved interaction between the nanotubes and the polymer resin. Ormsby *et al.*, (2010a) used MWCNT that were surface modified with a carboxyl grouping, as it has been reported that the static mechanical properties of PMMA polymer resin can be significantly improved with this arrangement (Pande *et al.*, 2008). Ormsby *et al.* (2010a) observed that surface modification of the MWCNT with carboxyl groups did not result in significant improvements in the compressive or bend properties of the PMMA cement on a consistent basis. However, the fracture toughness of the PMMA cement was significantly enhanced (p-values<0.001) when the MWCNT were surface modified with carboxyl groups. It is unclear currently as to whether the improvements in performance of the MWCNT-PMMA cements are a direct consequence of good MWCNT dispersion within the PMMA matrix, providing mechanical reinforcement, or is due to a chemical interaction between the MWCNT and PMMA matrix (Ormsby *et al.*, 2010a). Eitan *et al.*, (2006) used strain dependent Raman spectroscopy to show that there is load transfer from the matrix to the nanotubes, and that the efficiency of the load transfer is improved by surface modification of the MWCNT.

It is also interesting to observe that significant improvements in fracture toughness did not correlate to improvements of the same magnitude for strength and modulus of the different cement combinations tested. Ormsby *et al.* (2010a) postulated that the methods adopted for specimen preparation, specimen configuration and the different modes of loading employed during testing could account for this. It has been reported that different loading regimes evaluate differing reinforcement mechanisms within the specimen microstructure, therefore dissimilar responses are expected (Lewis and Mladsi, 2000; Wagner and Chu, 2006). Wagner and Chu (2006) also found distinctions in mechanical properties when testing three dental core ceramic based materials. They found significant differences in the biaxial flexural strength, but reported no significant difference for the indentation fracture toughness for the materials tested (Wagner and Chu, 2006).

Subsequent to this investigation, Ormsby *et al.* (2010b) also published a study investigating the efficacy of adding different concentrations of MWCNT to PMMA bone cement of varying functionality as a means of improving MWCNT dispersion and thus augmenting the mechanical properties of the PMMA bone cement further. The bone cement was prepared using the optimal method for MWCNT incorporation, as determined in their previous study (Ormsby *et al.*, 2010a). Ormsby *et al.* (2010b) reported that adding MWCNT at low loadings (≤0.25 wt. %) to MMA monomer, prior to cement mixing with a proprietary mixing system, improved the mechanical properties of the resultant nanocomposite cement. Adding carboxyl and amine functional groups enhanced the dispersion of the MWCNT within the cement matrix and potentially increased the interaction between the carbon nanotubes and the cement, thereby improving the mechanical integrity of the resultant nanocomposite cement. These improvements in mechanical strength are potentially significant as mechanical failure of the bone cement mantle remains a prevalent issue in total joint replacement surgery often leading to revision surgical procedures. Adding MWCNT at higher loadings (≥0.5 wt. %) provided a negative effect on the mechanical performance of the nanocomposite cement. This was attributed to poor dispersion of MWCNT resulting in agglomerations forming within the cement matrix. In contrast, low loadings (≤ 0.25 wt. %) of MWCNT were more readily disentangled by the application of ultrasonic energy and homogenously dispersed in the resulting nanocomposite. The presence of well-dispersed MWCNT in PMMA cement with their anticipated strong nanotube-matrix bonding and high tensile properties, suggests that a percentage of the MWCNT would be orientated with their longitudinal axis perpendicular to the crack wave. Such MWCNT were effective in bridging the initial crack and preventing crack propagation, further enhancing the mechanical integrity of the cement mantle. These improvements could have clinical benefits for the application of MWCNT-PMMA nanocomposite cement in TJR surgery, due to a reduction in the rate of crack propagation through the reinforced nanocomposite cement mantle. This effect may have greatest significance for misaligned femoral implants resulting in areas of thinner cement mantle thickness, which continues to be cited as a main factor of cement mantle failure(Ormsby *et al.*, 2010b).

Gojny *et al.*, (2003) also reported that the addition of chemical functional groups to the MWCNT can provide a negative charge to the MWCNT and thus reduced agglomeration and improve interaction between the nanotubes and the host polymer. The results of this study by Ormsby *et al.*, (2010b) concurred with the findings of Gojny *et al.* (2003). The PMMA bone cement with MWCNT-UNF exhibited least significant improvements (p-value<0.1) for all mechanical properties measured. This reduced improvement in mechanical properties was attributed to poor dispersion of MWCNT within the cement matrix, resulting in the occurrence of MWCNT agglomerations. The MWCNT-UNF provided a degree of mechanical reinforcement at lower loading (≤ 0.25 wt. %), largely due to the reduced tendency for MWCNT agglomerations. MWCNT-COOH provided the most significant (p-value<0.001) improvements in all mechanical properties of the PMMA cement. It is proposed these significant improvements are a result of a homogenous dispersion of the MWCNT within the PMMA matrix aided by the negatively charged carboxyl groups. This homogeneous dispersion in tandem with interfacial interactions between the functionalised MWCNT and PMMA matrix could provide improved mechanical properties of the resultant nanocomposite. The bone cements incorporating amine functionalised MWCNT ($MWCNT-NH_2$) also improved mechanical properties. These improvements were less significant p-value<0.01 when compared with the addition of MWCNT-COOH. It is postulated that this is due to the lower level of functional groups present on the $MWCNT-NH_2$ when compared with the MWCNT-COOH (that is 0.5% vs. 4.0%, functional groups, respectively). This lower concentration of $MWCNT-NH_2$ functional groups may result in a more heterogeneous dispersion of the MWCNT within the cement matrix, therefore resulting in a less successful transfer of stress through the cement mantle.

Thermal Properties

PMMA bone cement is produced by a free radical reaction on mixing the polymer powder and liquid monomer constituents. The polymerisation reaction is a highly exothermic chemical reaction and as a consequence the peak temperatures typically reach 80-100° C. It has been reported that polymerizing bone cement has the potential to cause thermal necrosis of the surrounding bone cells, which is one of the mitigating factors for aseptic loosening of an implant fixed with PMMA bone cement (Dunne and Orr, 2002).

Reducing the polymerisation reaction of PMMA bone cement, therefore lowering the extent of thermal necrosis has been investigated by many research groups. Meyer et al. (1973) reported reducing the temperature (22° C) prior to bone cement mixing had a significant influence on the polymerisation reaction of the PMMA cement. They concluded that mixing PMMA cement at a temperature of 4° C resulted in a peak temperature (T_{max}) of 53° C, while mixing the same cement at 37° C increased the peak temperature to 125° C. Meyer et al. (1973) also investigated the effects of pre-chilling the femoral prosthesis prior to implantation into the bone cavity; they found adopting this approach did not influence the peak temperature. Larsen et al. (1991) also investigated the effects of pre-chilling the femoral prosthesis, however, they reported a 5° C reduction in the peak temperature at the bone–cement interface. Additionally, Lidgren et al.(1987) found using chilled water to pulse-lavage the bone cavity prior to cement delivery had a significant effect on the extent of the polymerisation reaction, the peak temperature was subsequently reduced from 59° C to 45° C. The mixing method used to prepare the PMMA bone cement prior to delivery into the bone cavity also has a role in its polymerisation reaction.Dunne and Orr (2002) reported the level of heat generated for bone cement prepared under the application of a vacuum was significantly reduced when compared to the same cement prepared under atmospheric conditions using a bowl and spatula mixing arrangement. Other methods can be used to reduce the degree of polymerisation reaction of PMMA bone cement, such as altering the compositions or constituents of the cement. However, this can have a significant influence on the mechanical and handling performance of the bone cement (Lewis et al., 2007).

CNT incorporation has previously been reported to improve the thermal properties of a range of polymers, including polyethylene (McClory et al., 2010), polyurethane (Marrs et al., 2006), polystyrene (Andrews and Weisenberger,

2004),polyvinyl alcohol and methyl methacrylate-styrene copolymer (Xie*et al.*, 2005).

Andrews and Weisenberger (2004) proposed that the thermal property improvements for CNT-polymer composites are a function of CNT type, degree of dispersion, CNT loading, CNT alignment and polymer matrix. Xie *et al.* (2005) reported a significant improvement ($\approx$125%) in the thermal conductivity of an epoxy when 1.0 wt. % SWCNT powder was added. Choi *et al.* (2003) observed an increase ($\approx$300%) in the thermal conductivity of an epoxy for a SWCNT loading of 3.0 wt. %. The thermal properties of PMMA bone cement have been modified with MWCNT by Ormsby *et al.*, (2010a). Incorporating either unfunctionalised or carboxyl functionalised MWCNT into the PMMA powder or liquid monomer prior to mixing both components together had a significant effect on the exothermic polymerisation reaction. It was observed that maximum temperature and the setting properties exhibited during polymerisation were significantly reduced by the inclusion of 0.1wt. % (unfunctionalised or carboxyl functionalised) MWCNT into the PMMA cement, irrespective of the method of introduction. Other studies have also reported reductions in the thermal properties of PMMA cement on addition of 5-15 wt. % steel fibres (Kotha *et al.*, 2002). Dunne and Orr (2002) reported that reduction of the polymerisation exotherm will decrease the likelihood of residual stresses developing within the cement mantle, which can cause premature failure of the cement when subjected to mechanical loading.

The importance of minimising the bone cement exothermic reaction has been stressed, as it may result in a permanent cessation of blood flow and bone tissue necrosis, which shows no sign of repair after 100 days (Moritz and Henriques, 1947; Feith, 1975; Eriksson and Alberksson, 1983; Mjoberg *et al.*, 1984). The cumulative TNI (Thermal Necrosis Index) has been used previously to assess the level of irreparable damage bone cement caused by heat generation (Moritz and Henriques, 1947; Dunne and Orr, 2002). If TNI exceeds one there is the possibility of thermal damage to the living tissue cells. The thermal necrosis index is typically calculated at two temperatures; >44° C and >55° C, chosen because the temperature threshold for impaired bone regeneration has been reported to be in the range of 44-47°C (Moritz and Henriques, 1947; Eriksson and Alberksson, 1983). The incorporation of MWCNT to PMMA based bone cement may reduce the incidence of polymerisation induced hot spots and thermal necrosis of the surrounding tissue adjacent to the cement mantle, which is believed to be observed radiographically (Linder, 1977). Reducing the occurrence of such tissue damage may improve the mechanical integrity of the cement-bone interface, thereby promoting implant longevity.

Ormsby *et al.*, (2010a) report that the incorporation of unfunctionalised or carboxyl functionalised MWCNT assisted in the dissipation of the heat produced during the exothermic polymerisation reaction of PMMA bone cement, irrespective of the method of introduction. With unfunctionalised MWCNT, this reduction was not below the levels necessary to prevent thermal tissue damage as the TNI was greater than one. In contrast, surface modification of the MWCNT with carboxyl groups and subsequent addition to the liquid monomer using magnetic stirring did reduce the TNI values at >44° C and >55° C to levels below one.

In a subsequent study by Ormsby *et al.*, (2011)the incorporation of unfunctionalised, amine, and carboxyl functionalised MWCNT at increasing wt. % assisted in the dissipation of the heat produced during the polymerisation of PMMA bone cement. It was observed that any effect on the reaction exotherm was dependant on MWCNT loading. The greater reductions in exotherm were reported for the highest level of MWCNT loading (1.0 wt. %). Saha and Pal (1986) reported a similar finding when examining carbon fibre reinforced bone cement. The greatest reductions in peak exothermic temperature were associated with the highest levels of carbon fibre. It is important to note that the types of MWCNT used within the study by Ormsby *et al.*, (2011)had thermal conductivity values of >3000Wm^{-1} k^{-1}. It was therefore proposed that the MWCNT act as a heat sink within the PMMA bone cement and therefore assist in the dissipation of the heat generated during the polymerisation reaction (Ormsby *et al.*, 2011). This behaviour is also a function of the extent of MWCNT dispersion and distribution throughout the PMMA bone cement matrix, such that uniform dispersion of MWCNT within the cement will dissipate the thermal energy throughout the cement matrix. This is further aided by the interconnectivity of MWCNT entanglements and the very large surface area of MWCNT (600-1000 m^2/g) (Peigney *et al.*, 2009). Bonnet *et al.* (2007) found a similar effect on the addition of 7 vol. % of SWCNT to PMMA reporting a 55 % increase in the thermal conductivity. It is therefore hypothesised that the thermal conductivity of the PMMA bone cement described here will have also increased due to MWCNT addition.

It has been stated that for composites incorporating CNT to be thermally conductive, they must form a percolated network of overlapping or touching CNT for the transport of heat energy (Marrs, 2007). Therefore bone cements with relatively poor levels of MWCNT dispersion ($\geq$0.5 wt. %) within the PMMA matrix, due to agglomerations (Figure 26), demonstrated the greatest reduction in thermal properties.

It is possible to use this theory to explain why the MWCNT of different chemical functionality provided differing thermal properties. The addition of MWCNT-UNF and MWCNT-NH$_2$ provided more significant reductions in the polymerisation reaction when compared to the MWCNT-COOH. It is suggested by Ormsby *et al., (2011)* that this may be due to a less homogeneous dispersion of the MWCNT-UNF and MWCNT-NH$_2$ within the cement in comparison to the improved dispersion of the MWCNT-COOH.

Ormsby *et al.* (2010b) added MWCNT of various chemical functionality at increasing loadings to PMMA cement and assessed the mechanical properties of the resultant composites. They reported significant improvements in mechanical properties at low levels of MWCNT loading (≤0.5 wt. %).Ormsby *et al.* (2010b) showed that MWCNT-COOH provided the greatest improvement in mechanical properties, due to the improved MWCNT dispersion associated with improved interfacial interactions between these MWCNT and PMMA through enhanced van der Waals attraction and hydrogen bonding.

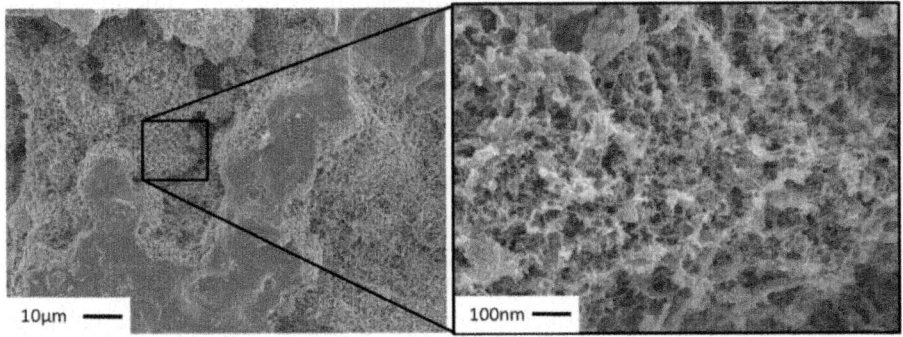

Figure 26. SEM image of 1.0 wt% MWCNT filled PMMA bone cement showing MWCNT-UNF.

It is noteworthy that the MWCNT inclusion altered the rate of PMMA polymerisation. A slower rate of polymerisation extended the time taken for the bone cement to fully polymerise, which in turn reduced the T_{max} and TNI values. It is postulated that the presence of MWCNT in the cement not only altered the kinetics of the polymerisation reaction, but additionally played a role dissipating heat energy. Incorporation of carboxyl and amine functionalised MWCNT had a greater influence on the polymerisation reaction of the bone cement used in this study, compared to the unfunctionalised (Ormsby *et al.*, 2011).

Rheology Properties

The efficacy of PMMA bone cement in anchoring a TJR is affected by many fundamental characteristics. Among these are the rheological, polymerisation, and handling properties, whose significance is two-fold (Ormsby *et al.*, 2011).

Firstly, the ease with which the cement flows into the intramedullary bone canal facilitates the controlled positioning of the prosthesis. This is critical as it has been reported that initial prosthesis position is a contributory factor to the longevity of the cemented implant (Jones *et al.*, 1992; Lewis and Carroll, 2001). Secondly, the rheological properties of the cement may play an important role in the development of pores in the cement during mixing and delivery. Such pores may act as sites for the initiation of cracks, which, in turn, can cause or contribute to aseptic loosening of the prosthesis (Jones *et al.*, 1992).

To date, there have been limited studies examining the viscoelastic properties of PMMA bone cement, with oscillatory shear rheometry (OSR) being the most common method employed. Harper et al. (2000) observed that the complex viscosity (η^*) of VersaBond ™ and Palacos® R cements increased from 1000 Pa.s at 2.5 min to 5000 Pa.s at 6 min. They defined this sharp increase in η^* as the onset of cure.Spiegelberg and McKinley (1998) determined the critical gel time of Simplex P™ cement as 9.7 min.Farrar and Rose (2001) investigated the initial polymerisation reaction of several commercial bone cements. They examined η^* over a range of temperatures and concluded the polymerisation of bone cement is strongly dependent on temperature. Ormsby et al., (2011) have assessed the influence of differing MWCNT (unfunctionalised, carboxyl functionalized or amine functionalised) on the rheological properties and cure kinetics of the polymerising PMMA bone cement. They investigated how the differing MWCNT systems influenced the time at which the onset of polymerisation occurred, as well as the time at which polymer gelation occurred. Ormsby et al., (2011) found that MWCNT addition significantly influenced the rheological behaviour of the polymerising cement. For each cement investigated, η^* increased with time. Ormsby et al., (2011) explained this trend applying the Krieger–Dougherty equation (Equation 1) (Krieger and Dougherty, 1959), which describes the viscosity of a concentrated suspension (η).

$$\eta^* = \eta_s \left(1 - \frac{\varphi}{\varphi_m} \right)^{-[\eta]\,\varphi_m}$$

(1)

where, $\eta_s$is the viscosity of the suspending medium, φ is the phase volume of the particles in the suspension, $\varphi_m$is the maximum packing fraction of those particles, and η is the intrinsic viscosity. This equation may be used to comment on the variation of the polymerizing bone cement's η^*as a function of time, although its application is limited as it primarily applies to Newtonian suspensions. During the initial stages of mixing the powder and liquid components, the high initial viscosity is attributed primarily to the swelling of the polymer beads within the cement powder (Lewis and Carroll, 2001). As elapsed time from start of mixing increases and swelling causes both φmand η to decrease. Thus, η*increases with t, a trend observed in the present results of the studies of Lewis and Carroll, (2001), andOrmsby et al., (2011).

Ormsby et al., (2011) found that the incorporation of chemically functionalised MWCNT (MWCNT-COOH and MWCNT-NH$_2$) into PMMA bone cement significantly extended the onset of cure. This effect was more pronounced as MWCNT loading was increased. Indicating the time delay before the onset of cure for these composite cements is in part due to the role the functional groups play in altering the polymerisation reaction, in addition to physically preventing cross-linking of the polymer chain. The onset of cure of the PMMA cements with MWCNT-UNF addition was also delayed, but to a lesser extent. In all cases, MWCNT addition to PMMA bone cement prevented macro-gelation from occurring. It was also significant to observe that on addition of MWCNT-COOH, gel-times increased up to a loading of ≤0.5 wt. %, but at 1.0 wt. % the gel-time decreased, compared to the control sample. This finding is commonly reported for heavily-filled polymers, as the cement may exhibit solid-like properties from the onset of mixing. Therefore, initially the filled bone cement will have a higher viscosity than the control, but the actual onset of polymerisation may not occur until much later in the reaction. Lalko et al. (2009) reported a similar behavior after incorporating increasing fractions of functionalised CNT into polycarbonate.

Lower loadings of MWCNT-COOH (≤0.5 wt. %) did extend gel-times, when compared to the control (MWCNT free bone cement), again supporting the hypothesis that the reduced rate of polymerisation is due to chemical interactions between functional groups present on the surface of the MWCNT and the polymer matrix, as the time before gelation occurs increased with level of loading (and thus concentration of functional groups). Ormsby et al., (2011) have suggested that the physical presence may indeed affect the rate of polymerisation, but the functional chemical groups may be the predominant influence.

This hypothesis is supported by the theory that if the functional groups on the MWCNT were indeed interrupting the polymerisation reaction by terminating polymer chains via formation of covalent bonds, then the onset of cure (sudden increase in complex viscosity) would never occur and the cement would never reach a hardened state. It is noteworthy though, for this to occur, the MWCNT loading would need to be significantly higher than 1.0 wt. % (Ormsby et al., 2011). Interestingly, the gel-times remain relatively unchanged for the bone cement with MWCNT-UNF, with no clear pattern evident irrespective of MWCNT-UNF loading. These results would indicate that the prolonged time before the onset of cure experienced in the bone cements with MWCNT-COOH is dependent on the carboxyl functional group.

SUMMARY AND CONCLUSIONS

As the number of primary TJR continues to increase each year and, even with the reported decrease in the proportion of cemented TJR performed, PMMA bone cement is still required for the majority of TJR procedures. At present with longer life expectancy and younger patient populations requiring TJR, an increase in cemented revisions seems inevitable. Aseptic loosening is continually cited as being the most common indication for revision. It is well established that for cemented implants a number of factors contribute to aseptic loosening, of which, fatigue damage of the cement mantle has been observed *in vivo*. Therefore, a crucial requirement exists for the development of new technologies and biomaterials for the treatment of traumatic injuries and chronic diseases, which allow less tissue damage and more tissue regeneration and are conducive to rapid patient recovery. Particularly for biomaterials and devices designed to replace a degenerated or diseased joint, bone structure, many questions need to be answered. Such devices and implants would benefit significantly from availability of a material that is multi-functional and can meet the biomechanical and biological requirements.

The conventional biomaterials available today are reaching their maximum capabilities, notwithstanding their successful application in treating and preventing different medical conditions. There is a need for the development of new biomaterials which must satisfy several requirements ranging from physical, mechanical, biological, toxicological and other characteristics, depending on the final clinical application.

Carbon is chemically inert and CNT not only demonstrate superior mechanical, chemical and electrical properties, but also have the potential to be biocompatible particularly when appropriately functionalised. Also, encapsulation of other materials within CNT could potentially create applications for therapeutic use in medicine. Incorporation of MWCNT into PMMA based orthopaedic bone is a case in point, whereby a high degree of MWCNT-polymer matrix interaction has been shown to increase the fracture resistance during mechanical loading. Furthermore, it has been reported that MWCNT-PMMA bone cement leads to increased viscosity and reduced polymerisation temperatures. Reducing the temperature generated during polymerisation could reduce the thermal cellular necrosis experienced *in vivo*, reducing the probability of aseptic loosening. Furthermore, a reduction in the exotherm of bone cement will reduce residual stresses within the cement mantle as a consequence of excessive shrinkage.

To fully exploit the use of MWCNT in PMMA bone cement further development and research is required. In particular a detailed investigation of the biocompatibility of the MWCNT composite cements is required. This would require exposing human osteoblast cells to the composite MWCNT-PMMA bone cements, ultimately leading to *in vivo* cell work. This would provide a clearer indication of the MWCNT composite cements potential integration into the body.

Regardless of this interest, there are many issues and limitations to be considered. The field of nanomaterials for biomedical and bioengineering applications is still very much in its infancy and many difficult questions remain unanswered, including manufacturing, safety and regulatory issues. Preliminary investigations substantiate the enormous potential of MWCNT systems for biomedical and bioengineering applications either as a structure, coating, scaffold or composite; although most of these are only at laboratory-scale and in vitro testing. There is a major requirement for interdisciplinary collaboration and exchange of knowledge at many levels to effectively address the current issues, before being able to fully understand and explore the true potential of CNT for biomedical and bioengineering applications.

REFERENCES

1.   American Society for Testing and Materials (ASTM), Specification 45195 Standard specification for acrylic bone cement, 1996 Annual Book of ASTM Standards, 13 01. Philadelphia, American Society for Testing and Materials (1996) 4945 .

2.   P. M. Ajayan, 1997 "Carbon nanotubes: novel architecture in nanometer space." Progressin Crystal Growth and Characterization of Materials 34(1-4): 37-51.

3.   D. Apple, 2003 "A pioneer in the quest to eradicate world blindness." Bulletin of the World Health Organization 81 10 756757 .

4.   R. Andrews, D. Jacques, D. L. Qian, T. Rantell, 2002 "Multiwall carbon nanotubes: synthesis and application." Accounts of Chemical Research 35 12 10081017 .

5.   R. Andrews, M. C. Weisenberger, 2004 "Carbon nanotube polymer composites." Current Opinion in Solid State and Materials Science 8 1 3137 .

6.   P. P. Anthony, G. A. Gie, C. R. Howie, R. S. Ling, 1990 "Localised endosteal bone lysis in relation to the femoral components of cemented total hip arthroplasties." Journal of Bone and Joint Surgery- British 72-B (6): 971-979.

7.   M. Baleani, L. Cristofolini, C. Minari, A. Toni, 2003 "Fatigue strength of PMMA bone cement mixed with gentamicin and barium sulphate vs. pure PMMA." Proceedings of the Institution of Mechanical Engineers, Part H (Journal ofEngineering in Medicine) 217 912 .

8.   A. H. Barber, S. R. Cohen, H. D. Wagner, 2003 "Measurement of carbon nanotubepolymer interfacial strength." Applied Physics Letters 82 23 41404142 .

9.   G. Baroud, M. Samara, T. Steffen, 2004 "Influence of mixing method on the cement temperature-mixing time history and doughing time of three acrylic cements for vertebroplasty." Journal of Biomedical Materials Research Part B-AppliedBiomaterials 68B(1): 112-116.

10. R. H. Baughman, A. A. Zakhidov, W. A. De Heer, 2002 "Carbon nanotubes- the route toward applications." Science 297 5582 787792 .

11. A. Bellare, W. Fitz, A. Gomoll, M. B. Turell, R. Scott, T. Thornhill, 2002 "Using nanotechnology to improve the performance of acrylic bone cements." TheOrthopaedic Journal at Harvard Medical School 4

12. N. E. Bishop, S. Ferguson, S. Tepic, 1996 "Porosity reduction in bone cement at the cement-stem interface." Journal of Bone and Joint Surgery- British 78B 3):349-356.

13. O. L. Blakslee, D. G. Proctor, E. J. Seldin, G. B. Spence, T. Weng, 1970 "Elastic constants of compression-annealed pyrolytic graphite." Journal of Applied Physics 41 8 337382 .

14. P. Bonnet, D. Sireude, B. Garnier, O. Chauvet, 2007 Thermal properties and percolation in carbon nanotube-polymer composites. Journal of Applied Physics Letters 91: 201910-1-201910-3.

15. BSI, British Standards Institution 1993 Non-metallic materials for surgical implants. Part 1. Specification for acrylic resin cement. BS 7253. ISO 5833.

16. M. Cadek, J. N. Coleman, K. P. Ryan, V. Nicolosi, G. Bister, A. Fonseca, J. B. Nagy, K. Szostak, F. Beguin, W. J. Blau, 2004 "Reinforcement of polymers withcarbon nanotubes: The role of nanotube surface area." Nano Letters 4 2 3536 .

17. W. D. Callister, 2000a Chapter 17: Composites. Materials Science and Engineering: An Introduction, John Wiley & Sons, Inc.: 520561 .

18. G. Chao, Z. Hailin, W. Yanping, P. C. P. Watts, K. Hao, C. Xiaowen, D. Yan, 2006 "In situ polymerization approach to multiwalled carbon nanotubes-reinforcednylon 1010 composites: Mechanical properties and crystallization behavior." Polymer47 1 11322 .

19. M. Chandler, R. S. Z. Kowalski, N. D. Watkins, A. Briscoe, A. M. R. New, 2006 "Cementing techniques in hip resurfacing." Proceedings of the Institution of Mechanical Engineers Part H-Journal of Engineering in Medicine 220(H2): 321-331.

20. A. L. Chun, J. G. Moralez, H. Fenniri, T. J. Webster, 2004 "Helical rosette nanotubes: A more effective orthopaedic implant material." Nanotechnology 15 4 2349 .

21. D. T. Colbert, 2003 "Single-wall nanotubes: A new option for conductive plastics and engineering polymers." Plastics, Additives and Compounding 5 1 1825 .

22. J. N. Coleman, M. Cadek, R. Blake, V. Nicolosi, K. P. Ryan, C. Belton, A. Fonseca, J. B. Nagy, Y. K. Gun'ko, W. J. Blau, 2004 "High-performance nanotubereinforcedplastics: Understanding the mechanism of strength increase." AdvancedFunctional Materials 14 8 791798 .

23. J. N. Coleman, S. Curran, A. B. Dalton, A. P. Davey, B. Mc Carthy, W. Blau, R. C. Barklie, 1998 "Percolation-dominated conductivity in a conjugated polymercarbon-nanotube composite." Physical Review B (Condensed Matter) 58 12 74925 .

24. C. A. Cooper, S. R. Cohen, A. H. Barber, H. D. Wagner, 2002 "Detachment of nanotubes from a polymer matrix." Applied Physics Letters 81 20 38735 .

25. D. Cui, F. Tian, C. S. Ozkan, M. Wang, H. Gao, 2005 "Effect of single wall carbon nanotubes on human HEK293 cells." Toxicology Letters 155 1 7385 .

26. R. F. Curl, R. E. Smalley, H. W. Kroto, S. O'Brien, J. R. Heath, 2001 "How the news that we were not the first to conceive of soccer ball C60 got to us." Journal ofMolecular Graphics and Modelling 19 2 185186 .

27. H. W. Demian, K. Mc Dermott, 1998 "Regulatory perspective on characterization and testing of orthopedic bone cements." Biomaterials 19 17 16071618 .

28. A. B. Dalton, S. Collins, E. Munoz, J. M. Razal, V. H. Ebron, J. P. Ferraris, J. N. Coleman, B. G. Kim, R. H. Baughman, 2003 "Super-tough carbonnanotubefibres." Nature 423(6941): 703.

29. M. Davoren, E. Herzog, A. Casey, B. Cottinerau, G. Chambers, H. J.

Byrne, 2007 In vitro toxicity evaluation of single walled carbon nanotubes on human A549 lung cells, Toxicol in Vitro21 438448 .

30.   S. Deb, G. Lewis, S. W. Janna, B. Vazquez, Roman. J. San, 2003 "Fatigue and fracture toughness of acrylic bone cements modified with long-chain amine activators." Journal of Biomedical Materials Research Part A 67A(2): 571-577.

31.   B. G. Demczyk, Y. M. Wang, J. Cumings, M. Hetman, W. Han, A. Zettl, R. O. Ritchie, 2002 "Direct mechanical measurement of the tensile strength and elasticmodulus of multiwalled carbon nanotubes." Materials Science and Engineering A334(1-2): 173-178.

32.   W. Ding, A. Eitan, F. T. Fisher, X. Chen, D. A. Dikin, R. Andrews, L. C. Brinson, L. S. Schadler, R. S. Ruoff, 2003 "Direct observation of polymer sheathing incarbon nanotube-polycarbonate composites." Nano Letters 3 11 15937 .

33.   N. J. Dunne, J. F. Orr, 2002 Curing characteristics of acrylic bone cement. Journal of Material Science 13(1), 17-22.

34.   N. J. Dunne, J. F. Orr, M. T. Mushipe, R. J. Eveleigh, 2003 "The relationship between porosity and fatigue characteristics of bone cements." Biomaterials 24 2 239245 .

35.   A. Eitan, F. T. Fisher, R. Andrews, L. C. Brinson, L. S. Schadler, 2006 "Reinforcement mechanisms in MWCNT-filled polycarbonate." Composites Scienceand Technology 66 9 11591170 .

36.   A. R. Eriksson, T. Alberksson, 1983 Temperature threshold levels for heat-induced bone tissue injury-A vital microscopy in the rabbit. Journal of Prosthetic Dentistry 50 1 101107 .

37.   B. Fadeel, V. Kagan, H. Krug, A. Shvedova, M. Svartengren, L. Tran, 2007 There's plenty of room at the forum: potential risks and safety assessment of engineered nanomaterials, Nanotoxicology1 (2), 73-84.

38.   D. F. Farrar, J. Rose, 2001 Rheological properties of PMMA bone cement during curing. Biomaterials 22 30053013 .

39.   R. Feith, 1975 Side effect of acrylic cement implanted into bone. Acta Orthopaedica Scandinavica 214;161.

40.   F. T. Fisher, R. D. Bradshaw, L. C. Brinson, 2002 "Effects of nanotube waviness onthe modulus of nanotube-reinforced polymers." Applied Physics Letters 80(24): 4647.

41.   P. Franklin, D. J. Wood, N. L. Bubb, 2005 "Reinforcement of poly(methyl methacrylate) denture base with glass flake." Dental Materials 21 4 365370 .

42. H. Fukushima, Y. Hashimoto, S. Yoshiya, M. Kurosaka, M. Matsuda, S. Kawamura, T. Iwatsubo, 2002 "Conduction analysis of cement interface temperature in total knee arthroplasty." Kobe Journal of Medical Science 48 6372 .

43. J. L. Gilbert, J. M. Hasenwinkel, R. L. Wixson, E. P. Lautenschlager, 2000 "A theoretical and experimental analysis of polymerization shrinkage of bone cement: A potential major source of porosity." Journal of Biomedical Materials Research 52 1 210218 .

44. J. L. Gilbert, D. S. Ney, E. P. Lautenschlager, 1995 "Self-reinforced composite poly(methyl methacrylate): static and fatigue properties." Biomaterials 16 14 10431055 .

45. J. L. Gilbert, J. M. Hasenwinkel, R. L. Wixson, E. P. A. Lautenschlager, 2002 Theoretical and experimental analysis of polymerisation shrinkage of bone cement: A potential major source of porosity.Journal of Biomedical Material Research 52 1 210218 .

46. M. P. Ginebra, L. Albuixech, E. Fernandez-Barragan, C. Aparicio, F. J. Gil, Roman. J. San, B. Vazquez, J. A. Planell, 2002 "Mechanical performance ofacrylic bone cements containing different radiopacifying agents." Biomaterials 23 8 18731882 .

47. D. Granchi, E. Cenni, L. Savarino, G. Ciapetti, G. Forbicini, M. Vancini, C. Maini, N. Baldini, A. Giunti, 2002 "Bone cement extracts modulate theosteoprotegerin/osteoprotegerin-ligand expression in Mg63 osteoblast-like cells."Biomaterials 23 11 23592365 .

48. H. W. Goh, S. H. Goh, G. Q. Xu, K. P. Pramoda, W. D. Zhang, 2003 "Crystallization and dynamic mechanical behavior of double-C60 -end-capped poly(ethylene oxide)/multiwalled carbon nanotube composites." Chemical PhysicsLetters 379(3-4): 236-41.

49. E. J. Harper, M. J. German, W. Bonfield, M. Braden, E. Dingeldein, H. Wahlig, 2000 A comparison of VersaBondTM, a modified acrylic bone cement with improved handling properties, to Palacos R, Simplex P. Trans Sixth World Biomater Cong, Kamuela (Big Island). 540.

50. J. G. E. Hendriks, J. R. Van Horn, H. C. Van Der Mei, H. J. Busscher, 2004 "Backgrounds of antibiotic-loaded bone cement and prosthesis-related infection." Biomaterials 25 3 545556 .

51. E. Herzog, A. Casey, F. M. Lyng, G. Chambers, H. J. Byrne, M. Davoren, 2007 A new approach to the toxicity testing of carbon-based nanomaterials. The clonogenic assay, Toxicol Lett174 4960 .

52. K. Y. Huang, J. J. Yan, R. M. Lin, 2005 "Histopathologic findings of retrieved specimens of vertebroplasty with polymethylmethacrylate

cement- case control study." Spine 30(19): E585 -E588.

53. D. Hull, T. W. Clyne, 1996a Fibres and matrices. An Introduction to Composite Materials. Clarke, D. R., Suresh, S. and Ward, I. M., Cambridge University Press: 938 .

54. D. Hull, T. W. Clyne, 1996b General introduction. An Introduction to Composite Materials.. Clarke, D. R., Suresh, S. and Ward, I. M., Cambridge University Press:18 .

55. G. L. Hwang, Y. Shieh, T. , K. C. Hwang, 2004 "Efficient load transfer to polymergrafted multiwalled carbon nanotubes in polymer composites." Advanced FunctionalMaterials 14 5 487491 .

56. S. Iijima, 1991 "Helical microtubules of graphitic carbon." Nature 354 5658 .

57. S. Iijima, 2002 "Carbon nanotubes: past, present, and future." Physica B: Condensed Matter 323(1-4): 1-5.

58. D. Janssen, R. Aquarius, J. Stolk, N. Verdonschot, 2005a "The contradictory effects of pores on fatigue cracking of bone cement." Journal of BiomedicalMaterials Research- Part B Applied Biomaterials 74 2 747753 .

59. D. Janssen, J. Stolk, N. Verdonschot, 2005b "Why would cement porosity reduction be clinically irrelevant, while experimental data show the contrary." Journal ofOrthopaedic Research 23 4 691697 .

60. M. Jasty, W. J. Maloney, C. R. Bragdon, D. O. Oconnor, T. Haire, W. H. Harris, 1991 "The initiation of failure in cemented femoral components of hiparthroplasties." Journal of Bone and Joint Surgery-British 73 4): 551-558.

61. Z. Jia, Z. Wang, C. Xu, J. Liang, B. Wei, D. Wu, S. Zhu, 1999 "Study on poly (methyl methacrylate)/carbon nanotube composites." Materials Science &Engineering A (Structural Materials: Properties, Microstructure and Processing) A271(1-2): 395-400.

62. P. R. Jones, D. W. L. Hukins, M. L. Porter, K. E. Davies, K. Hardinge, C. J. Taylor, 1992 Bending and fracture of the femoral component in cemented total hip replacement. Journal of Biomechanical Engineering 14 (5): 444.

63. V. E. Kagan, Y. Y. Tyurina, V. A. Tyurin, N. V. Konduru, A. I. Potapovich, A. N. Osipov, 2006 Direct and indirect effects of single walled carbon nanotubes on RAW 264.7 macrophages: role of iron, Toxicol Lett165 (1), 88-100.

64. J. D. Keener, J. J. Callaghan, D. D. Goetz, D. R. Pederson, P. M. Sullivan,

R. C. Johnston, 2003 "Twenty-five-year results after charnley total hiparthroplasty in patients less than fifty years old- a concise follow-up of a previousreport." Journal of Bone and Joint Surgery-American 85A 6): 1066-1072.

65. K. H. Khor, J. Y. Buffière, W. Ludwig, H. Toda, H. S. Ubhi, P. J. Gregson, Kim. P. And, L. Shi, A. Majumdar, P. L. Mc Euen, 2001 "Thermal transport measurements of individual multiwalled nanotubes." Physical Review Letters 87 21 2155021 .

66. I. M. Krieger, T. J. Dougherty, 1959 A mechanism for non-Newtonian flow in suspensions of rigid spheres. Transaction of the Society of Rheology 3 137152 .

67. K. Konnecke, G. Rehage, 1981 "Crystallization and stero association of steroregular PMMA." Colloid and Polymer Science 259 10621069 .

68. S. P. Kotha, C. Li, P. Mc Ginn, S. R. Schmid, J. J. Mason, 2006 "Improved mechanical properties of acrylic bone cement with short titanium fiber reinforcement." Journal of Materials Science: Materials in Medicine 17 8 7438 .

69. S. P. Kotha, C. Li, S. R. Schmid, J. J. Mason, 2004 "Fracture toughness of steelfiber- reinforced bone cement." Journal of Biomedical Materials Research- Part A70 3 514521 .

70. K. D. Kuehn, W. Ege, U. Gopp, 2005a "Acrylic bone cements: compositions and properties." Orthopedic Clinics of North America 36 1728 .

71. S. M. Kurtz, M. L. Villarraga, K. Zhao, A. A. Edidin, 2005 "Static and fatigue mechanical behavior of bone cement with elevated barium sulfate content for treatment of vertebral compression fractures." Biomaterials 26 17 36993712 .

72. S. T. Larsen, S. Franzen, L. Ryd, 1991 Cement interface temperature in hip arthroplasty. Acta Orthopaedica Scandinavica 62 2 102105 .

73. M. P. Lalko, L. Rakesh, S. Hirschi, 2009 Rheology of polycarbonate reinforced with functionalized and unfunctionalized single-walled carbon nanotubes. Journal of Thermal Analysis and Calorimetry 95 1 203206 .

74. R. R. Lee, M. Ogiso, A. Watanabe, K. Ishihara, 1997 "Examination of hydroxyapatite filled 4-META/MAA-TBB adhesive one cement in in vitro and invivo environment." Journal of Biomedical Materials Research 38 1 1116 .

75. W. Leelapornpisit, M. Ton-That, T. , F. Perrin-Sarazin, K. C. Cole, J. Denault, B. Simard, 2005 "Effect of carbon nanotubes on the

crystallization and propertiesof polypropylene." Journal of Polymer Science, Part B: Polymer Physics 43 18 24452453 .

76. A. B. Lennon, P. J. Prendergast, 2002 "Residual stress due to curing can initiate damage in porous bone cement: experimental and theoretical evidence." Journal ofBiomechanics 35 3 311321 .

77. G. Lewis, 1997 "Properties of acrylic bone cement: state of the art review." Journal of Biomedical Materials Research 38 2 155182 .

78. G. Lewis, 2000 "Relative roles of cement molecular weight and mixing method on the fatigue performance of acrylic bone cement: simplex-p versus osteopal." Journal ofBiomedical Materials Research 53 1 119130 .

79. G. Lewis, 2003 "Fatigue testing and performance of acrylic bone-cement materials: stateof- the-art review." Journal of Biomedical Materials Research Part B-AppliedBiomaterials 66B(1): 457-486.

80. G. Lewis, M. Carroll, 2001 Rheological properties of acrylic bone cement during curing and the role of the size of the powder particles., Journal of Biomedical Material Research (App Biomaterials) 63, 191199 .

81. G. Lewis, S. Janna, M. Carroll, 2003 "Effect of test frequency on the in vitro fatigue life of acrylic bone cement." Biomaterials 24 6 111117 .

82. G. Lewis, S. I. Janna, 2004 "Effect of fabrication pressure on the fatigue performance of cemex acrylic bone cement." Biomaterials 25(7-8): 1415-1420.

83. G. Lewis, C. S. J. Van Hooy-Corstjens, A. Bhattaram, L. H. Koole, 2005 "Influence of the radiopacifier in an acrylic bone cement on its mechanical, thermal, and physical properties: Barium sulfate-containing cement versus iodine-containing cement." Journal of Biomedical Materials Research- Part B Applied Biomaterials 73 1 7787 .

84. L. Lidgren, B. Bodelind, J. Möller, 1987 Bone cement improved by vacuum mixing and chilling. Acta Orthopaedica 58 1 2732 .

85. L. Linder, 1977 Reaction of bone to the acute chemical trauma of bone cement. Journal of Bone Joint Surgery 59 1 8287 .

86. C. Liu, S. M. Green, N. D. Watkins, P. J. Gregg, A. W. Mc Caskie, 2001 "Some failure modes of four clinical bone cements." Proceedings of the Institution ofMechanical Engineers, Part H (Journal of Engineering in Medicine) 215(H4): 359- 66.

87. W. Luo, B. , T. Yang, Q. , X. Wang, Y. , 2004 "Time-dependent craze zone growth at a crack tip in polymer solids." Polymer 45 10 35193525 .

88. J. F. Mandell, D. D. Huang, F. J. Mc Garry, 1980 Crack propagation modes in injection molded fibre reinforced thermoplastics. Cambridge,

Massachusetts, School of Engineering, Massachusetts Institute of technology: 134 .

89. B. Marrs, R. Andrews, T. Rantell, D. A. Pienkowski, 2006 "Augmentation of acrylic bone cement with multiwall carbon nanotubes." Journal of BiomedicalMaterials Research Part A 77(A): 269276 .

90. B. Marrs, R. Andrews, T. Rantell, D. Pienkowski, 2006 Augmentation of acrylic bone cement with multiwall carbon nanotubes.Journal of Biomedical Material Research 77 2 269276 .

91. B. A. O. Mc Cormack, P. J. Prendergast, 1996 "Interface failure in implants cemented with different bone-cements- a fracture mechanics approach". 2nd International Symposium on Computer Methods in Biomechanics and Biomedical Engineering, Swansea, Gordon and Breach.

92. B. A. O. Mc Cormack, P. J. Prendergast, 1999 "Microdamage accumulation in the cement layer of hip replacements under flexural loading." Journal of Biomechanics 32 5 46775 .

93. B. A. O. Mc Cormack, C. D. Walsh, S. P. Wilson, P. J. Prendergast, 1998 "A statistical analysis of microcrack accumulation in PMMA under fatigue loading: applications to orthopaedic implant fixation." International Journal of Fatigue 20 8 581593 .

94. C. Mc Clory, T. Mc Nally, G. Brennan, J. Erskine, 2007 Thermosetting polyurethane multiwall carbon nanotube composites. Journal of Applied Polymer Science 105 10031011 .

95. C. Mc Clory, T. Mc Nally, M. Baxendale, P. Pötschke, W. Blau, M. Ruether, 2010 Electrical and rheological percolation of PMMA/MWCNT composites as a function of CNT geometry and functionality. European Polymer Journal 46 5 854868 .

96. T. Mc Nally, P. Potschke, P. Halley, M. Murphy, D. Martin, S. E. J. Bell, 2005 Polyethylene multiwall carbon nanotube composites by melt blending. Polymer. 468222 .

97. P. R. Meyer, E. P. Lautenschlager, B. K. Moore, 1973 On the setting properties of acrylic bone cement. Journal of Bone Joint Surgery 55(A): 149156 .

98. B. Mjoberg, H. Petterson, R. Roseqvist, A. Rydholm, 1984 Bone cement, thermal injury and radiolucent zone. Acta Orthopaedica Scandinavica 55 597600 .

99. L. N. Molino, L. D. T. Topoleski, 1996 "Effect of BaSO4 on the fatigue crack propagation rate of PMMA bone cement." Journal of Biomedical Materials Research 31 1 131137 .

100. A. R. Moritz, F. C. Henriques, 1947 Studies of thermal injury-The relative importance of time and surface temperature in the causation of cutaneous burns. American Journal of Pathology 23 695720 .

101. W. F. Mousa, M. Kobayashi, S. Shinzato, M. Kamimura, M. Neo, S. Yoshihara, T. Nakamura, 2000 "Biological and mechanical properties of PMMA-basedbioactive bone cements." Biomaterials 21 21 21372146 .

102. B. P. Murphy, P. J. Prendergast, 2000 "On the magnitude and variability of the fatigue strength of acrylic bone cement." International Journal of Fatigue 22 10 855864 .

103. B. P. Murphy, P. J. Prendergast, 2002 "The relationship between stress, porosity, and nonlinear damage accumulation in acrylic bone cement." Journal of BiomedicalMaterials Research 59 4 646654 .

104. R. K. Nalla, J. J. Kruzic, R. O. Ritchie, 2004 "On the origin of the toughness of mineralized tissue: microcracking or crack bridging?" Bone 34 5 790798 .

105. K. K. Narva, L. V. J. Lassila, P. K. Vallittu, 2005 "Flexural fatigue of denture base polymer with fiber-reinforced composite reinforcement." Composites Part A: AppliedScience and Manufacturing 36 9 12751281 .

106. T. L. Norman, V. Kish, J. D. Blaha, T. A. Gruen, K. Hustosky, 1995 "Creep characteristics of hand-mixed and vacuum-mixed acrylic bone-cement at elevated stress levels." Journal of Biomedical Materials Research 29 4 495501 .

107. N. Nuno, M. Amabili, 2002 "Modelling debonded stem-cement interface for hip implants: Effects of residual stresses." Clinical Biomechanics 17 1 4148 .

108. N. Nuno, G. Avanzolini, 2002 "Residual stresses at the stem-cement interface of an idealized cemented hip stem." Journal of Biomechanics 35 6 849852 .

109. D. O. O'Connor, D. W. Burke, M. Jasty, R. C. Sedlacek, W. H. Harris, 1996 "In vitro measurement of strain in the bone cement surrounding the femoral componentof total hip replacements during simulated gait and stair-climbing." Journal of Orthopaedic Research 14 5 769777 .

110. R. Ormsby, T. Mc Nally, C. A. Mitchell, N. Dunne, 2010a Incorporation of Multiwall Carbon Nanotubes to Acrylic Based Bone Cements: Effects on Mechanical and Thermal Properties. Journal of Mechanical Behaviour of Biomedical Materials 3 2 136145 .

111. R. Ormsby, T. Mc Nally, C. A. Mitchell, N. Dunne, 2010b Influence of multiwall carbon nanotube functionality and loading on mechanical

properties of PMMA/MWCNT bone cements.Journal of Material Science- Materials in Medicine 21 8 22872292 .

112. R. Ormsby, T. Mc Nally, C. A. Mitchell, P. Halley, D. Martin, N. Dunne, 2011 Thermal and Rheological properties of PMMA/MWCNT bone cements. Carbon, DOI:10.1016/j.carbon.2011.02.063.

113. J. F. Orr, N. J. Dunne, J. C. Quinn, 2003 "Shrinkage stresses in bone cement." Biomaterials 24 17 29332940 .

114. S. Pal, S. Saha, 1982 "Stress relaxation and creep behaviour of normal and carbon fibre reinforced acrylic bone cement." Biomaterials 3 9396 .

115. B. Pascual, B. Vazquez, M. Gurruchaga, I. Goni, M. P. Ginebra, F. J. Gil, J. A. Planell, B. Levenfeld, J. S. Roman, 1996 "New aspects of the effect of size and size distribution on the setting parameters and mechanical properties of acrylic bone cements." Biomaterials 17 5 509516 .

116. J. U. Park, S. Cho, K. S. Cho, K. F. Ahn, S. J. Lee, S. J. Lee, 2005 "Effective insitu-preparation and characteristics of polystyrene-grafted carbon nanotube composites." Korea-Australia Rheology Journal 17 2 4145 .

117. A. Peigney, C. Laurent, E. Flahaut, R. R. Bacsa, A. Rousset, 2009 Specific surface area of carbon nanotubes and bundles of carbon nanotubes. Carbon 39 4 507514 .

118. R. M. Pilliar, R. Blackwell, I. Macnab, H. U. Cameron, 1976 "Carbon fiber reinforced bone cement in orthopedic surgery." Journal of Biomedical MaterialsResearch 10 6 893906 .

119. P. J. Prendergast, B. Murphy, 2000 "On the magnitude and variability of the fatigue strength of acrylic bone cement." International Journal of Fatigue 22 10 855864 .

120. P. J. Prendergast, 2001a Chapter 35: Bone prostheses and implants. Bone Mechanics Handbook. Cowin, S. C., CRC Press LLC.

121. P. J. Prendergast, 2001b "The functional performance of orthopaedic bone cement." Key Engineering Materials 198-199: 291-300.

122. B. Pukanszky, 2005 "Interfaces and interphases in multicomponent materials: past, present, future." European Polymer Journal 41 4 645662 .

123. G. C. Pulos, W. G. Knauss, 1998a "Nonsteady crack and craze behavior in PMMA under cyclical loading. I. Experimental preliminaries." International Journal ofFracture 93(1-4): 145-59.

124. G. C. Pulos, W. G. Knauss, 1998b "Nonsteady crack and craze behavior in PMMA under cyclical loading. II. Effect of load history on growth rate and fracture morphology." International Journal of Fracture 93(1-4):

161-85.

125. G. C. Pulos, W. G. Knauss, 1998c "Nonsteady crack and craze behavior in PMMA under cyclical loading. III. Effect of load history on cohesive force distribution on the craze." International Journal of Fracture 93(1-4): 187-207.

126. R. P. Robinson, T. M. Wright, A. H. Burstein, 1981 "Mechanical properties of poly(methyl methacrylate) bone cements." Journal of Biomedical Materials Research 15 2 203208 .

127. A. Roques, M. Browne, A. Taylor, A. New, D. Baker, 2004 "Quantitative measurement of the stresses induced during polymerisation of bone cement." Biomaterials 25 18 44154424 .

128. S. L. Ruan, P. Gao, X. G. Yang, T. X. Yu, 2003 "Toughening high performance ultrahigh molecular weight polyethylene using multiwalled carbon nanotubes." Polymer 44 19 564354 .

129. K. P. Ryan, M. Cadek, V. Nicolosi, S. Walker, M. Ruether, A. Fonseca, J. B. Nagy, W. J. Blau, J. N. Coleman, 2006 "Multiwalled carbon nanotube nucleatedcrystallization and reinforcement in poly (vinyl alcohol) composites." SyntheticMetals 156(2-4): 332-335.

130. S. Saha, S. Pal, 1986 "Mechanical characterization of commercially made carbonfibre-reinforced polymethylmethacrylate." Journal of Biomedical Materials Research 20 6 817826 .

131. J. A. Sauer, G. C. Richardson, 1980 "Fatigue of polymers." International Journal of Fracture 16 6 499532 .

132. J. Scheirs, 2000a Chapter 15: Failure of fibre-reinforced composites. Compositional and Failure Analysis of Polymers. A Practical Approach, John Wiley & Sons, Ltd.: 449481 .

133. J. Scheirs, 2000b Chapter 12: Mechanical failure mechanisms of polymers. Compositional and Failure Analysis of Polymers. A Practical Approach, John Wiley & Sons, Ltd.:304362 .

134. M. K. Seo, J. Lee, R. , S. Park, J. , 2005 "Crystallization kinetics and interfacial behaviors of polypropylene composites reinforced with multi-walled carbon nanotubes." Materials Science and Engineering A 404(1-2): 79-84.

135. K. Serbetci, F. Korkusuz, N. Hasirci, 2004 "Thermal and mechanical properties of hydroxyapatite impregnated acrylic bone cements." Polymer Testing 23 2 14555 .

136. B. D. Shannon, J. F. Klassen, J. A. Rand, D. J. Berry, R. T. Trousdale, 2003 "Revision total knee arthroplasty with cemented components and

uncemented intramedullary stems." Journal of Arthroplasty 18 7 2732 .

137. Z. Shi, Y. Lian, F. H. Liao, X. Zhou, Z. Gu, Y. Zhang, S. Iijima, H. Li, K. T. Yue, S. Zhang, L. , 2000 "Large scale synthesis of single-wall carbon nanotubes byarc-discharge method." Journal of Physics and Chemistry of Solids 61 7 10311036 .

138. S. Shinzato, M. Kobayashi, W. F. Mousa, M. Kamimura, M. Neo, Y. Kitamura, T. Kokubo, T. Nakamura, 2000 "Bioactive polymethyl methacrylate-basedbone cement: Comparison of glass beads, apatite- and wollastonite-containing glass ceramic,and hydroxyapatite fillers on mechanical and biological properties." Journalof Biomedical Materials Research 51 2 258272 .

139. A. A. Shvedova, E. R. Kisin, R. Mercer, Johnson. V. J. Murray, A. I. Potapovich, 2005 Unusual inflammatory and fibrogenic pulmonary responses to single-walled carbon nanotubes in mice, Am. J. Physiol289 L698 -L708

140. A. A. Shvedova, J. P. Fabisiak, E. R. Kisin, A. R. Murray, J. R. Roberts, Y. Y. Tyurina, 2008 Sequential exposure to carbon nanotubes and bacteria enhances pulmonary inflammation and infectivity, Am J Respir Cell Mol Biol38 (5), 579-590.A.A.

141. A. A. Shvedova, E. R. Kisin, D. Porter, P. Schulte, V. E. Kagan, B. Fadeel, Castranova, 2009E., Fadeel, B., Castranova, 2009 Mechanisms of pulmonary toxicity and medical applications of carbon nanotubes: Two faces of Janus? Pharmacology and Therapeutics 121 (2), 192-204.

142. N. Sinha, J. T. W. Yeow, 2005 "Carbon nanotubes for biomedical applications." IEEE Transactions on Nanobioscience 4 2 180195 .

143. S. B. Sinnott, R. Andrews, 2001 "Carbon nanotubes: synthesis, properties, and applications." Critical Reviews in Solid State and Materials Sciences 26 3 145249 .

144. S. B. Sinnott, R. Andrews, D. Qian, A. M. Rao, Z. Mao, E. C. Dickey, F. Derbyshire, 1999 "Model of carbon nanotube growth through chemical vapor deposition."Chemical Physics Letters 315(1-2): 25-30.

145. M. D. Skibo, R. W. Hertzberg, J. A. Manson, S. L. Kim, 1977 "On the generality of discontinuous fatigue crack growth in glassy polymers." Journal of MaterialsScience 12 3 53142 .

146. S. K. Smart, A. I. Cassady, G. Q. Lu, D. J. Martin, 2006 "The biocompatibility of carbon nanotubes." Carbon 44 6 10341047 .

147. S. H. Spiegelberg, G. H. Mc Kinley, 1998 Characterization of the curing process of bone cement with multi-harmonic shear rheometry. In: Trans

24th Annual Meeting of the Society of Biomaterials, San Diego, CA. 283.

148. G. R. Starke, Birnie, and van den Blink, P. A. 2001 Numerical modelling of cement polymerisation and thermal bone necrosis. Computer methods in biomechanics and biomedical engineering, Gordon & Breach, London.

149. M. Stanczyk, B. van Rietbergen, 2004 "Thermal analysis of bone cement polymerisation at the cement-bone interface." Journal of Biomechanics 37 12 18031810 .

150. J. Stolk, N. Verdonschot, B. P. Murphy, P. J. Prendergast, R. Huiskes, 2004 "Finite element simulation of anisotropic damage accumulation and creep in acrylic bone cement." Engineering Fracture Mechanics 71(4-6): 513-528.

151. S. Suresh, 1998 Chapter 12 Fatigue crack growth in noncrystalline solids. Fatigue of Materials, Cambridge University Press: 408431 .

152. M. T. Takemori, 1984 Polymer fatigue. Annual Review of Materials Science. 14 Annual Reviews: 171-204.

153. The Royal Society and the Royal Academy of Engineering 2004 Nanoscience and nanotechnologies: opportunities and uncertainties. London, The Royal Society and the Royal Academy of Engineering.

154. E. T. Thostenson, T. Chou, W. , 2003 "On the elastic properties of carbon nanotubebased composites: modelling and characterization." Journal of Physics D: AppliedPhysics 36 5 573582 .

155. E. T. Thostenson, R. Zhifeng, C. Tsu-Wei, 2001 "Advances in the science and technology of carbon nanotubes and their composites: A review." Composites Scienceand Technology 61 13 1899912 .

156. L. D. T. Topoleski, P. Ducheyne, J. M. Cuckler, 1990 "A fractographic analysis of in vivo poly(methyl methacrylate) bone-cement failure mechanisms." Journal ofBiomedical Materials Research 24 2 135154 .

157. L. D. T. Topoleski, P. Ducheyne, J. M. Cuckler, 1993 "Microstructural pathway of fracture in poly(methyl methacrylate) bone-cement." Biomaterials 14 15 11651172 .

158. L. D. T. Topoleski, P. Ducheyne, J. M. Cuckler, 1998 "Flow intrusion characteristics and fracture properties of titanium-fibre-reinforced bone cement." Biomaterials 19 17 15691577 .

159. C. I. Vallo, T. R. Cuadrado, P. M. Frontini, 1997 "Mechanical and fracture behaviour evaluation of commercial acrylic bone cements." Polymer International 43 3 260268 .

160. C. Velasco-Santos, A. L. Martinez-Hernandez, F. Fisher, R. Ruoff, V. M.

Castano, 2003 "Dynamical-mechanical and thermal analysis of carbon nanotube-methylethylmethacrylate nanocomposites." Journal of Physics D (Applied Physics) 36 12 14238 .

161. N. Verdonschot, R. Huiskes, 1997a "Acrylic cement creeps but does not allow much subsidence of femoral stems." Journal of Bone and Joint Surgery-British 79B 4): 665-669.

162. N. Verdonschot, R. Huiskes, 1997b "The effects of cement-stem debonding in THA on the long-term failure probability of cement." Journal of Biomechanics 30 8 795802 .

163. T. J. Webster, M. C. Waid, J. L. Mc Kenzie, R. L. Price, J. U. Ejiofor, 2004 "Nano-biotechnology: carbon nanofibres as improved neural and orthopaedic implants." Nanotechnology 15 1 4854 .

164. E. W. Wong, P. E. Sheehan, C. M. Lieber, 1997 "Nanobeam mechanics: elasticity, strength and toughness of nanorods and nanotubes." Science 277 5334 19715 .

165. T. M. Wright, R. P. Robinson, 1982 "Fatigue crack propagation in poly methylmethacrylate bone cements." Journal of Materials Science 17 9 24638 .

166. X. L. Xie, Y. W. Mai, X. P. Zhou, 2005 Dispersion and alignment of carbon nanotubes in polymer matrix: A review. Material Science Engineering 49 4 89112 .

167. J. M. Yang, P. Y. Huang, M. C. Yang, S. K. Lo, 1997 "Effect of MMA-g-UHMWPE grafted fiber on mechanical properties of acrylic bone cement." Journal ofBiomedical Materials Research 38 4 361369 .

168. Y. Zhang, H. Gu, S. Iijima, 1998 "Single-wall carbon nanotubes synthesized by laser ablation in a nitrogen atmosphere." Applied Physics Letters 73 26 38279 .

169. Y. Zhang, S. Iijima, 1998 "Microscopic structure of as-grown single-wall carbon nanotubes by laser ablation." Philosophical Magazine Letters 78 2 13944 .

170. B. Zhao, H. Hu, S. K. Mandal, R. C. Haddon, 2005 "A bone mimic based on the self-assembly of hydroxyapatite on chemically functionalized single-walled carbonnanotubes." Chem. Mater. 17 12 32353241 .

CITATION

CHAPTER 1

Kris N. J. Stevens, Yvette B. J. Aldenhoff, Frederik H. van der Veen, Jos G. Maessen, and Leo H. Koole, "Bioengineering of Improved Biomaterials Coatings for Extracorporeal Circulation Requires Extended Observation of Blood-Biomaterial Interaction under Flow," Journal of Biomedicine and Biotechnology, vol. 2007, Article ID 29464, 10 pages, 2007. doi:10.1155/2007/29464

CHAPTER 2

S. Mondal, B. Mondal, A. Dey and S. Mukhopadhyay, "Studies on Processing and Characterization of Hydroxyapatite Biomaterials from Different Bio Wastes," Journal of Minerals and Materials Characterization and Engineering, Vol. 11 No. 1, 2012, pp. 55-67. doi: 10.4236/jmmce.2012.111005.

CHAPTER 3

Yang Cao and Bochu Wang, Biodegradation of Silk Biomaterials, Int. J. Mol. Sci. 2009, 10(4), 1514-1524; doi:10.3390/ijms10041514

CHAPTER 4

M. Türk, G. Kahraman, S. Khalilova, Z. Rzayev and S. Oguztüzün, "Bioengineering Functional Copolymers. XVII. Interaction of Organoboron Amide-Ester Branched Derivatives of Poly(Acrylic Acid) with Cancer Cells," Journal of Cancer Therapy, Vol. 2 No. 2, 2011, pp. 266-275. doi: 10.4236/jct.2011.22034.

CHAPTER 5

Lopez-Lopez MT, Scionti G, Oliveira AC, Duran JDG, Campos A, Alaminos M, et al. (2015) Generation and Characterization of Novel Magnetic Field-Responsive Biomaterials. PLoS ONE 10(7): e0133878. doi:10.1371/journal.pone.0133878

CHAPTER 6

Kasoju N, Kubies D, Kumorek MM, Kříž J, Fábryová E, Machová L, et al. (2014) Dip TIPS as a Facile and Versatile Method for Fabrication of Polymer Foams with Controlled Shape, Size and Pore Architecture for Bioengineering Applications. PLoS ONE 9(10): e108792. doi:10.1371/journal.pone.0108792

CHAPTER 7

George Z. Kyzas, Jie Fu, and Kostas A. Matis, New biosorbent materials: selectivity and bioengineering insights, Processes 2014, 2(2), 419-440; doi:10.3390/pr2020419.

CHAPTER 8

M. Arnal-Pastor, J. C. Chachques, M. Monleón Pradas and A. Vallés-Lluch (2013). Biomaterials for Cardiac Tissue Engineering, Regenerative Medicine and Tissue Engineering, Prof. Jose A. Andrades (Ed.), ISBN: 978-953-51-1108-5, InTech, DOI: 10.5772/56076.

CHAPTER 9

Nicholas Dunne and Ross W. Ormsby (2011). MWCNT Used in Orthopaedic Bone Cements, Carbon Nanotubes - Growth and Applications, Dr. Mohammad Naraghi (Ed.), ISBN: 978-953-307-566-2, InTech, DOI: 10.5772/20317.

INDEX